MW00453177

# Breathe

## Surviving the Storm
### Through the Power of Prayer

Eileen Hornback

Quantity sales special discounts are available on quantity purchases by corporations, associations, and others. For details, contact the publisher at the address above.

Orders by U.S. trade bookstores and wholesalers. Email info@BeyondPublishing.net

The Beyond Publishing Speakers Bureau can bring authors to your live event. For more information or to book an event contact the Beyond Publishing Speakers Bureau speak@BeyondPublishing.net

The Author can be reached directly at BeyondPublishing.net

Manufactured and printed in the United States of America distributed globally by BeyondPublishing.net

**BEYOND**
PUBLISHING

New York | Los Angeles | London | Sydney

ISBN Softcover: 978-1-952884-44-3

ISBN Hardcover: 978-1-952884-43-6

# Dedication

To my husband Scott, the keeper of my heart, the one who walked with me through a tragedy that shreds many marriages. I have seen your faith grow while your emotions were laid bare, exposed to the world. Thank you for holding our family together, wiping away the tears of our little ones and allowing me to stay with Zack throughout his recovery. I cherish those moments when we held each other and depended solely on God to get us through each moment.

To my children, Dylan, Kyle and Logan. Thank you for forgiving my failures, for understanding when my absence was painful but necessary and using those trying times, when our world revolved around Zack's recovery, to develop perseverance that will carry you through life. Each of you have a unique perspective that heralds how God molded you into amazing servants. Hold onto the power of prayer and remember, everything I do, I do for you.

To my miracle Zack, thank you for giving me a glimpse of heaven as I witnessed God answer prayers. Watching you struggle to get your life back, never giving up, taught me how to trust God's perfect plan. Your positive outlook and thirst for life is contagious. You taught me to appreciate every sunset as a spectacular gift from a loving creator. As desperate as those times were, I never felt closer to God than during your recovery. That is a gift, the reflection of God's grace, that I can never repay.

"In *Breathe*, Eileen Hornback takes the reader into a deep, emotional ride. Based on her own true story, *Breathe* is the journey of a mother who will not give up, her son's struggle between life and death, and the power of love, God, and prayer. A must read!

**Rosa Salazar** *Arenas Award-winning Screenwriter*

"Recovery from a TBI is unique for all individuals, as no two brain injuries are identical. Zack's story is an account of one survivor's extraordinary journey. It demonstrates what is achievable when all facets of brain injury recovery are implemented impeccably, in combination with profound spiritual strength and a will to persevere."

**Dr. Greg Perri** *Psy.D/MBA Clinical Neuropsychologist*

"Fasten your seatbelt to walk with Eileen through Zack's horrific accident and traumatic brain injury. When doctors warned he might not survive, Eileen held onto Jesus. I doubted after seeing Zack's broken body, swollen head, and empty eyes. She did not. I looked at the tiniest improvement and thought it was too little. Eileen looked at it like a miracle leap forward. Journey with Eileen, and you'll see white-knuckle faith that refuses to give up. And you'll see that miracles are happening all around us."

**Ruth Schenk** *Award-winning Journalist*

*Breathe*, the epic journey of Zack and Eileen Hornback is an inspiring story of triumph over adversity, hope over despair, and perseverance over long and dark odds. It is a bright light in a cold and uncertain world. It should serve as an eternal roadmap of the path to overcome any obstacle in life, whatever the challenge. You will never know how much fight you have left....until someone tells you that you are all done. Bravo, Zack and Eileen!

**Duane W. Densler, MD,** *FAANS, FACS Neurological Surgeon*

# Acknowledgements

Thank you to the dedicated staff at University Hospital, Dr. Densler, Dr. Mutchnick, Kim Meyer, the Critical Care Team, and the nurses in Neuro ICU. The many tearful nights I spent waiting for Zack to wake up are also filled with memories of small victories on 5West. Your expert care helped to save my sons life and I am eternally grateful.

Thank you, Frazier Rehab, and Dr. Mook, for taking a chance on Zack when he didn't meet your criteria for admittance and giving him his life back. You saw the potential in my son when others couldn't and embraced my role, and Gods, in his recovery. God planted you in just the right place to ensure the best possible outcome for Zack and your commitment to his recovery is our reward.

To Mary Beth, Amy, and Kathy, his Rockstar therapy team that recognized Zack's competitive nature could be used in rehab to conquer obstacles. Thank you for allowing me to see you at your best and comforting me when I couldn't see Zack's progress. The genuine love you showed for my son are precious memories forever stored in my heart.

To the Frazier nurses, especially Kendra, Dana, Jennifer, and Kelly for your expert care of not just my son but our whole family. Thank you for pretending not to notice when we broke every rule on visitation. Zack may not remember you but I will never forget each tender touch or precious words of encouragement. Never underestimate the value you bring to those in recovery and their families.

To Dr. Kraft, who took the time to explain the amazing ability of the brain to recover and the importance of family support, helped me through some of the most difficult times in rehab. Your message is one I give to every family struggling with TBI.

To Suzanne and Leslie at Frazier East for recognizing the resiliency in my son and using it in outpatient therapy to ensure success when he returned to school. Thank you for stepping out of your comfort zone and adapting techniques to keep him engaged in therapy. He has confidence today because you believed in him.

To Dr. Perri, no one made a bigger personal impact on Zack as an outpatient. You not only helped him recognize his deficits but instilled in him the belief that those shortcomings didn't have to define who he was or what he could accomplish. His days were better when he could spend time talking with you and those conversations molded his outlook on his future. Thank you for helping me to understand the complexity of his unique injury and for embracing Zack's humor as a successful coping mechanism. I don't know quite when your relationship evolved from doctor/patient to endearing friendship but I'm grateful that you continue to be part of our lives. Thank you for believing his story needed to be told and encouraging me to write it.

To my pastors, Bob Russell, Dave Stone, and Kyle Idleman your leadership at Southeast Christian Church came to life for our family during Zack's recovery, but especially in those desperate days at University Hospital when we faced life and death decisions. Thank you for building a congregation that believes in the power of prayer and encouraging those people to lift up our family. I have no doubt that this is how God intended his church to respond. The miracle of modern medicine can accomplish nothing apart from the Great Physician and although we had expert care from dedicated professionals, I believe that it is the prayers of many believers that are responsible for Zack's miraculous recovery. Well done good and faithful servants.

To Mrs. Rafla, Mr. Greener, the staff, and teachers at Christian Academy of Louisville, I couldn't ask for a better place for Zack to continue his education after the accident. Thank you for graciously accommodating his special academic needs and tolerating the initial disruption of his return to school. Our family was surrounded by the prayers of faithful students who were nurtured in your classrooms.

To Carol Britton and Jalynn Speaks we are so blessed that God placed you at Christian Academy in positions to make a difference in Zack's education. Your dedication to helping those with learning differences made a challenging education successful for Zack. Thank you for being there when he needed you the most.

To Janet Smith thank you for reaching out over the years to encourage me to write this book and believing our story needed to be told. Who could have imagined when you were teaching Zack science in 8th grade that only two years later, he would face traumatic brain injury? We have cherished your prayers, your support and our continued friendship.

To my niece Sharon Jones, thank you for setting up the blog, faithfully uploading pictures and bringing me the comments of readers. Many times, those remarks were the encouragement I needed and they enabled me to stay focused on Gods perfect plan through Zack's recovery. The blog became the outline for this book, so your foresight enabled me to capture many aspects of his recovery that might have otherwise been lost. *Breathe* is coming to fruition in part due to your insistence that I blog.

To my forever friend Teri Carrico, I know I can always count on you to look out for me. Thank you for commandeering my phone and answering a million questions in those early days at University Hospital. For stepping in when I needed a break and staying late to walk me to my car. We have traveled many years together, through the best and worst times of our lives and our friendship means the world to me.

To my beloved friend Donna Jaha, you always underestimate the role you played in Zack's recovery. Without you stepping in at Frazier Rehab so I could return to work, I would have lost my mind and my job. You have loved my children as your own, but with Zack you embraced that role wholeheartedly. You gave up your peaceful mornings to assist with therapy and took detailed notes so I wouldn't miss a single word or accomplishment. Thank you for keeping me awake with those late-night phone calls while I drove home. Thank you for your prayers, your faith, your friendship and your love.

To Zack's friends, especially Andrew, Tiffany, Rob, Brittany, Trey, and Dan, thank you for never giving up on your friend. For spending all your summer nights at the hospital, encouraging Zack and playing silly games so he knew how to be a teenager. None of his therapist could teach him that, so your role in his recovery was invaluable. Thank you for your prayers, for spreading the word around the world so that others would lift him up as well. You embraced the power of prayer.

To our family, my sisters and brother, Scott's brothers, Grandpa, Penny, and Jay, thank you for your prayers and support when we needed it most. I am thankful that my Mom and Grandma Rita got to witness Zack's remarkable recovery and I know they would be proud of the amazing person he has become. What a fabulous family reunion we will have one day, dancing on streets of gold in heaven.

To my dear friend de de Cox, my partner in writing adventures, the catalyst that pushed me to finally write this story. Thank you for coaching me through all things technical, for your endless connections and for blazing the trail as a new author and dragging me along. Sailing the seas at the Winter Story Summit, being mentored by the amazing Rosa Salazar Arenas and signing with Michael Butler would not have been possible without you. Thank you for believing in me, for talking me off the ledge when I was overwhelmed, for listening every morning and sharing in my excitement. You have been my inspiration as an author and *Breathe* is finally a reality.

Life seemed close to perfect approaching the summer of 2005. Every parent's nightmare began for us one evening when Zack came home earlier than expected. Of course, we never imagined that he would sneak out after midnight when he was certain we were asleep. Nor that we would be awakened to the news that a car accident had placed him precariously on the edge of death. It shattered our idyllic world and changed the course of our lives.

In this profoundly moving book, readers will experience the emotional faith of a mother and witness the amazing recovery from traumatic brain injury. Faced with the daunting news that her son may never walk or talk again and forced to consider the rest of his life in a nursing home, she turned to the only person who had the power to restore him. Within the desolate walls of the ICU, she cried out to God for healing, and saw prayers answered in miraculous ways. God was in control, and through the power of prayer, they would discover his perfect plan was more than they could hope or imagine.

Looking back to that fateful day, there has always been that one word. The word his doctor warned us with. The word God whispered to me in my desperation. That one word that stalked us – my son just needed to breathe. Walk the journey of a miracle with my son and my family, and I dare you not to breathe.

I can hear the phone ringing in my dream. It is not even 5:00 a.m. I roll over, pretending to be asleep, so Scott would have to answer. He mumbles something and abruptly hangs up. Seconds later, the phone rings again, and I can hear an authoritative voice on the other line identify himself as an officer with the Jefferson County Police.

*"This is not a joke. Don't hang up."* He asks if we have a son, Zack Hornback, and explains that he has been in a car accident, and we need to get to University Hospital right away. Was I dreaming? Scott turns on the light and instructs me to stay calm.

*"Zack's been in an accident; we need to go. We need to go right now."* I jump out of bed and start opening drawers, trying to shake the fog from my head as the phone rings again. It is the emergency room, clarifying that Zack Hornback had been Stat Flighted to University Hospital, and we need to get there immediately. I am confused. Now wide awake and getting dressed, I keep thinking that Zack had come home early last night, before his curfew, and was sleeping in his room in the basement.

My thoughts are interrupted with the doorbell buzzing. My sister-in-law, Robin, still in her pajamas, is nervously volunteering to watch the girls. Apparently, the police had mistakenly called her house first, since we have the same last name and live on the same street. Our nine-year-old daughter, Kyle, stumbles sleepily out of her room, rubbing her eyes and asking what is wrong. I hug her, nudging her back towards her room.

*"Zack was in an accident, and we need to go to the hospital. He's going to be fine. Robin is here, so go back to bed, and we will be home later."* I sound much more secure than I feel. I hurry down the stairs and can hear Scott honking the horn in the driveway. This is all surreal and very confusing. I jump in Scott's truck, and we head downtown. Fumbling for my phone, already feeling a panic rising within me, I call my sister, Rosemarie, and get her answering machine. I leave a message that Zack had been in a car accident, and we were on our way to the hospital. "Call Mom", I plead. "I will let you know more later. And pray, please pray."

I hang up and dial Scott's Aunt Penny. I need her to get in touch with his parents, who are in Hilton Head, vacationing with our other son, Dylan. I know she can contact Dave Stone, the pastor at Southeast Christian Church who baptized all my children, to let him know that Zack was badly injured, and we are on the way to the hospital. Scott grabs my phone and tells me no more calls, because it is making him nervous. I lean my head on the passenger side window and peer out into the darkness. Thoughts are racing through my mind about what we might find when we get to the hospital. Picturing Zack broken and bloodied, I can't stop the tears from sliding down my cheeks. I glance at Scott, wanting to ask a question, but not knowing what to say. He seems determined, in control, and I reach for his hand. Speeding towards downtown, it isn't until we exit the freeway that we realize neither of us know exactly where the University Hospital is located. We must look frantic, pulling to the curb at such an early hour and asking a stranger, a homeless man, to point us in the right direction.

We arrive at the emergency room entrance and find the staff waiting for us at the door. They usher us into a small waiting room. It is dimly lit, and I nervously take a seat as Scott paces the room. A sliver of light pierces the shadows as the door opens, and the ER nurse says we have a visitor. She quietly ushers in our pastor and slips out of the room. Dave Stone admits that our situation is dire and puts his hands on our shoulders to pray as I crumble into a chair in tears. Abruptly, his whispered prayer is interrupted when another door slides open and several residents approach us.

Dr. Densler, a neurosurgeon, informs us how grim our situation actually is. He explains that they aren't sure if Zack has any internal injuries, but he has suffered a serious traumatic brain injury, and they didn't expect him to live. What! NO! This can't be real. I am clinging to Scott's hand as they lead us through a busy emergency room to his gurney. The area is brightly lit, and I am not prepared for what I see as the curtain is pulled away. My knees buckle, and my wail pierces the chaos. There is my baby with a tube down his throat and his clothes cut away. There is dried blood on his face, and he looks…broken. Dr. Densler proceeds with little emotion as he explains what they have already discovered. A CAT Scan revealed that Zack has a blood clot on the right side of his brain and a bruise on the left. He also has a deep laceration on the top on his head that cuts through his skull to his brain. This area was full of glass and debris from the accident. And his brain is swelling.

Up until this point, Scott had been in control, driving us to the hospital and keeping me calm. But seeing his son lying there, he suddenly realizes he can't fix this. He turns, pounds his fist against the wall in anguish, and slides to his knees, weeping. He is inconsolable. I reach for him, but can't pry myself from the gurney. Zack has been given drugs to paralyze him, and every hour, as they wear off, he shakes uncontrollably. I don't know what to do; how to comfort Scott or stop Zack from shaking? I begin to pray out loud. Holding Zack's hand, sobbing, I recite the 23rd Psalm, *"The Lord is my Shepherd; I shall not be in want. He makes me lie down in green pastures, he leads me beside quiet waters, he restores my soul. He guides me on paths of righteousness for his name's sake. Even though I walk through the valley of the shadow of death, I will fear no evil, for you are with me. Your rod and your staff, they comfort me. You prepare a table before me in the presence of my enemies. You anoint my head with oil… you anoint my head with oil…you anoint my head with oil."* I can't get past that verse, repeating it over and over again. I am consumed with grief, at times unable to breathe. They give us only that moment before tearing us away as they prepare to take Zack into surgery.

We are sent to a large, second floor surgery waiting room, where news of the accident has quickly spread, and friends have started to arrive. Everyone is asking questions, and we have no answers, only the foreboding message that Zack might die. The anxiety of the unknown and awareness that we have no control leaves me feeling helpless and abandoned. I jump to my feet, consumed with a sense of panic each time the surgery doors open and dissolve back into my chair with a whimper when the news is for someone else.

Finally, Dr. Densler, still in scrubs, approaches us. He is serious, with a detached professionalism you would expect from a surgeon. He methodically describes how a shunt was inserted in Zack's head to drain the excess fluid and monitor the pressure building up inside his brain. This Inner Cranial Pressure, or ICP, was at 28 and rising. This number would haunt us for the next several days as he explains its significance. They are treating him with drugs and have him on a respirator, but they can't seem to get his ICP to an acceptable reading under 20. I sense the blood drain from my face, and I feel as though I might faint. Soon, the waiting room is full of Zack's friends from Christian Academy, our family, and other people from our church. Periodically, someone would approach us and offer to pray, which only made me realize how dismal our situation has become.

When his ICP reaches an alarming 36, Dr. Densler tells us to prepare for another surgery. He explains that they need to remove part of Zack's skull, so his brain can swell outside of his head. He admits that it is a risky surgery with many complications, so we decide to seek a second opinion, and several friends with connections start making phone calls. At 2:00 p.m., his ICP has reached 40, and the bruise on the left side of his brain has grown. Although we are still waiting for a second opinion, Dr. Densler impatiently states that surgery has to be performed immediately, or Zack will certainly die. My heart is pounding, and it feels as though the room is spinning in slow motion. Paperwork is shoved at me, and I realize we can't wait any longer. My hand is shaking, and tears stream down my face as I approve the procedure, reading the possible complications— including death. They take the consent form and rush back into surgery, the door sliding shut like a prison. My baby, my firstborn, might die. I may never hold him in my arms again. How could I go on without him?

Hours pass in a blur, and visitors continue to comfort us, offering gentle hugs and prayer. I am terrified when finally, the surgery doors slide open, and Dr. Densler approaches us cautiously. He describes how they successfully removed his right bone flap and the blood clot. In the process, they discovered that he had glass in his brain from the deep laceration to his head.

Zack is alive, but far from being safe from death's grasp. I can hardly breathe. Choking. Silently begging for a nugget of hope that is never offered. Tears cloud my vision as the doctor's feet, wrapped in blue shoe covers, seem to be swallowed up by the floor as he walks away. I want to feel grateful, but this isn't over. Time is not on our side, and I glare at the clock as if it were the enemy. We wait, anxiously jumping to our feet each time the surgery doors slide open. We are surrounded by family and dozens of Zack's friends, when Dr. Densler informs us that another CAT scan will be done to show whether the bruise on the left side of his brain has grown or begun to bleed. These conditions could result in his left bone flap being removed, which Dr. Densler does not want to do.

They had intentionally removed his right bone flap, even though the more serious injury was the bruise on his left side. The left side of the brain controls speech and motor skills, and they do not want to risk damaging any brain cells on that side during surgery. By removing the right bone flap, they are forcing his brain to swell on that side, which is more easily retrained. It makes sense, but provides little comfort. I sit with my mind racing, my hands trying to stop my legs from nervously shaking as I grasp what has happened over the last 12 hours.

Trying to comprehend what the doctors had just revealed, I am approached by a staff member who hands me a plastic bag. With trepidation, she explains that these were my son's clothes. The ones he'd had on when he was brought in. I sense all eyes in the room are on me, piercing the silence, like shards of glass cutting through the pain. I open the bag and carefully remove a tattered sweatshirt stained with blood. My son's blood. I hug it to my chest. Here are Zack's jeans, cut off of him, bearing witness to his injury, and one white tennis shoe. Just one.

A strange prayer escapes my lips. *You can have his other shoe, Lord, just please give me back the feet that walked across my heart for the last 15 years.*

I look up and see a group of tired, confused teenagers, all searching for answers. Clinging to his clothes, tears sliding down my checks, I look from one face to another. These were the kids who saw Zack every day, and now, I see them as a part of him. I need to comfort them, to correct them, and to give them the hope I so desperately need to feel myself. Abruptly, I tell my friend, Teri, to get me some scissors. I have known Teri since high school, and we attended college together. Her daughter, Katie, is only six weeks older than Zack, so we have raised them, sharing our fears as new mothers often do. She kneels down to eye level with me, and I repeat, "Just get me some scissors." She looks around the room, searching for a reason to question my request, her eyes landing back on my face as I whisper, "Please." Squeezing my hand, she looks towards the nurse's station and heads off on her mission. I examine his garments, feeling my heart beat as I hold them tightly to my chest.

Zack's closest friends slowly move towards me as Teri returns with borrowed scissors and cautiously hands them to me. As if in slow motion, my mind flashing back to those precious photos I neatly trimmed to place in his baby book. I start carefully cutting up his clothes. A tear wells up in the corner of my eye and drips off the tip of my nose when I look up at the anxious faces waiting for me to speak. I place a precious square of Zack's grey sweatshirt in Andrew's hand, whispering, "This is a symbol of what has happed to Zack. Let it be a reminder to make good decisions and never stop praying for him." A line forms, and desperate hands reach for a little piece of Zack as they hug me and promise to pray. When I finish passing out all the pieces of my heart, our large group gathers together in the middle of that tearful room. We hold hands in a circle, and Dale Mowery, an elder from Southeast Christian Church, begins to pray. Prayers from our church family, and all those waiting with us literally hold us up. Others begin calling their churches, and soon, thousands of people are praying for Zack. Time stands still as I will myself not to think about my son's future that I see slipping away.

Finally, Dr. Densler brings promising news. The CAT scan reveals that his brain has shifted back to the center, and there is no additional bleeding. The room explodes in praise, but our brief moment of celebration is quickly dampened when he confesses that this is only the beginning. Zack's brain will continue to swell, and he has no idea what damage has been done, or if Zack will recover. He cautions that the next 24 hours are critical. My thoughts drown out the long list of facts he rattles off. He slips away, promising to report on the ICP readings as they change. We live hour by hour by those numbers, each decline giving us a glimmer of hope Zack could survive. And each minute, I have to remind myself to breathe.

Zack is moved to Neuro ICU on the fifth floor. This area requires you to ring a buzzer and announce what patient you are there to see in order to gain admittance. A large nurses' station is surrounded by private rooms. The humming of machines echoes off the walls. We are ushered to his room, and I feel nauseous as my gaze lands on the bed. His face is purple, the right side engorged from surgery, and his eye is swollen shut. Most of his head is shaved, and he looks like Frankenstein with staples holding his scalp over his brain.

There is no skull on the right side, and his brain has swelled, making his head oddly shaped. I notice the cuts on his face and whimper as the nurse says in a soft voice that they are mostly superficial. Zack is sedated with a fast-acting drug by a continuous IV drip hanging from a pole next to his bed. There are several monitors with an immense amount of information flowing onto the screens. I'm transfixed at the blinking numbers, my eyes clouding with tears. His nurse gently explains everything that they have to do.

Every hour, they turn the drip off to access his condition. Holding a flashlight, she shines it in his eyes to see if his pupils dilate. He doesn't like it, and tilts his head away from the light. Because his right eye is swollen shut, she has to pry it open, but nods in satisfaction and explains that both eyes are responding. Then, she pinches him near his armpit to get a reaction. This is done on both sides of his chest. My hands are clenched together, pressed to my lips to suppress a cry as I watch her continue to pinch his tender skin. She coaxes him to reach up to make her stop. His reflexes are slow, but he consistently reaches his hand up to where she is pinching him. She sees me grimace and explains that his reaction is very good, because, although he is not conscious, he is responding to pain. She makes a notation on his chart and quietly shuts the door, leaving me alone with Zack for the first time.

I'm almost afraid to approach his bed and glance at the flashing green numbers on the monitor. I remember what Dr. Densler said about the significance of the ICP number and recognize that it has dropped since I first entered the room. This gives me courage as I move closer to his bed, my heart aching. Suddenly, he is that little boy who fell off his bike, his chin quivering, trying to be brave as I fuss over a skinned knee. Memories swirl around my mind, and I swallow a lump in my throat. I whisper his name. I tenderly stroke his arm and hold his hand. He doesn't respond, but I can't let him go. I want him to know that I'm here. Forcing a smile, I kiss his hand, then his swollen face, and soon, my tears drench the arm of his hospital gown. *"I'm here, Zack. God will take care of you. He is holding you in the palm of His hand."* Sobbing, my temples throbbing, I return again to the 23rd Psalm. I bow my head, placing my forehead on his arm and pray out loud.

That is how Scott finds me when he is ushered into the room. He comes to the side of the bed and pulls me towards him, holding me tight, his shoulders quivering with each sob. He looks at Zack and can't find the words to express his pain. We silently stare at our boy, each lost in our own thoughts until I feel my knees going weak, and I melt into the chair.

Through the open door, I can see the nurses watching us, compassion splashed across their faces as their gaze bounces from our room to the hallway where the buzzer announces other visitors. I look at the clock and realize we have left concerned people downstairs expecting an update. I wipe my eyes and kiss Zack's hand again. Scott hugs me and says he needs some time alone with his son. I hear his voice crack as he begins his own familiar prayer, and I head to the second floor waiting room.

Amongst all our friends in the waiting room are Dan and Mary Rivard. Their son, Matt, was the driver of the car the night of the accident. I didn't know the Rivards, but Matt had briefly played baseball with Zack before leaving Christian Academy. He was several years older and not someone we were aware Zack was hanging out with. He hadn't been injured in the accident, but had been taken from the scene to jail, after showing signs of intoxication. His parents were devastated, mourning Zack's injuries alongside our family, and now, his mother cautiously approaches me. Matt would be released today and wants to come to the hospital to see Zack. Since many of Zack's friends don't appreciate having the Rivards at the hospital, they generally sit by themselves or with members of their church who have come to offer prayer and support. I know these teenagers will not want to see Matt, but I quickly agree, reasoning that he needs to see the result of his decisions and hoping I can find out more about what happened that night.

The Rivards have already left when Scott comes down from Zack's room. I quietly tell him Matt is coming to the hospital, and he is angry. No, livid. He holds Matt responsible for putting us in this situation and doesn't want him anywhere near his son. He insists that I call the Rivards and cancel the visit. I argue that it will be helpful for Matt to see Zack's condition, and it is too late, because they are on the way. He storms out and leaves me standing in the waiting room with most of Zack's friends agreeing that it is a bad idea.

Scott rushes to the first floor lobby and tells the guard at the front door that his son is upstairs dying, and the man responsible is coming to the hospital. He must look half crazy, as he explains that he wants to see him but not be seen. The guard tells him to pull his truck up to the curb, and he will be able to watch them as they approach the entrance. For the next 10 minutes, he sits in the emergency lane, chain smoking, his eyes glued to the sidewalk where they have to pass. Finally, he sees the Rivards, heads down, walking determinedly towards the entrance. Between them is not the monster he expects, but an overgrown teenager. The agony and despair Scott felt over the last two days suddenly turns to intense hatred. As they enter the hospital, he slams on the gas pedal and pulls into traffic with an overwhelming sense of evil. He pictures himself plucking the flesh off the bones of Matt Rivard. He wants to inflict the same pain that he feels on the person he deems responsible for taking his son away. He is outraged at the mere sight of him.

Earlier, I had planned for Scott to meet Donna and Buddy Jaha at Pat's Steakhouse, so he could eat dinner, and even though it is early, he heads in that direction. When he arrives at the restaurant, there are only a few people at tables, so he takes a seat at the bar. He is seething with rage and feelings he can't explain. In anguish, he reaches out to a young man in an apron coming from the kitchen. Crying out in desperation, Scott asks if he could give him a word of encouragement, because he just saw the man he holds responsible for putting his son in the hospital. The young man's eyes widen, but before he can even say a word, Scott apologizes for putting him in such an uncomfortable spot. He looks at Scott's tear-stained face. "No, hold on. I'll be right back," says the young man and disappears into the kitchen.

Scott places his elbows on the bar, his hands covering his face, trying to hide his hopelessness. A moment later, the guy returns with a man wiping his hand on his apron. He looks at Scott, places his hand on the boy's back and explains that this is his son. Then, he puts his arm around Scott's shoulder and tells him an incredible story. He describes how, years ago, his son had also been in an accident and suffered a traumatic brain injury. He promises everything will be okay and encourages Scott not to lose hope. They speak for only a few minutes before he has to rush back to the kitchen.

Scott was pondering the aura the man seemed to have around him as he walks numbly to the front door. Then, he sees it. Hanging on the wall next to the entrance is the framed article about the accident. The man who comforted Scott was none other than Pat, the owner of Pat's Steakhouse. And the young man he asked for an encouraging word was this boy in the accident. After reading the article, he steps outside and is overcome with a sense of peace. His shoulders feel as if a sudden burden has been lifted. The anger and need for revenge are gone. Divine forgiveness floods over him, and he sits on the front steps and sobs. He calls me from his truck. Through tears mixed with laughter, he begs me to tell Matt Rivard that he forgives him.

Before the day is over, Dr. Densler reports that it is "very strange" that the CAT Scan today showed no change…the bruise has not grown as they had all anticipated. He is guarded and emphasizes that this result is not typical. They can't explain it, and he cautions us not to be too optimistic. Straightening his back, he rubs his chin, as if puzzled, and shoves his hands in his coat pockets. Taking a deep breath, I smile and look up, shaking my head. Not bewildered, but grateful. He's taken aback when I embrace him in a hug before striding towards the surgery doors. I feel a warmth envelope me as I thank God for His healing touch. We know the power of prayer, and Zack is placed carefully in the hands of God.

W e have been fighting these pesky little ants for weeks in our kitchen at home, and although we have tried everything, we can't get rid of them. This morning when I wake up and go downstairs, I see the food that Scott has left out on the counter and know the ants will be having a field day. But no ants. Not one anywhere in sight. God knew that I had enough going on, and I could not bear those pesky ants another day. He took care of them for me. Thank you, Lord!

It's nearly 6:00 a.m. as I head out the door for my 20-minute drive in the dark to the hospital. Our neighborhood is still asleep, and I don't want to break the silence by turning on the radio. I can't bear to listen to news or music that confirms the rest of the world is going on without us. My thoughts are racing as I imagine my son's condition. Tears well up in my eyes as I consider that he might be in pain. My silent prayers become vocal as I cry out to God, seeking His presence. Pleading for strength that will see us through whatever lies ahead. The sun is peeking over the parking garage as I make my way into the hospital. Anxious to get up to the fifth floor, I intentionally jab the elevator button several times, rushing in as soon as the doors slide open. Nervously tapping my foot, I ring the buzzer to be let into Neuro ICU and immediately gain entrance.

This area seems to never sleep, and several nurses glance up as I slip into Zack's room. Moving to the opposite side of the bed, I survey his face and decide that he looks bludgeoned. The swelling on the right side of his face has improved, but I'm alarmed that the left side has started to protrude and now that eye is swollen shut. He tends to turn his head to that side, and fluid is settling there, so that his neck is also starting to puff up. Feeling distressed that I no longer have a good side of his face to focus on, I lean forward and caress his arm, trailing my fingers around the tubes that puncture his skin. "This is still my baby;" I whisper to myself. The beeping of the monitors catches my attention, and I notice how low his ICP number has registered. My peace is shattered when the lights flick on, signaling that rounds have begun.

Our nurse scrambles into the room just ahead of the residents and starts checking all the hookups. Zack appears to be moving around more, and when Dr. Densler assesses him, his hand quickly creeps to where he is pinched. The doctors are more aggressive, almost twisting as they pinch him, so Zack opens his right eye halfway to peek at who is hurting him. They remove the bottom of the bedsheet and expose his feet. When they stick his toe with a pin, he moves his legs. He appears to be closer to consciousness, even though he is still in a coma and unable to breathe on his own.

As quickly as they arrive, the residents march out of the room, hardly taking notice of me. The nurse replaces one of the bags hanging from the pole next to his bed, adjusts the pic line and secures all the wires monitoring his vital signs. She dims the lights and slides out of the room, quietly closing the door halfway. I take my seat next to his bed and stroke his arm as I watch the numbers blinking on the monitor. I listen to his respirator and softly pray out loud, my pleas falling in step with his rhythmic mechanical breathing, as tears slide silently down my cheeks.

It is Sunday, and Scott manages to get the girls dressed for church, but becomes increasingly frustrated dealing with their hair. Logan pouts that her ponytail is crooked, so Kyle attempts to correct it, succeeding only in making her complain louder. The tension in the air can be cut with a knife. We had signed Dylan up for summer camp at Country Lake before the accident, and he was looking forward to celebrating his 12th birthday there with friends. Knowing that our church family will quell his anxiety, we agreed that camp would be the best place to shield him from the turmoil going on at home. Dylan adores his brother and doesn't know how to reckon the serious nature of Zack's condition with the superman athlete he admires. With Dylan at camp, Scott is left alone to wrangle the girls into the truck. Arriving at church, he is grateful to pass the girls off to his mom.

Feeling overburdened and not up to answering the concerned inquiries of those we share a pew with every week, he decides not to sit in our usual spot on the first floor at Southeast Christian Church. Instead, he wanders into the second-floor balcony and finds an empty cry room. Typically sprinkled with fussy babies, this one is vacant and provides a place to hide. Through the soft lighting, he focuses on the stage below, where songs of praise pierce his heart. The worship team shuffles offstage, and our senior pastor steps to the pulpit. He begins his sermon, suddenly halting in mid-sentence. His heart aching with grief, Scott listens as Bob Russell urges the congregation to pray for Zack Hornback. Our megachurch becomes eerily solemn, bowing their heads in appeal for God's mercy. Scott is overcome with emotion, suffocating, unable to summon a word, tears streaming down his face. As the sermon continues, he hears nothing but his own sobbing. An usher gingerly approaches to ask if he needs help or wants to talk with someone. He chokes out, "That's my son dying in the hospital, pray for him."

Scott arrives at the hospital, but before I can finish filling him in on the morning assessment, the nurse reports that they have begun to take Zack off sedatives. She is guarded, explaining that now he could "wake up" at any time. And so, we wait, watching the number blinking on the monitor as hours pass. I'm emotionally drained, but can't fathom leaving his bedside, for fear he may wake up without me there. Or worse, that he won't wake up at all. Restlessness settling in, we take turns reporting to our friends congregating in the hall, hoping they are allowed a brief visit in his room. It is agonizing waiting for him to wake up. The doctors don't offer much hope, only statistics, which has the opposite effect. The waiting for answers and praying for Zack to show any positive change is exhausting, but we are lifted up by many visitors. Acquaintances from church who pledged to pray this morning offer their sentiments, and the parents of kids who are here every day graciously plan to bring food to the house.

Dave Stone arrives with the youth ministers from Southeast Christian Church. They pray with us, and, in an attempt to breathe life back into him, I read the letter that Zack had written us about a month earlier. He was presenting a compelling case on why his curfew should be later than 11:00 p.m. It is well-written, and his points are clearly made. It gives those who don't know Zack very well a glimpse of his personality. Of course, agreeing to an 11:00 p.m. curfew doesn't mean anything if you intend to sneak back out at 1:00 a.m. My lip quivers as I struggle to make it through his note, recognizing the irony that his message proclaimed what good decisions he makes, and yet, here he is. A motionless witness to the decisions that led to his accident. His typewritten letter started:

> I wrote you this note, so that I can express my thoughts about the situation to you, without my emotions taking over and another fight breaking out. Please, be open-minded while reading it.

*None of my friends have an 11:00 curfew. I know you and Dad don't like to compare with other kids or other parents, but sometimes, one must look at another with more experience. Parents such as Jeremy's and Andrew's have already raised teenagers and have learned from their experiences. As you look at the parents who have more experience, you will see that the curfews are slightly later, and the parents are more relaxed. You and Dad are great parents, but you still don't have the experience with teenagers and are still striving for agreeable rules.*

*To me, or someone who doesn't work, the weeknights and the weekends seem no different. I feel silly having to come in at 11:00 when everyone else is doing their normal thing. Not only does it make me feel silly, but it is hard to go out with my friends. I know they do not want to take me home at 11:00 and interrupt their night, and if I spend the night with friends and my curfew is 11:00, then that makes their curfew 11:00. They will no longer want me to spend the night, because I will seem like a burden to them.*

*When spending the night out, why does the curfew have to be 11:00? From research, the city-wide curfew for Louisville teens is 1:00 a.m. I'm not asking to stay out till 1:00, but 11:00? Maybe we can talk it over and set it back a little bit. If the parents of the guy I'm spending the night with wait up for us at 11:30 or 12:00, then why does it affect you so much? You are fighting for a curfew of 11:00 that benefits neither of us, and from recent experiences, usually leads into a fight. When spending the night out, I felt that my curfew should not be 11:00, especially because my friends will get irritated, and I will be looked at as the international loser of the world and, eventually, end up getting shot or something.*

*Parents do not always tell the truth. Because of my wisdom (gag), I know that parents have an inner circle in which they try to impress other parents by flaunting how strict they are.... when actually it's all an act. Sure, a parent can say their child's curfew is strictly 11:00, but when the next day they say sure that its fine be in by 12:00... you know something is up. One thing I see in you and Dad is that you stick to the rules way too strictly. You aren't even willing to change them in certain circumstances. Off the subject, but you call me constantly when going out. I'm not going to lie to you and Dad. I'll tell you where I'm going, and if I don't feel comfortable in situations, I will leave. I'm not out to rebel against you and Dad. I just want to go out with my friends, and when I'm receiving phone calls all night, telling me that I cannot spend the night or I can't be there, or you don't trust me, it ends up ruining my night. BE RELAXED. I'm not a bad kid. I really never have gotten in trouble going out. I make the right decisions and strive to put myself in the right situations. I haven't been arrested, beaten up, taken drugs, drank, etc. How many times have you received a phone call saying that your son is in trouble, you need to come pick him up?* (The tears are now streaming steadily down my face and blurring my vision, but I continue). *I have it under control... I know that may be scary for you, but I really do. I love you and Dad, and I'm out to make you proud. I get good grades and do the right things. It would be different if I were a big troublemaker... then my curfew could be earlier. But think about it... I have never gotten in trouble going out. Fighting over curfews and what I'm doing does nothing but hurt the relationship between us. I'm not running wild, but I'm just out trying to have fun with my fellow Christian friends. Try to realize where I'm coming from.*

*Love your son, Zachary*

I carefully fold the letter and clutch it to my chest while my heart is feeling as if it's shredded to tiny pieces. Vivid images of Zack before the accident flood my mind, and my hands tremble as I place his note carefully back in my Bible. I am grateful for the presence of my pastor and his sincere prayers, but I suddenly feel the need to be alone with Zack. Sensing my change in demeanor, my guests excuse themselves, and I move closer to his bed. *"You don't look like you have it all under control now, Zack,"* I whisper. I flash back to the phone call, and my arms bristle aching to hold him. *I love you, please wake up. God, please, wake him up.* I caress his hand, trying to make his limp fingers curl around mine. A beeping sound alerts the nurse that I've loosened the finger monitor registering his oxygen level, and she rushes into the room. Opening her mouth to chastise me, she hears my whimper and gently places her arm around my shoulder. "Have you eaten? You should get some rest." I halfheartedly smile and wipe my eyes on my sleeve. For a minute, we both stand silently gazing at Zack, caught up in the moment. A shrill alarm sounds from another room, and she hurries away. I gently pat his hand, muttering a prayer as I slip out the door and head to the waiting room.

Even in the midst of the pain we are experiencing, we see God bringing good from it. Several strangers cautiously approach us when I'm standing with Scott and a flock of his friends. They describe being in the surgery waiting room on Friday when Dale Mowery gathered our group together to pray. They saw the huge circle of teenagers, friends, and family bow their heads and tearfully lift Zack up, silently witnessing to other hurting people who don't know him. Extremely touched, they found themselves pleading for the life of a boy they knew only by name. They continue to pray for him.

I receive several messages from parents, saying they are hearing their teenagers talk about the power of prayer. The entries these kids scribble in the notebook we started for Zack express how they don't pray enough, but they are now. They recognize that any one of them could be in his situation, and they have a front row seat to the agony it would cause their family. And no one ever imagined it would happen to Zack. He had life under control. God got their attention. God is in control.

Zack's countenance is different with the sedatives no longer clogging up his veins. He appears calm, in spite of his bloated face and tubes running every which way, connecting him to life. I scan the readings as his body registers new information, satisfied that the pressure in his brain is diminishing and his heart rate is steady. The rhythmic beeping of the monitor is almost soothing as I lean in and grasp his hand. Softly, I begin to recite the 23rd Psalm, our mantra that I have clung to since we first laid eyes on his broken body in the emergency room. I pray with him, and in the tranquility of the moment, tears well up in the corners of his eyes. I sense that he hears me and knows that we are here praying for him. Soon, I am lost in my thoughts, absently staring at the respirator that coaxes a breath every few seconds.

The door opens and Karen introduces herself as Zack's physical therapist. She is friendly, with an upbeat attitude, as she explains her role. He is unable to move much more than a finger or toe in response to pain. She manually manipulates his arms and legs to facilitate muscle memory, retraining his brain to learn how to move his arms and legs on his own. Zack is calm at first while she works with his legs, her voice turning melodic as I focus on his expressionless face.

However, when she starts shifting his arms around and over his head, he gets very agitated. The monitor loudly announces when his blood pressure shoots up, and he starts trembling uncontrollably. Karen steps aside as the Critical Care Team rushes into the room in crisis mode, injecting seizure medication into the pic line. Within minutes, he is quiet and tranquil again, but my heart is pounding wildly, and my white-knuckled hands grip the railing of his bed. Sensing my anxiety, Karen smiles, and, with a soothing voice, promises to return tomorrow. Only briefly left alone to regain my composure, I am greeted by another member of Zack's medical team.

Dr. Lenhardt, the anesthesiologist, strides in with his gaggle of residents to analyze the oxygen levels and recorded information from the monitor. He announces that his team would like to keep him on the respirator for five more days before considering a tracheostomy, since Zack might regain consciousness. On the other hand, Dr. Densler, the neurosurgeon, would like to move to a trach immediately, to avoid any potential complications. Depleted oxygen would cause the pressure in his brain to build up and could, ultimately, impair brain function. They reach a compromise, agreeing to defer the procedure for two days to see how he is responding. The back and forth between the doctors is excruciatingly frustrating. We want to ask questions, but don't know who to ask, or even if they will agree. Scott shrugs his shoulders, rolling his eyes in confusion and signals that he's headed downstairs.

Drained and exhausted, Scott wanders into the lobby, absentmindedly twirling a cigarette. His brain flooding with questions, he goes outside to smoke and clear his head. He stumbles onto a concealed spot around the left side of the building behind an oversized rock. Overwhelmed by the thought that his son may never wake up, he drops to his knees, begging

God to save Zack. He mourns for the boy whose laughter filled the air while he was teaching him to master the game of golf. His heart aching, he adjusts the brim of his cap to cover his tear-stained face and returns to the lobby. Waiting for the elevator, he pushes the button, hangs his head, and tears stream down his face. A woman from behind the front desk approaches him. Compassionately, a maternal, southern voice inquires, "What's wrong, baby?" Feeling like a broken record, Scott chokes out the words that his son is upstairs dying. She embraces him, steps back with a smile, and whispers, "Oh, everything is gonna be fine, baby. I have a direct line to Jesus." The doors slide open, and she nudges him into the elevator. As the doors close, he looks back and sees her beautiful, smiling face.

Comforted by her revelation, Scott comes bounding into the waiting room and proclaims that he believes Zack will wake up. Enthusiastic, launching into a description of the wonderful soul that just altered his outlook, he pulls me towards the elevator. He urges me to be introduced to the messenger responsible for his epiphany, but there are a lot of visitors vying for my attention. I assure him that I will make time to meet her, and with a tired smile, I continue my conversation with concerned relatives patiently waiting to be updated.

As I take a seat, I am approached by a couple I don't recognize. Monica Key introduces herself as a friend of my niece and explains the reason for her visit. Her husband had been in a motorcycle accident, suffered a traumatic brain injury, and nearly died. My attention is drawn to Mark. His smile lights up his entire face as he hands me a small notebook and explains I should write down my questions. "You don't get to see the doctors very much, and if you don't write them down, you may forget to ask important questions," he sputters. I accept the notebook, and he feels around in his pocket, disappointed when he cannot locate a pen. Monica instructs him to ask at the nurse's station, and Mark slowly shuffles towards the desk.

"I know what you're thinking," she says sympathetically. "He's not right... not... perfect." I start to protest, but she interrupts. "Mark is different. He's still recovering, but he won't ever be the same. And I couldn't love him more. It's hard to explain, but I feel very blessed to have this version of him."

 I watch as he makes his way back to us. He takes tiny steps and seems almost robotic. But it's his engaging smile and the adoring way his wife looks at him that captivates me. He presents me with the pen, reminding me to write my questions down, so I won't forget. It's worthy advice, since the 10 minutes during rounds in the morning leave little time for contemplation. As I stand to say goodbye, they promise to stay in touch, and we embrace. Monica hugs me and whispers, "You'll see." I slide the notebook into my back pocket, and they amble to the elevator, holding hands like high school sweethearts.

We are receiving cards at the hospital with words of encouragement from people we have never met; strangers who were here for other reasons and came across us circled in prayer or saw all his friends in the second floor waiting room. They are amazed that teenagers would prefer to spend their time hanging around a hospital, rather than enjoying their summer vacation. There is so much love and prayers flowing around Zack, I don't see how he can "sleep" much longer.

I settle in Zack's room for the evening, and Scott leaves to tend to the kids at home. He bristles with anticipation, striding through the lobby, searching for the angel with divine wisdom and engaging smile. Plopped behind the information desk, a young girl with her face buried in a magazine barely looks up when he describes who he is looking for. He calls me from his truck, confident he will find her tomorrow and arrange for us to meet. It is well past midnight when I finally arrive home, and the house is asleep. I will be gone, standing vigil at Zack's bedside, before anyone wakes up.

Rushing to the hospital in the rain, traffic piling up even at this early hour, has me fretting that I won't get to see Zack before rounds at 7:00 a.m. My tires squeal on the wet pavement as I enter the garage, and I quickly bounce out of the car. Fumbling, I drop my keys in a hurry to get stuff out of my car, and they careen down the sewer grate. Crying tears of frustration, realizing that now I will have to wait until 8:30 to get into the ICU, I collapse to my knees in a desperate attempt to fish them out. The parking attendant, like a knight in polo and khakis, comes to my recue and quickly retrieves them with a hanger.

I rush through the hospital corridor, taking the stairs, rather than having to wait for the elevator. The doors to Neuro ICU are closed, and no one will be allowed in until after doctors make their rounds. Finding a comfortable way to sit on the floor, I decide not to take any chances and remain right outside the ICU doors. It was worth the wait to see Zack doing so well.

His face is still bloated, but his eyes aren't as swollen, and I notice that something *sounds* different. The familiar methodical rhythm is frequently interrupted, and the nurse explains that he is breathing over the ventilator. The staff has come to expect me here during morning rounds, so she fills me in on what I missed while key fishing in the garage. She describes how when the doctor called him by name, his blood pressure shot up, which indicates he is aware of things going on around him. When Dr. Densler pinched him, he opened his eyes and quickly moved his hand to that spot. I've witnessed that twisted tweak. I coax an opening in his gown and place a kiss from my fingertips on the purple bruises forming near his arm pit.

Forcing a smile as tears slip slowly down my cheeks, I thank her for being so patient and sink into my chair. Intently staring at the monitor, I whisper his name, wondering which blinking number indicates his blood pressure. With a mother's intuition, I sense that he knows I've been here by his side, and now, I want the monitor to validate my feelings. I squeeze his hand and murmur that I don't need some stupid machine to confirm that he is mindful of my presence. I inhale deeply as I close my eyes, steeple my fingers, and announce that God is in control.

Throughout the day, Zack's friends arrive to take their places in the waiting room. The hospital has become a gathering place, and I often get to sit with teenagers and listen to their stories. Witnessing the turmoil of what our family is going through has opened their eyes and many express guilt over things they were doing. They compete with stories about Zack, and at times, I can't help but cry, which in turn, makes them choke up. Listening as they describe various tales of adventure and giggling at their antics makes me feel closer to Zack. But as the surgery doors slide open, and doctors bring disheartening news to other families, we are jolted back to reality. We are humbled, vulnerable. It feels healing.

Then, at 6:30 p.m., my whole world ignites. Escorting the next troop of friends up to visit Zack, I see the overhead lights on in his room and a frenzy of excitement. Zack was giving the thumbs up! His eyes were open! Those big, brown eyes, refusing to blink, pierce my heart, until I think it will explode. As his nurse gives a command, he delivers. Before long, the room is bursting with the entire nursing staff celebrating this momentous occasion. Zack gives us quite a show. It is intentional and spectacular. He presents his thumb, wiggles his toes, and sticks out his tongue on command. It is the most exhilarating moment, filled with lots of tears. Scott has to sprint from the room, because he is so overwhelmed. Scott's mom and numerous friends are dashing in, and the staff is gracious to allow many people to share our experience. We wear Zack out.

Needless to say, my emotional state is entirely different than when I arrived at the hospital early this morning. I am practically skipping down hall when we leave him. My face is beaming with joy. None of this would be possible without the prayers of so many people over the last four days. I have never asked why this happened. I know why it happened…it was an answered prayer. For the last several years, every morning in my prayers for my children, I ask that they be caught in their disobedience, so bad behavior can be corrected. I didn't expect the discipline to be quite so harsh, but only God knows how to get Zack's attention. In the process, many of his friends have learned a valuable lesson, and it's spreading across our community as other teens hear about his accident. Many know him only casually through other friends, yet they arrive in droves, hoping to see him and sheepishly request a piece of his sweatshirt. They recognize the significance. GOD ANSWERS PRAYERS!

Some prayers have been answered quietly, and others, God throws at us like thunder!

# *Wednesday*

When I step into Zack's room this morning, I know something is different. His night nurse, Stephanie, quietly follows me into the room. Grinning ear to ear, she excitedly reveals that he has been breathing on his own all night. She draws my attention to the monitor, and I peer at the rapidly changing numbers. His ventilator is set at 14 breaths per minute, but the screen displays 18, 20, 23, and remarkably, 28; indicating that the ventilator was assisting him, but he is also taking several breaths on his own. Moving closer to the bed, I notice an obvious difference in his demeanor. He appears relaxed, almost as if he has grown accustomed to the frenzy of the ICU. My gaze returns to his monitor, and I take note of other critical statistics: his ICP was low, and his heart rate was strong. A smile spreads across my face, and I clutch his hand in both of mine. This patient is starting to resemble my boy again.

Just before lunch, Dr. Mutchnick, part of the neurological team, strides into the room. Pulling on surgical gloves, he removes the dressings and examines Zack's head. He reports that the laceration on the top of his head is "a mess", and he will have to remove all the stitches, clean it out, and re-stitch it to eliminate any leaks. I begin to ask questions when he interrupts me, turns on the overhead light, and adjusts the bed. I'm standing there with a puzzled look when he tells me to talk to Zack and hold his hand. Flabbergasted that this is going to happen in his room, right now, I swallow the lump forming in my throat, maneuver around the cords, and grab his hand. My palms are sweating and my pulse is quickening as he starts removing tiny sutures. I can hear him nonchalantly babbling, but I intently focus on Zack, trying my best to comfort him. He is sedated and loaded with morphine, but he definitely feels it. His body stiffens, and his heart rate climbs sharply. Dr Mutchnick scrubs his head like an old boot. I can't even watch surgery on TV, and never thought I could handle it live, but I hold it together for Zack, silently wiping the tears on my sleeve. When it is finally over, I feel like I just appeared on a dramatic episode of *ER*.

Zack is out for several hours while the sedatives continue to work their magic. I take the opportunity to call Scott and fill him in on my chance opportunity to be part of his bedside surgery. He is so disappointed he wasn't there to comfort Zack, and no matter what I say to relieve his guilt, he feels like he had failed his son.

It seems only a short time later that Scott hurries into the room, breathless, with tear-streaked cheeks. Proudly holding up a baseball, he presents it to Zack, stating, "This homerun was hit for you!" Then, he describes how he was driving past the baseball stadium, feeling dejected and frustrated that he had let Zack down, when suddenly a baseball came out of nowhere and bounced in front of his truck. Without thinking, he slammed his truck into park and bounded out into the street in the middle of a busy intersection. He held up his hands up to stop traffic, with horns blaring, as he chased after the ball that had rolled underneath a parked car. After retrieving it, he held it up like a trophy for the other commuters to see, jumped back into his truck, and raced to the hospital to deliver it to Zack. He places it in Zack's right hand and curls his fingers around the ball. *"This was hit for you. God sent this for you"*. I don't know if Zack understands what he is saying, but it doesn't matter. This gift is just what Scott needed.

I am amazingly grateful that when we feel defeated and alone, God sends us something to let us know He is always there. He could have chosen numerous ways to make us feel His presence, but today, it was a baseball, hit at just the right time so Scott would see it. No small coincidence. Scott delights in repeating his baseball story for several visitors, and before long, his demeanor became one of confident assurance that God is in control.

At 6:00 p.m., a nurse informs us of the decision to turn off the ventilator, since Zack was breathing on his own. Although the vent is not assisting him, he still has the tube down his throat, and as he breathes, he gets additional oxygen. The sedatives wear off, and he starts to respond to verbal commands. Not quite so quick with the thumbs up, but still responding. His nurse agrees that he is much farther along than anyone expected, considering the severity of his injury. Drawing close to him, I stroke his brow, and he flinches. I'm torn between two emotions: delighted that he is breathing on his own, but cautious, since he seems uncomfortable and somewhat agitated.

As darkness starts to swallow up his room, I get the opportunity to speak with Dr. John Hill, one of the critical care team. I confess that I'm concerned about the tube still clogging up his throat, reiterating that it seems to bother him, and ask when they might remove it. He wrinkles his forehead and studies Zack's appearance, scanning the monitor as it continues to register his oxygen stats. Nodding and careful not to overpromise, he says, "Probably in four or five days." Not the answer I want, but then, I smile to myself as I consider our outwardly impossible situation.

We ride a roller-coaster of emotions, life-threatening decisions, and unbearable circumstances. But I have felt His presence and witnessed His mercy. God has broken all the rules with Zack. I am starting to feel honored that God has chosen Zack to glorify Him with daily blessings in the form of healing. God is the great physician, and if Zack got up and walked out of here tomorrow, I would be elated, but not surprised.

A nxious for my update from Stephanie, his night nurse, I arrive at the hospital at 6:30 a.m. She grins and follows me to the foot of Zack's bed and says that Zack had a great night. She describes that hours earlier, he had given a thumbs up, so feeling encouraged, Stephanie asked for two fingers. She coaxed him several times, but he wouldn't oblige. Then, as she turned to leave the room, she happened to glance back at him. There he was tapping two fingers on his chest. It just took him a little longer than she anticipated, explaining that it is typical after a traumatic brain injury for reactions to be slower as the neurons in his brain struggle to make connections. Satisfied with her clarification, she adjusts his bedding, and we stand side by side, our gaze stuck on Zack's face, just silently watching him breathe.

I relish the time I have alone with Zack in the morning. Taking my place on the side of the bed, always facing the door, I notice that he is alert. He has stopped the shaking. Stephanie agrees that he is beginning to get used to what they have to do to assess him every hour. I try to get a thumbs up from him, slightly disappointed when I get no response. I am holding his right hand when he starts very purposefully rubbing the top of mine with his thumb. From the beginning as I keep vigil, I stroke his hand or caress his arm. Now, it feels as though he is returning that love. My hand rests on his chest as the moment envelopes me. Suddenly, out of the blue, he snaps his fingers twice. Startled, I call out towards the nurse's station, catching Stephanie's attention. As she enters the room, I take her arm to draw her next to the bed. Excitedly pointing and dancing my feet around, I exclaim, "Zack just snapped his fingers! Twice!" We repeatedly try to get him to do it again, but that seems to be a trick only for Mom.

Throughout the morning, he repeatedly taps his upper chest with two fingers. Not by command, but as though he's trying to communicate. He appears restless, rolling his shoulders. Breathing on his own, unassisted by the ventilator, but still with this thick plastic tube shoved down his throat. His eyes are open. I study his face. I feel as though he speaks to me through those pleading eyes. This is my boy. Memories flash across my mind of that precious baby gazing up at me, trusting, totally reliant on my care. We are connected, and without words, I understand his pleas. I know that he doesn't want that tube clogging his throat. It brings tears to my eyes. I entwine my fingers into his, murmuring a prayer, not really knowing what to request. Our door faces the nurses' station, and they perceive my distress. Nodding in my direction, the sympathetic staff allows me to stay with him through rounds.

At 9:00 a.m., Dr. Mutchnick arrives to remove the bolt implanted in his head that measures the pressure inside his brain (ICP). He greets me with a sideways glace, washes his hands at the sink, and the staff starts to prep the room. Bright lights flood overhead, and the hairs on the back of my neck stand on end. I hear him snap his latex gloves and realize I will witness another surgery. Mutchnick watches over her shoulder as the nurse injects a syringe into the pic line. They discuss his reaction during the procedure yesterday, and I picture his writhing torso. Concluding that he seems to be very resistant to pain medication, they decide to dose him heavily with morphine and sedatives. He looks at me as if I do this every day, nods, and says, "Take his hand." I cradle Zack's left hand in both of mine, and my legs tremble. I can't watch. I mumble incoherently as Mutchnick makes small talk. He removes the bolt and takes a few stitches. It didn't take long, but I felt every minute as I counted the heartbeats echoing in my ear. Heavily medicated, I think Zack came through this one better than I did.

I recover in time to have a consult with the plastic surgeon, who comes in to examine the stitch job done the day before to close his laceration. He reports that it is sealed tight and looks good, but because of the trauma to that area, Zack will not grow hair on a patch a little bigger than a quarter. The sutures from the bolt will heal fine without noticeable scarring. Additional staff arrive and fit him with a rubber helmet that he must wear to protect his brain until his skull is reattached. Flooded with morphine during his bedside surgery, he is quiet most of the day, not really responding to verbal commands.

As his friends arrive, I take several in to see him at a time. There are stringent regulations in the ICU, but the staff accommodates our constant parade. I gather them in the hall outside, reviewing with a group of about 12 or 15 teenagers the plan for the next several days. We believe it is vital to Zack's recovery that his friends be able to visit him. These moments are crucial for them as well. Our message on the power of prayer resonates when they are able to witness each small victory. We need to keep him stimulated during the day, but resting at night, so in the afternoon, we turn on the TV and open his blinds. As evening approaches, Scott comments that Zack looks uncomfortable and tells him to wiggle his toes if he wants to sit up. Immediately, he moves his toes. A very positive sign, since most of the day he was not consistently following commands.

My thoughts wander as I have a conversation with our night nurse. Marca claims Zack is trying very hard to "wake up". His eyes are open, but he's not all the way there. He is not in a coma, but he is not awake either. Stuck in a land somewhere in between. He keeps squeezing my hand and purposefully pointing to the tube. He is not restrained, and at times, tears fall from his eyes. My heart aches, I am overcome with emotion, and I pledge that the tube will come out tomorrow. Less than confident that I can fulfill my promise, hunched over his bed, I sob as if the air is too thick to breathe. I feel as though I am giving birth to him all over again, only this time, he is the one experiencing the pain. It is excruciating, knowing there is little I can do to comfort him. I know that he is cognizant of what's going on and asking me to help him. I beg God for the peace that I had earlier. I turn again to the 23rd Psalm and pray with Zack, hoping he can understand me through choked-backed tears. In my mind, I search for words that can bring me comfort and dwell on the scripture that God disciplines those he loves. Blinking through the tears, I look up and see the button someone pinned above his bed that says, "I am loved."

He is loved…by me, his dad, his family, and countless others. But most significantly, he is loved by God. I cannot fathom how anyone can make it through this kind of tragedy without faith in God. The peace that passes all understanding is a gift of love from God to those who believe and trust in Him.

It is exactly one week since we were awakened in the middle of the night by a call that turned our world upside down. I'm replaying that fateful moment in my mind as I arrive on 5West. A nurse trails me as I enter his room, seeming less than enthusiastic to provide the morning report. Zack has a fever of 100.1, which means his body is fighting something. He is less responsive today than yesterday. She explains that the critical care team will assess him during rounds to determine whether they can extubate him. Pointing to the new apparatus strapped to his mouth, she informs me that at 4:00a.m., they put him on T-Piece (TP). This is a smaller tube that gives him humidified oxygen as he breathes. They rotate this treatment with TP for two hours and then return to CPAP, which provides only pressure to encourage him to take a breath. This is in preparation for his critical 7:00 a.m. exam. He has to perform well for the doctors in order for the tube to be pulled.

The team makes their rounds, and I'm heartbroken. Zack does not do well. Refusing to give a thumbs up or even wiggle his toes, his assessment is over in minutes. Dr. Lenhardt says he is not ready. Hugely disappointed, remembering my commitment to Zack last night that we would get that tube out today, I plead with Dr. Lenhardt. Justifying Zack's lack of response to his rough night sleep and elevated temperature, I beg for another opportunity. Recognizing my determination, the team agrees to reevaluate him later. He makes a notation on his chart and departs to address other ICU patients, leaving me to wallow in despair. I'm immediately shuttled back to last night, watching his feeble finger pointing to this foreign object gagging up his throat. My spirits are low, and I am very emotional. We have been so blessed with how fast he has been recovering that we expect new progress every day.

Zack looks tired, his eyelids drooping, but it appears as if he is watching the golf match on TV. I'm focused on the clock, its jerky hands reminding me that time is ticking away. Finally, the critical care team returns to give Zack a second chance, but he repeats his pitiful morning performance. Dr. Lenhardt is very cautious and doesn't want to extubate him yet. He explains that the important thing is that Zack is off the ventilator and breathing on his own. I can't wrap my mind around that attempt at consolation, arguing internally. I scream in my head that the important thing to me is that Zack is tortured by that tube clogging his throat, so we want it out. I'm trembling, my legs feeling the strain of an uncertain attempt to fight for my son. It's so difficult to go from Dr. Lenhardt's cautious approach when we have become accustomed to Dr. Densler's aggressive one. Finally, he agrees to give Zack another assessment tomorrow, and I breathe a sigh of relief.

Kim Myre, the nurse practitioner for the Neuro Team, confers with ICU nurses, Tom, and Christy, about putting Zack in a chair, reasoning that he will be more alert sitting up. They also decide to put him back on TP. We are gathered at the nurses' station, but my attention is drawn to his room. I slip in to talk with Zack, and, for the first time, I am frustrated with him. I speculate that he is being stubborn, and I lecture him on the importance of his consistent response to verbal commands in order to be rid of the tube. I'm desperately begging for the slightest sign of cognition.

After much coaxing, he gives me a small thumbs up, but nothing else. I fight back tears. My shaking hands grip the bedrails. I feel as though we need a Lazarus miracle, and I pray for one.

At 2:00p.m., they put his helmet on and prepare the chair, a special type of stretcher that adjusts into a sitting position. Dr. Densler and Dr. Mutchnick are made aware of my incessant appeals and stride in, just as they are moving him to the chair. It is notably obvious how upset I am. They command his room and discuss options with the nursing staff, requesting his blood gases be checked. They want to examine how his body is processing carbon dioxide, which is an indicator of how well he will do when they extubate. Dr. Densler reminds me that a trach could be the next step, and it is not necessarily a bad thing. His voice exudes confidence, and it's strange that a trach does not evoke fear in me.

While I have been managing the current crisis, a herd of his friends have been forming at the entrance to 5West. Tom tells me I need to control them, so we have a poignant conversation in the corridor on the role they play in his recovery. I succeed in bringing a dozen of Zack's classmates into his room. We close the door, and they talk with him. Their sincerity is stirring, and I am encouraged by the amazing team of people praying, urging Zack to respond. He struggles, but his friends are able to get a thumb wiggle out of him, which heightens all our spirits. Throughout the day, Zack remains inconsistent in following verbal commands. He still localizes to pain, but that is not sufficient. I am an emotional wreck, waiting for miracles that don't come. God is giving me lessons in patience, because it is certainly not one of my virtues.

Coach Woods, one of Zack's baseball coaches, announces his arrival. As he addresses him, it appears Zack is listening intently. Intuitively, Coach keeps giving him baseball signals until Zack responds to the "wipe off" sign. He intentionally moves his arms several times, reassuring us that he's still in there. At this point, we will accept whatever miniscule action resembles our son. Scott and I are both on edge, at times snapping at each other and subsequently riddled with guilt for not considering the other's distress. A pained look in his eye, Scott kisses my cheek and asserts that he is staying the night, and I need to leave earlier, so I can get more sleep. His tone is admonishing as he reminds me that Dylan and the girls need to see their mom.

From the beginning of this ordeal, I have spent all my waking hours at the hospital, while Scott has managed things at home. The girls, in particular, don't understand why I'm not there to help with summer reading or tuck them into bed. Last night, Scott had gathered all three of them together and explained that Zack isn't doing well, and right now, he needs his mom more than they did. Kyle and Dylan listened quietly at his feet, but Logan is only six and cries as she sits in her daddy's lap. It is difficult for Scott not to cry himself as he explains that he misses me, too, but we have to be strong for Zack. He promises them that their mom still loves them, and if they were in the hospital, I would be with them, too. Often, after he gets them in bed, he sits in the dark on the deck, watching the puddle of tears grow between his feet. At his lowest, he drowns his sorrows in a bottle of bourbon. Sometimes, he feels as if he has no wife and his children have no mother. I have had the grim job of learning to be an advocate for Zack, but at times, I think it has been tougher for Scott. He anxiously calls for updates and gets concerned when I don't answer my phone. Every minute that he waits for me to return his call, he imagines something terrible has happened. He has had to learn how to fix little girls' hair, get them dressed for day camp, and make sure that all three do their summer reading. He has been forced to be both Mom and Dad during a very traumatic time for our family.

Before leaving, I request that Zack have no more visitors, so he can get some rest and be ready for his assessment in the morning. We need to get the tube removed, but he must consistently respond to verbal commands for that to happen. Deep in thought, my muscles quivering with tension, I hurry to the parking garage. When I left his room, I noticed that Zack looked so tired. I can't get this image out of my mind on the ride home. A light illuminates the kitchen as I pull into the driveway. Dylan and Kyle are watching TV with our neighbor, Morgan. Not quite a year older than Dylan, she has championed the evening hours when both of us are at the hospital. Logan has fallen asleep on the couch and awakens at the sound of my voice. Both my girls rush to hug me, while Dylan hangs back with a sheepish grin on his face. It is good to be home, but there is a hole in my heart where my eldest child is missing. I watch as Dylan walks Morgan across the lawn to her house, the girls fighting for my attention. I promise a slumber party with all of us in my bed, and they scurry off to claim their spot. Dylan returns, and I finally get his hug as he informs me that he will be sleeping in his own bed. The house is dark as I climb the stairs to our bedroom. Logan is already asleep, and Kyle takes up more than her share, so I make do with my sliver of bed. I try to relax but can't help dwelling on the notion that Zack seems to have taken steps backwards in his recovery. I pray that he will be giving the thumbs up again, that he can fight off infection, that I will get my peace back and not be so restless. Our God is so powerful, but sometimes, he needs to slow things down, so we can hear His whispers and feel His healing touch.

Arriving at 6:30 a.m. to the distressing news that Zack had been unresponsive all night, was not the ideal way to start the morning. Scott describes his periodic attempts through the night to get Zack to follow verbal commands to no avail. As he rambles on, seeming to apologize for the failure, I notice he looks nearly as bad as Zack. He is visibly distraught, dark circles under his eyes, and a disheveled appearance. Repeating that Zack would be assessed during morning rounds, and he fears disaster, he hangs his head in defeat. After speaking with the nurse, I had a better understanding of why Scott seemed so out of sorts. It is impossible to obtain a moment of sleep when every two hours, the staff interrupts the night to check vitals and change IV bags. The in-line suction of his lungs is a grotesque, disturbing sound that echoes in your ears long after the procedure is over. The guidance the staff gave me early on, to go home to sleep, proves to be excellent advice. Zack's temperature has continued to climb, necessitating further tests. They obtain blood, urine, and sputum cultures, discovering that his white count is elevated, further indicating he is fighting infection. The lab must identify the infection to know what type of antibiotic to prescribe. Our only positive report was that the latest CAT scan shows no change, a good sign.

The neurosurgeon, Dr. Harpring, arrives to report that Zack has pneumonia, so they will keep him on the tube through the weekend and trach him on Monday. The good news is that we now have an explanation for his lack of response. He doesn't feel well. He doesn't want to do anything, which is natural, considering his condition. But the bad news is that annoying tube remains. I feel so helpless. Why can't they just go ahead and remove it today? The nurses have described that once they trach him, it will be a lot easier to suction his lungs; he will start feeling better and be more responsive. They help me visualize an optimistic future that has Zack advancing into rehab, detailing the steps that must occur for a patient to be accepted. They explain that when he recovers from pneumonia and no longer presents a fever, they will remove the NG tube from his nose and insert a gastric tube into his stomach. He needs more fuel to repair his brain and stave off further infections. Most importantly, he also cannot be transferred to Frazier Rehab until the feeding tube is out of his nose, and that is the ultimate goal... to start rehab.

I am doing my best to relay all of this information to his friends who were gathered in the corridor for a group visit, when Rita informs me that Scott wants to spend time alone with Zack. He is feeling guilty for pressuring Zack throughout the night to follow verbal commands, only to find out this morning that he has pneumonia. Desperate to apologize, he requests that I take the group back downstairs to wait. On Saturdays, we crowd the waiting room with visitors, and today is no exception, with most of them there to see Zack. Only minutes later, our chattering is interrupted when Rita comes panting downstairs, claiming they are removing the tube. Rushing upstairs, I shake my head in confusion. The Neuro Team had just declared this morning that they wouldn't proceed until Monday. Dr. Lenhardt is instructing the staff when I enter the room.

I nervously relay how baffled I am that they are doing this now, after what Neuro had told me this morning. Very nonchalantly, he reminds me that this is what I had wanted yesterday, but Zack wasn't ready and now he is. Just like that.

It is early afternoon, the overhead light obnoxiously bright as Scott and I stand anxiously at the foot of his bed. The room is a fury of activity with various medical personnel dashing around in preparation. This frenzy just added to the turmoil blowing up my brain. Dr. Lenhardt explains that when they remove the tube, Zack has to breathe, or we will go through the traumatic experience of reinserting it. He pauses, looking us solemnly in the eyes, to be sure we grasp the gravity of what he just revealed. My heart thumping wildly, I back towards the wall and grab onto Scott's arm. Time seems to move wickedly in slow motion. A resident on each side guides Zack to a sitting position, supporting his back with their elbows. Hearing what I perceive as a muffled countdown, Lenhardt grasps the tube and pulls. I stare at Zack's face. His eyes bulging as though they would burst from their sockets, his mouth gaping as they abruptly yank the tube from his throat. It seems ridiculously long and slimy, covered with mucus.

I bury my head into Scott's chest, my legs shuddering. Immediately, startling the staff, Scott starts screaming, "Breathe Zack, breathe!" I begin to sob, gasping, as if unable to breathe myself. Suddenly, Zack coughs, and a big glob of something gross shoots out of his mouth. All eyes intently bounce back and forth between his face and the monitor. He is breathing on his own! He collapses onto the pillow, the fear draining from his face as his color returns to normal. There are celebratory high fives among the staff. Scott holds me; our arms draped around each other as we cry tears of relief.

Zack is instantly put on an oxygen mask. His eyes are completely open, his face flushed as if he just completed a marathon. With an almost quizzical look, he stares at something or someone, his eyes glazing over. Several of the superficial cuts on his face have begun to heal, the pink scars contrast against his clammy skin. Without a bone flap, his brain expands the right side of his bulbous head, which is slowly growing peach fuzz around the massive train tracks that mark his surgery. His arms are limp beside his shrinking torso, his legs numb with exhaustion. Nurses move about the room, adjusting the monitor cables and calling out vital information for the record. An aide cleans up, discarding the mucous plug that catapulted from Zack's mouth, landing at my feet like an alien. I lower the bed rail and lean forward. My skin is tingling, and my whispered voice cracks, "You did it, Zack." I inhale sharply, exhaling loudly through pursed lips. "Breathe." It's a bizarre feeling to be traumatized by witnessing an event that you had lobbied for so vigorously. A nurse gets our attention and explains that Zack must continue to cough and swallow. He needs to be able to maintain his airway and move fluids from his lungs. In the blink of an eye, we have new numbers haunting us … his respiratory rate. She identifies the blinking light on his monitor, currently fluctuating between 18 and 23. If this number were to climb over 30, they would consider him in respiratory distress.

We are elated that there is no longer a gruesome tube violating his mouth. As the evening wears on, Zack looks much more like himself, except when they remove his mask, and I remark on his big, swollen lip. His nurse gives me a lopsided smirk and describes the first time they attempted to suction some mucus from the back of his throat. He clamped down on his teeth, his eyebrows narrowing. There was no way he was letting anyone put anything back into his mouth. Unfortunately, his lip got in the way, and he bit it until blood was running down his chin. I smile. Perhaps a little of the stubborn teenager has returned.

So much has transpired that it seems like we've been here much longer than nine days. Our world is so confined to these walls. I don't watch the news, read any magazines, or even listen to the radio in my car. I don't want to think that the world carries on without him. Time flies when I am at the hospital. We are forced to live in the moment and not think much beyond tomorrow, because we don't know what the future holds. I have faith that God will heal Zack, but I know it will be in His timing, and sometimes, that doesn't seem to move fast enough. Just when I am frustrated to the point of tears, the right person shows up. They pray with us and listen to my never-ending accounts of what has occurred during the day. Many seek prayer requests, and I'm grateful that our needs seem to be made abundantly clear to me. Our petition now is for Zack to cough and swallow, that he gains enough strength to battle pneumonia. I request peace for Scott, who struggles now with having to leave the hospital in order to work a few hours. We appeal to all the kids out there who just haven't gotten the message yet, and hope that their parents aren't sitting here someday.

As I mindlessly walk through sterile corridors to the parking garage, I think about how odd it is that I have adjusted to spending my days in a hospital room, instead of constantly being on the go, running kids to the next practice. I am grateful that God has given me the necessary forte to make what feels life and death decisions every day for Zack. But I feel guilt-ridden that my other children don't get any of my time. I shake my head, intentionally trying to push those thoughts out of my mind. Zack needs me now more than any other time in his life, and I will make sure my kids understand that I love them just as much.

I arrive home to Scott in his usual spot in the dark on our deck, and he seems anxious to talk with me. He begins to recreate the scene where he coaches Zack to breathe, reliving it as he weeps. My mind drifts back to that paralyzing moment, but fatigue gets the best of me. I'm tired and just need to get some sleep. Absentmindedly patting his back, I turn to go inside, trying not to feel guilty for denying him my attention. *There's only so much of me to go around,* I think to myself. Climbing in bed, I drift off to sleep, hearing God's gentle whisper, prompting me to breathe.

This morning, I step into an intense flurry of activity. Zack's respiratory rate is a very high 33 to 38. The grave expression from his nurse has me feeling nauseated, even before she points out that Zack is not moving at all. His white count is up, and he is still running a fever. He refuses to cough, even though his lungs rattle. Although his chest x-ray looks better today than yesterday, he has a lot of fluid in his upper respiratory, and it sounds like he has the croup. As he struggles to breathe, you can see his rib cage expanding. His frightened eyes flutter as he gasps for air. It is like he is breathing through a straw. It is an ugly sight. Nurse Kelly compassionately explains that his blood gases are presently good, but should they become compromised, the Neuro Team foresees his brain swelling. I am distraught, and tears stream down my face.

Frantically, I call Scott, barely capable of stringing two words together that make any sense. Choking back tears, I plead with him to get in touch with Southeast Christian Church and have everyone pray. Not able to concentrate, my entire body shivering with fear, I keep wiping Zack's brow and clutching his hand. I nudge closer and envision us in the valley as I recite the 23rd Psalm. Repeating the 4th verse, I whisper, "Even though I walk through the darkest valley, I will fear no evil, for you are with me." I echo the final verse, my head buried into his chest, "and I will dwell in the house of the Lord forever." Acutely aware that respiratory distress would require them to intubate him again, I cry out to God. I can't bear the thought of that tube jammed down his throat, but this is worse.

The critical care team starts him back on Vancomycin, an antibiotic to treat his pneumonia. They consult with Dr. Reed, a respiratory therapist, who adopts an old school approach. He introduces an anti-inflammatory in Zack's oxygen mask, hoping to shrink the swollen airway passage. It helps, but it's only temporary. I pace aimlessly, the sound of my son straining to breathe fills my ears. We have garnered the attention of most of the ICU staff, each one intent on tracking his vitals, as the neon green numbers mock their attempts. Dr. Miller, resident anesthesiologist, draws the short straw and delivers the news.

Zack can't continue like this. They will have to intubate. Oh, please, God, no. I beg for other options and tearfully request a second opinion, explaining that I would rather have him trached. Suddenly uncomfortable, he confesses that a tracheotomy won't be done on a Sunday and leaves the room. Ever present, Nurse Kelly overheard the impassioned conversation. She glances at the door, and although they are not supposed to voice their opinions, she quietly tells me to stand my ground. "The squeaky wheel gets the oil," she rumbles. I consider her admonition, grasping his excuse is that it's Sunday. Well, I can't allow that to be the deciding factor on whether he is trached or if another tube invades his mouth.

I can't stay seated and stomp around the room, pleading with God to show me what to do. My prayers are interrupted when my second opinion arrives. Dr. Parker, ENT, becomes my knight in shining armor as I whimper my concern about damage to Zack's vocal cords and trauma to his throat if they intubate. He listens patiently, agrees to review the x-rays, and discusses it with the critical care team to devise a plan. Within 20 minutes, they start him on Glycopyrrolate to decrease the secretions in his airway. They announce the decision to perform a bronchoscopy to suction the fluid from his lungs. At that time, they will look at his vocal cords, and if they are swollen, or if his throat is ulcerated, they will trach him. The procedure is scheduled for 2:00 p.m.

The afternoon church service at Southeast Christian Church has ended, and people flock to the hospital. Teenagers, parents, family, and friends congregate, offering support. There are 15 of us, encircled in prayer, in the second-floor surgery waiting room. It is an emotional stretch that seems to do little to comfort the foreboding feeling enveloping me. I sit off by myself, my hands covering my ears to drown out the sound that accompanies the vivid images parading across my mind. *Click, click, click.* I close my eyes and envision my white-knuckled hands gripping the bar of a roller-coaster as it inches its way to a sharp peak. Unconsciously, I hold my breath as I feel myself plummet down the other side. In reality, this coaster would slide smoothly into its berth at the bottom.

In my horrid fantasy, it crashes off a cliff. That describes my state of mind for several agonizing hours. The surgery doors slide open, and I jump to my feet when I recognize members of our critical care team. They inform us that the procedure was successful, and Zack now has a trach. There was not much swelling to his vocal cords, but he has an ulcer on his bronchi that became inflamed and irritated when he coughed. This explains his behavior. The sore would not have healed as long as the tube annoyed his throat. Everyone agreed that a trach was the best approach. Prayers of thanksgiving drastically alter the mood in the room and my imaginary roller-coaster careens with the cross.

I am relieved that we made the right decision and feel empowered that I had stood my ground requesting a second opinion. I had barely finished patting myself on the back when I was approached by staff with more information. Further test results reveal that in addition to pneumonia, Zack has MRSA, a bacterial infection rampant in hospitals. This seems to be causing more problems than the pneumonia.

I am introduced to Dr. Raff, from Infectious Decease Control (IDC), who is brought in to consult. He will be a crucial part of the team that will determine the best antibiotic to fight both infections. Dr. Raff explains that he has started the approval process for a powerful new drug that only IDC can prescribe.

By 6:00 p.m., Zack is back in his room, breathing on his own again, no longer laboring like before. The night shift nurses fuss over who will get to take care of him. Sandy indulges Stephanie, writing her name on the wall chart, since she has become attached to us. Scott believes Stephanie has a special way with Zack, and it's apparent that he is currently her favorite patient. Before I leave, Stephanie gets him to squeeze her hand. A tiny glimmer of hope that all will be well. Despite my attempt not to cry, she hears my whimper. Placing her arm around my shoulder, she comforts me with the promise that he will be responding again tomorrow. This is the roller-coaster many have warned we would be riding throughout Zack's recovery. Two steps forward, one step back. I had prepared for frequent ups-and-downs, but not the coaster that his doctors keep throwing us on.

Heaven received an abundance of petitions today and responded with God's perfect timing. Southeast Christian Church was praying and at just the right time, Dr. Parker gallops in with his second opinion. We cover him in prayer in the waiting room, and Zack's procedure goes smoothly. Reflecting that our train is back on track, I recognize that our next obstacle is his battle with pneumonia and MRSA. God is in control, and we must wait for His timing. I'll probably say that a million times this month.

Zack's white count is up slightly from yesterday as his frail body battles serious infections. Dr. Raff confirms that he qualified for a new antibiotic called Linezolid, developed to aggressively attack MRSA. He says it kills everything but the patient. It is an expensive drug with strict criteria for which patients are allowed in the program. Now, we will have Dr. Vanmeter from IDC monitoring Zack's infection.

Stephanie finishes reading the written report, lowers her clipboard, and stands next to me at the bed, our shoulders touching. Her fingers trail along the bedrail, her eyes fondly resting on Zack's face. Her expression turns serious as she describes the panic attack he had last night. His heartrate reached 150 and the quick jump in his respiratory rate set off alarms. I explain that I witnessed one of these attacks days earlier and remember it well. Fear fills his eyes; his body trembles; he breaks out in a sweat, and you can see a sense of panic. Instinctively, she reaches for his hand and continues. "We just hold his hand, talk to him quietly, and he settles down." She nods her head, "Fevers can trigger these panic attacks." Patting his hand as if to indicate all is well, she slips out the door and briefs the next shift.

I move to my position on the left side of his bed and consider his appearance. Except for his bulging head where his brain is swelling, all the puffiness is gone. No bruises are apparent, and only a few cuts are still visible. The teenage stubble on his chin helps his face to look normal. They only shaved a portion of his head for surgery, so from my view, he has hair, even if it's only on one side. His eyes are open, but seem to stare off at nothing. He still isn't considered awake, but he is not in a coma. Nurse Yolanda gives me the best description of his condition. It is like he's perpetually daydreaming. I like that better than the medical term for this phase—which is "unresponsive".

It is late afternoon when they put his helmet on and move him to the chair for physical therapy. He is sitting higher than his bed allows and can see out the window. His head is turned in that direction, and the final rays of sunshine bounce off the glass, giving the room a soft glow. It's the perfect setting for my conversation with Karen, his physical therapist. As she manipulates his legs, she engages me with stories of other patients she has seen recover from head trauma. She delights in revealing that Zack is in the "miracle room". Given that designation because of the unforgettable patients who recovered here that were thought to be hopeless. Her softening tone promises encouragement, and I listen intently.

Not long ago, there was a 60-year-old teacher who was totally unresponsive for two months. His devoted wife wouldn't give up on him, even when they discussed turning off life support. One day, he just woke up, and today, he is teaching again. Or the young man who was here just last February, and this month is trying out as the place kicker for his high school football team. A warm smile spreads across her face. She slowly surveys the room, lifting her gaze to the ceiling, as if beholding angels. Her eyes meet mine; she lifts one finger, pointing towards heaven and repeats, "Miracle room." How could I ever doubt that God's path would lead Zack to the bed 4 where miracles happen?

Karen hugs me, pats Zack on the knee, and comments how alert he appears. She suggests that he stay in his chair a little longer for additional physical stimulation. As she strolls out the door, Yolanda catches my attention and gestures with her head toward the entrance of ICU. She buzzes in two female classmates, eager for their 10 minutes. Their chatter lightens the mood, and Zack seems to appreciate the change in voices. They coax him for a response, and his hand shudders at their request for a thumbs up. He struggles unsuccessfully several times, and the effort exhausts him. I take a moment to quietly explain that Zack is fighting serious infections, which gives him very little energy for anything else. As I usher the girls out, they look sheepishly at one another and request a piece of his sweatshirt. Our situation has been the focus for days, and teens have clipped these precious reminders to their keychains or dangle them from rearview mirrors. It motivates them to make wise decisions while prompting them to pray for Zack. I retrieve a piece for each and promise them future visits. Moving to Zack's side, I lean in until we are almost face to face. His forehead glistens with sweat. I take his hand in both of mine and vow that tomorrow will be better. Whispering a prayer, I ask God for His healing touch and supernatural strength for Zack to grapple with the poison racking his body.

I barely settle in my chair when another guest is ushered in, bearing a gracefully wrapped package. Appointed by Epiphany Church to deliver a healing blanket, she presents me with a beautiful, handmade covering and a letter from the Parish Nurse, expressing that Zack was covered in prayers. I am astonished that they are even aware of our situation, as she clarifies, "When confronted with fear and uncertainty, we sometimes feel like we can't go on. In the midst of that darkness, remember that you are never alone. God is always with you, helping you through these difficult times. Know that you are covered by the prayers of the Community of Epiphany. In Jesus' name, we pray that Zack will be healed." I could no longer contain the tears that had been bottled up since Stephanie's panic attack rendition. I had held it together through Karen's miracle stories, but now, I was unexpectedly overwhelmed. The booklet tucked neatly inside the blanket, I squeeze it to my chest and let the pent-up waterworks flow. Wiping my eyes, I express my gratitude as I follow her to the door. Undoubtedly, this sweet messenger will report to her parish that their offering was well-received.

God has carried us through every moment, knowing what we seek before we ask. Praying for His healing touch just moments before He sends a blanket, a sacred reminder that we are covered in prayer. I receive daily messages from strangers who are praying for Zack. The ripple effect as his story seems to travel on the wind. Students who have never met him, families at the dinner table, entire churches miles away, missionaries meeting secretly on foreign soil, soldiers serving in dangerous countries…all petition Heaven on his behalf. How is it that so many people who don't even know him are diligently praying for his recovery? We have felt God's presence and witnessed his merciful healing. The power of prayer cannot be denied. Prayer does not change God; it changes us.

The sunrise is barely visible over the garage when I arrive at the hospital. Zack appears rested, but is perspiring profusely; his hospital gown drenched in sweat. Concerned that his fever may have spiked, I hover in the doorway, searching for Stephanie. Rationalizing that we aren't her only patient, I turn my attention back to Zack, wiping his forehead and around his neck. My back is turned, and Stephanie slips in behind me and calmly states that this is normal. He doesn't register a fever. She describes this phenomenon as "storming"—his body trying to decide to fight the infection or just flow with it. She flashes an encouraging smile and announces that he gave her a thumbs-up last night.

Dr. Vanmeter from Infectious Decease Control makes rounds at 7:30 a.m. She reports that his blood cultures were negative for MRSA, which suggests they are keeping it contained. His chest x-rays indicate we are clearing up the pneumonia. She explains that Zack will continue with the new drug Linezolid until there are no indicators of infection. I recognize how fortunate we are to have IDC managing his infection after discovering they only come to 5West to see him. Another set of hands and eyes doing God's work to heal him. The Neuro Team—Dr. Densler, Dr. Mutchnick, and Dr. Harpring—arrive for a brief assessment. They tell me not to be concerned, but they ordered another CAT scan for today, just to check things out. They discuss that when Zack has no "nursing issues" for 24 hours, they will move him out of ICU. This sounds promising, but brings new concerns.

Between visitors yesterday, I took a stroll around the other floors in anticipation of his move from the ICU. I discovered that University Hospital can be a scary place. There were police standing guard outside several rooms where gunshot victims were recovering. Patients bellowed towards an empty nurses' station while their repeated requests were ignored. I felt uncomfortable with each sideways glance, and the scowling staff confirmed my suspicions. I would never be satisfied with the reduced nurse-to-patient ratio on the floor. I returned to the elevator lobby, punching both the up and down buttons as I waited. The cab seemed a safer place to me, and I just wanted to return to 5West. Mulling over my impromptu investigation, I come to the quick conclusion that my precious boy did not belong on "the floor". I conclude that I want him transferred to Kosair Children's Hospital. I buzz into my ICU cocoon and relay my findings to a sympathetic staff. I sense some apprehension when I tell them to inform the Neuro Team of my decision to leave University.

Late in the afternoon, a somber Dr. Mutchnick crosses the threshold of our room. Apparently, he is tasked with convincing me to keep Zack at University Hospital. He interrupts my description of life outside of 5West and rambles on about the excellent medical staff commissioned at this teaching hospital. When I continue to protest, he explains that they are concerned with "continuity of care" and wants the same team of doctors to continue to follow his progress. I agree that the neuro team and critical care team are excellent, but I see them sporadically during the day and rarely at night. I reiterate that it is the nursing situation, the patient-to-staff ratio on the floor, that troubles me. Frustrated with his failed attempt to change my mind, he stomps out of the room, mumbling about Zack's gastric surgery scheduled for tomorrow afternoon.

Nurse Marca waits until Dr. Mutchnick has left 5West before entering our room. She checks Zack's vitals and swaps out an IV bag, pretending not to listen to my phone conversation with Scott. I replay my discussion with Mutchnick and his reluctance to cooperate with the move to Kosair. Scott tells me how much the girls miss me, begging for me to come home early tonight. We hang up as I slide next to the bed and stroke Zack's arm. Marca approaches the opposite side of the bed and with a concerned expression comments that it "didn't go well," referring to my debate with Dr. Mutchnick. She points out that continuity of care is important, especially for someone with a serious traumatic brain injury. Pausing, she considers my previous emotional state, her tone softens. She gently reminds me that Zack is scheduled to have a G-tube placed in his stomach tomorrow afternoon, giving me more time to decide what to do. My voice cracks as I explain how strange it is to think he might be moved from bed four in the miracle room. I have come to love the staff here, their excellent care of Zack and compassion for our family. I know that leaving ICU is a positive step, but right now, I'm experiencing joyous fear. We have developed such a familiar pattern, and a glimpse into the future is uncertain and, at times, unnerving. Marca is understanding and says that prolonged isolation in the ICU often has families reluctant to advance to other units. She promises to make the transition smooth for us, but I still feel apprehensive.

As night approaches, I am alone with Zack and experience a calm serenity. The beeping of his monitor matches my heartbeat, and we can practically inhale the peacefulness. I notice the small stack of papers placed neatly beside my purse and remember my niece, Sherry, delivering them earlier. Reclining on the couch, I begin to pour over the messages posted on the blog where I keep everyone updated on Zack's recovery. With all the turmoil, I haven't had an opportunity to read them, so I am a week behind. This is where God rescues me again. I am captivated as I read of how Zack is surrounded by prayer. I am deeply touched by how people describe him and emotionally uplifted by the thought that while Zack sleeps, God is talking with him, holding him in the palm of His hand. That He is revealing himself to Zack, expressing how much He loves him. I close my eyes and envision this spectacular scene. Moving to the bed, I gaze at Zack without that anxious feeling of wanting him to wake up. My fingers brush his cheek tenderly as I imagine God whispering to him. What a perfect way to be directed back to God's timing. Thank you, Lord, for your perfect plan.

Driving home, I realize that I stayed much longer than I had intended. Silently chastising myself for not heeding Scott's advice, I pull up to a dark house that signals that everyone is asleep. Quietly entering through the garage, I tiptoe up the stairs. At the top landing, I see a torn piece of paper with a note scribbled in pencil. My sweet Kyle writes that she hasn't seen me in a long time, to please wake her, no matter how late it is, so she can give me a hug. I creep to her room and watch her as she sleeps. I kiss her cheek and whisper that I love her. She stirs and rolls over, sound asleep. I can't wake her this late. I go down to the kitchen and write her a simple message. "I love you. Zack needs me, but he's getting better, and I will be home again soon." I crawl into bed trying not to wake Scott, consumed with guilt. Then, I cry myself to sleep.

Zack had been fever-free for almost 24 hours. Throughout the night, his heart rate and respiratory remained steady. The results from yesterday's CAT scan showed no change, and even some improvement. Dr. Vanmeter explains that MRSA was not discovered in his lungs, indicating that we are only battling this infection in his upper respiratory. I am encouraged by his progress, but disturbed by an uneasy feeling. I catch myself wringing my hands every time a doctor approaches me.

During morning rounds, I venture a discussion with Dr. Mutchnick on what would make me more comfortable about Zack moving from ICU to the Critical Care unit here. I explain that I was concerned about his care being managed by interns and them cooperating with my busy visiting schedule. He reminds me that University is a teaching hospital, so there is no way to avoid being cared for by interns, and my visitors will have to learn to follow the rules. As tears well up in my eyes, he realizes this direction is not making me feel any more confident. Abruptly, he tells me that Zack is scheduled to have the feeding tube put into his stomach at 2:00p.m. and briskly walks away. I'm so tired of crying after every discussion with this man. I return to Zack's room, looking for someone more compassionate who can give me hope.

Christian is our nurse today, and he notices how troubled I am. Physically, Zack is improving, but neurologically, he has regressed, not following commands as consistently as last week. As Christian cleans around Zack's stoma and adjusts his trach collar, he casually explains, "We are taught that the body's resources are divided: 1/3rd to fight infection, 1/3rd to repair damage, and 1/3rd to maintain basic functions. Right now, Zack has to use more than 1/3rd of his energy to fight this infection, so he has less to spend on repairing his neurological functions." He grins, satisfied with his explanation, and I nod in agreement. It seems logical that once we have cleared him of this infection, he will have more energy to repair his brain. Christian has me focusing on Zack again, and not the fear of moving from our little home in ICU.

Mid-morning arrives, and Karen comes for physical therapy. Always positive, she declares that he is right on the verge of waking up, and we discuss what Zack was like before the accident. It is comforting to recall how smart he is, telling baseball stories and how the ladies love him. Our conversation has me smiling as I head downstairs to meet with a representative from the Brain Injury Alliance of KY. Eddie Reynolds gives me information on the Brain Injury Trust Fund and explains how to apply for grant money to assist with medical bills not covered by insurance. Eddie is gracious with guarded optimism as he offers his card and assistance maneuvering through insurance potholes. We are exchanging information when my niece arrives, and he politely excuses himself. Seizing the opportunity, I enlist Sherry in a field trip to Kosair Hospital to check out the Pediatric Critical Care Unit.

We chatter nervously on our brisk walk to the renowned Kosair Children's Hospital. I explain the purpose of my visit to a front desk aide, and she directs us to the Critical Care floor. The atmosphere at Kosair is very different. Sterile, but not so serious; an aura of hope, instead of frenzy. A young nurse shows us a cheery room that would be Zack's new haven, should we transfer him there. I am quite impressed, since the comparison was an uncomfortable vision of "the floor" at University Hospital.

Sherry is falling right in step with me on our way back to the hospital, supportive of my wish to relocate Zack, yet understanding how difficult that might prove to be. We arrive on the second floor waiting room to several visitors and describe our quick trip to Kosair, discussing the options. Since exploring the world outside of ICU, I have been praying that God would give me direction on the next step for Zack. Still conflicted, I resolve to change my plea, asking, instead, for Him to shut doors to Kosair if Zack is meant to stay here. In reality, I had already made up my mind. I want to move to the nice, warm, fuzzy place that Kosair represents to me. By chance, I see Dr Mutchnick leaving surgery and inform him of my decision to transfer Zack. Obviously frustrated, he shrugs his shoulders and says he would get the ball rolling, so I settle down happily, planning the move in my mind.

At 12:00 p.m., I return to our room, anxious to spend some time with Zack before his procedure. Before long, it is 5:00 p.m., and the staff informs me that it is unlikely that he will get his G-tube tonight. It will be Friday before they can reschedule it. Discouraged from waiting four hours, with no reward, and frustrated that Zack is still not responding to verbal commands, I deliver the disappointing news to our supporters in the waiting room. Most were reassuring, pointing out that meant he would remain on 5West, but an ominous feeling filled my gut. The waiting room is thinning out, allowing for an intimate circle to gather in prayer. Squeezing my eyes in concentration, I listen as others petition God on our behalf, and I silently beg for reassurance.

Settling into our evening routine, I dim the lights and perch myself next to the bed. Zack's hand remains limp as I entwine our fingers and rub my thumb in circles on his palm. A sliver of his eye peeks out under heavy lids, but he lays unresponsive to my touch. I stare at familiar, blinking statistics as his monitor indicates he is stable, but visibly, he seems lifeless. I tap my foot impatiently on the vinyl floor and glare at the clock. It is after 10:00 p.m. when I call Kim Myers to be sure they got my message about the transfer. As the nurse practitioner for the Neuro Team, she is a frequent liaison between distraught family and unavailable surgeons. Accustomed to the drama, she calmly informs me that they had run into a roadblock. Dr. Moriority has refused him as a patient at Kosair, stating that he felt Zack would be better served at University Hospital. My heart sinks, and in my despair, I didn't even recognize this is an answer to earlier prayers. God closed the door to Kosair, just as I had asked. We talked at length through my tears as Kim clarified our situation.

Soon, Zack will have no medical issues keeping him in the hospital, and his present condition indicates that he doesn't meet the requirements for admittance to Frazier Rehab. "You need to consider the possibility of a nursing home." Dear God, no! This can't be part of His plan. My shoulders fall forward, and my head rests between my knees as tears drip on the floor between my feet. She breaks the silence. "Zack must be able to go three hours with no nursing issues before Frazier will accept him, and he isn't there yet. Far from it, actually."

Desperate, I interrupt her with an unrealistic request to consult with a different doctor at Kosair, thinking that is the solution. She inhales sharply and answers in clipped words. "Mrs. Hornback, that's not possible. Kosair will not take him." I respond with only a choked back sob. Her tone remains professional as she explains that I was suffering from ICU psychosis, which isn't uncommon, but that did little to comfort me. Instead, a vivid image flashes across my mind of me trying to pry the door open that God had slammed shut.

Feeling as if a rug was just pulled out from under my feet, I return to the waiting room with my dismal report. This is proving to be our worst night since the shrill ring of that phone call at the break of dawn heralding the news of Zack's accident. Scott is extremely depressed, absorbing the update while feeling guilty over having to return to work. His mom, Rita, is crashing. Nothing can console us. I keep thinking how pitiful it is that God has answered my prayer by closing doors, yet I still doubt him. Scott escorts his mom to the garage, and I return to 5West to see Zack one last time before leaving for the night. Quickly buzzed into ICU, I shuffle slowly towards his room, despair written all over my face. Word has spread among the staff, and they sympathetically attempt to reassure me that he will be fine here at University on the Critical Care floor. Wisely. No one mentions a nursing home.

The room is dark, illuminated only by the hall lights and a neon glow from the monitors. Zack's gown is open, exposing the EKG leads stuck to his bare chest. His clenched fists are pulled to an unnatural position near his shoulders, drawing my attention to his face. His blank eyes stare off at nothing, his misshapen head twisted to the left. I pry open his fingers and place the open hands palm down on his stomach. Stroking his skinny arm, my fingertips trace over each knuckle, pressing his hand flat. My mind mulls over the day's events as the weight of every decision feels enormous.

My train of thought is interrupted when Dr. Mutchnick unexpectedly arrives. The purpose of his visit not apparent, he stands casually with his hands clasped behind his back, just staring at Zack. He is wearing scrubs and a lab coat, his expression restrained as I tearfully express my fears, rambling on about Kosair and Frazier. No doubt, he has had enough of me today, questioning his decisions, and his demeanor cools.

Very matter-of-factly, he looks at me, spreads his arms, gesturing towards the bed where Zack lay motionless, and says, "You better get used to the idea that this may be all you ever have." I flinch, as if a knife has been plunged through my heart. I'm shattered, unable to summon a response. He turns and walks out the door as I crumble onto the bed. I want so desperately to hear God whisper to me, yet I fill my ears with my own sobbing. Fear envelopes me. Fear that Zack will be left in a hospital bed for the rest of his life. Fear that he will linger in a nursing home amongst those just waiting to die. Fear that he will never have the future we dreamed of, nor any future at all. I caress Zack's face, closing his eyelids, so he won't see the cruelty I imagine mocking him from the dark shadows of his room. Moaning in prayer, I cry out, begging God to hear us. I wipe my tears on the sheet and raise his hand to my lips, a muffled cry escaping with my kiss.

Somehow, I manage to drag myself to the door. My toes scrape the floor, my feet turning to lead, suddenly too heavy to lift. It is hard to breathe. There doesn't seem to be enough oxygen to cut through the thick veil of fear that grips me. Glancing back one more time, I choke back tears and walk reluctantly out of his room. As I stumble down the hall, my heart physically aching, I clearly hear God say, "Oh, Eileen, if only you knew what I have in store for you tomorrow." It is so real, even audible, that I look around to see if anyone else had heard it. The corridor is empty, and the busy staff at the nurses' station never looks up. At first, it was difficult to move, but soon, I found myself running towards the elevator. I wanted it to be tomorrow. I fervently desired peace again with whatever the outcome. For healing, even if it is only to get his smile back.

Emboldened by God's message, I allow myself to think about the future. I envision Zack standing before other teenagers and preaching on how the decisions they make today could affect them for the rest of their lives. Describing how God rescued him from the most difficult circumstances through the power of prayer. It is a lesson slowly seeping into my consciousness. I know He hears me, but I often don't know what to ask of Him or recognize when my prayers have been answered. As always, I drive home in silence, not wanting to let the rest of the world interrupt my thoughts. I need to be still to hear God. On a dark highway, He faithfully responds with Psalm 27:14, "Wait for the Lord, be strong, and let your heart take courage."

I found it difficult to shut off my brain and hardly slept a wink last night, wondering what miracle God has in store today. There is not much traffic coming downtown at 6:00 a.m., and I'm traveling much faster than the speed limit allows, anxious to get this day started. I vow to stay positive, to remember God's promise. I plaster a half-hearted smile on my face and stroll into the ICU. Zack looks rested, and Tom confirms his stats have improved. I notice his eyes. Certainly not my imagination, but he is looking at me, not through me. "Hey buddy...you feeling better?" I move closer, so our eyes meet. "I know you're in there." Undaunted by his silence, I squeeze his hand, expecting a response. His gaze shifts, and we lose eye contact. I pat his hand reassuringly. *"That's okay...I love you."*

Morning rounds offer yet another tough conversation with Dr. Mutchnick. He reminds me that Zack can't be transferred to Kosair, and I nod my head that I understand. Sensing my next question, he carefully continues. He refers to a prior discussion about Frazier and his belief that Zack is not ready for rehab, but he has requested their assessment. Encouraged, I ask for a consultation with a neurologist, which instigates a lengthy explanation on why they do not deal with traumatic brain injuries. Finally, he concedes to placing my request with the neurologist on call. It was a rare, 20-minute chat, and Dr. Mutchnick grows sympathetic, agreeing to keep Zack in ICU for as long as possible. I acknowledge that it's not for him, but to pacify me.

A short time later, Dr. Schaeffer comes for the neurologist consult and basically confirms what Dr. Mutchnick told me. He is polite, but to the point. There is nothing he can do to improve Zack's condition. I shrug off his disheartening news, knowing deep down he is right. Hope arrived twofold. Dave Kennedy, a minister from Southeast Christian Church, answers an earlier request for a visit. He says he will help me be still and listen to God. He prays with me, placing a hand on Zack's chest and my shoulder. Before leaving, he reminds me, "If it flows, it's God's will; if it's forced, it's from man." Then, at noon, Karen arrives for physical therapy. She is always optimistic, and today is no different. She proclaims, "All kids wake up." She is absolutely certain that Zack will wake up.

I am nervously excited when Dr. Mook and his team from Frazier Rehab knock on our door. He explains the process while a resident looks official taking notes on her clipboard. I quickly turn into a cheerleader, telling them all the progress Zack had made before the pneumonia and MRSA set in. It is a desperate attempt to make him see something in Zack that the neurosurgeons didn't. I had done some research and discovered that Dr. Mook is a baseball fan, so I had Scott bring Zack's baseball glove, and we decorated his room with team pictures.

While I am chattering on about his prime physical condition during the season, I place our special homerun baseball in his hand, curling his fingers around the ball, like he is about to throw a pitch, all with the hope it would influence Dr. Mook in our favor. Then, I give him the letter that Zack had written about a month before his accident, trying to convince us to change his curfew. He scans it briefly, but a slight smile reassures me the letter had its desired impact. He asks a lot of questions about the accident, itself, and our home situation: how many stairs, siblings, bathrooms he had. Each of my answers is checked off the form by the intern. I am trying not to cry, but my voice is shaky. They examine Zack, but he barely responds. I keep repeating that before becoming infected, he was consistently cooperating. Dr. Mook looks at his staff, then they all look at Zack. No one speaks as my eyes dart from one to the other. He steps back, his arms crossed with one finger tapping his chin.

His lips part into a gracious smile, and he announces that once Zack gets his feeding tube placed tomorrow and goes to the Critical Care Unit for 24 hours, they will accept him at Frazier. I am ecstatic! Only 12 hours earlier, I had felt hopeless. I cried out to God to help me accept whatever condition Zack would be left in. Now, Dr. Mook is talking about getting his books from school, so they can use them in therapy. Someone is finally giving us a glance beyond today, where we have had to focus for so long.

He continues explaining that Zack will likely remain at Frazier Rehab for six to eight weeks, then graduate to the Neuro/Psych outpatient center at Frazier East. He will continue therapy as an outpatient while he lives at home. Oh, dear God, he's talking about when Zack comes home. Tears just won't stop flowing now. I practically fall over myself thanking each of his staff as they trail him out the door. Smiles beam from all the faces at the nurse's station as the Frazier Team parades out of our room, and I shake a fist in celebration. I careen with the bed, taking Zack's hand in mine and folding them in prayer. Praise replaces my earlier pleas as I thank God for His grace and favor.

We begin making plans for our exit from Neuro ICU. Tears of joy are shared with family and friends as I relive our visit from Dr. Mook and the Frazier staff. Mrs. Thompson and Mrs. Fenwick from Christian

Academy share my excitement when they arrive to see Zack, and he squeezes both their hands in response to their greeting. He spends an extended amount of time in passive therapy in his chair, briefly holding his head up, supporting the weight of his helmet. This physical exertion takes a lot of effort, and once settled back in bed, he sleeps peacefully.

As I watch the rhythmic rise and fall of his chest, I consider how wonderfully God closes doors, so we can trust in His perfect plan. A vivid picture dances through my mind: It is of God on his throne, looking down on me last night as I cried out in despair and his gentle reply, "Oh, Eileen, if you only knew what I had in store for you tomorrow." He is faithful, and I know we will never be the same. We will never be able to sit in church, listen to the word of God and not be impacted due to His timing, His grace, His plans for us, His drawing us near to Him. In the last 14 days, we have surrendered to them all. My thoughts turn to Zack's many friends who have lived through this with us. I whisper a prayer on their behalf, hoping they recognize what tragic consequences can come from decisions that seem harmless at the time. I slip out of his room, eager to announce our impending transfer to Frazier.

Several friends and church family greet me in the waiting room and rejoice at our news. We gather together, hold hands, and pray. I ask specifically that we are not bumped by new trauma cases, that Zack gets his feeding tube tomorrow, and that a private room will be available when we need it. I pray that teens get the message we share of obedience and trust that God has this under control. Then I remember the date, July 21st. Happy birthday, Scott! God has given you a gift greater than anything I could ever buy…an answered prayer. The mood is festive with people making plans to visit Zack at Frazier Rehab. A friend approaches and whispers in my ear to check out a message on the blog. It reads:

*To the family and friends of Zack:*

*It was suggested to me that I might share some of what I have heard from Matt, the driver in the accident. I am Matt's youth minister and love him very much and have seen a profound change in him as he prays for and watches his friend, Zack.*

*The Sunday after the accident, Matt and his family came forward for prayer at church. As I sat next to Matt, he held out a piece of a blood-stained sweatshirt. He looked me in the eye and with tears streaming down his face, said, "Look what I did to my friend."*

*Last week, Matt attended church camp and asked if he could address the camp. He spoke of choices. He confessed to everyone there that he had made some awful decisions, and the cost has been terrible. Matt chose to share all this with people, because he wants to prevent it from happening to someone else. His decision to be out too late, drinking, lying to his parents, and ultimately, getting behind the wheel of his car with some friends, has changed his life forever. It has changed Zack's life forever, and it has changed the many people who are involved in this tragedy as family and friends.*

*I know there are several who have posted, who have hoped and prayed for something good to come out of this situation. I don't pretend to know what God has in store for any of those involved, but I can say, His hand is at work. Our prayers continue to rise up on behalf of Zack and his family. May God's blessings pour out on this tragedy and bring peace, healing, comfort, and a resolve to let Him lead our lives.*

## Third Friday

Exactly three weeks ago, we frantically arrived at University Hospital to the terrifying reality of traumatic brain injury. I'm struck by how time seems to have swallowed up our life. Reflecting on recent answered prayers, I can attest that God's rescue wasn't confined only to Zack. The evidence of His mercy has rippled across our community with thousands acknowledging the power of prayer.

My demeanor is one of surrender as Dr. Mutchnick orders another CAT scan to check for fluid on his brain. It is a cautious step to ensure that there is no neurological cause for Zack's lack of response to verbal commands. I'm at peace, the fear of the unknown squashed, as I place my trust in God's perfect plan. The morning stretches into afternoon before we finally get the news that the CAT scan and an additional chest x-ray are clear. I'm content just watching Zack sleep, daydreaming of his revealing conversation with God. The staff comes to prepare him for surgery, and I return to the second floor waiting room, where his friends share positive stories of the impact our situation has made in the lives of others. God has unraveled the previous dread of facing surgery by focusing my thoughts on His grace. At 3:30, Dr. Rodriquez places the feeding tube in his stomach. The past anxiety each time the surgery doors slide open has been replaced with confident assurance that God has this under control. Scott arrives in work clothes just as an intern reports that the procedure was completed without complications, and Zack is recovering in his room. We retrace our familiar trail to 5West. Neika is reattaching the cables to his monitor and checking his vitals. We settle in his room, patiently waiting. By 6:00 p.m., the sedatives have worn off, and Zack opens his eyes. It is glorious to see him with no tubing in his nose or mouth and to stare into those big brown eyes with ridiculously long eyelashes.

Scott is entertaining the staff with comical tales of life with demanding daughters, when an aid says someone wishes to speak with me in the hallway outside of ICU. I had barely greeted our visitors when the nurse at the front desk pages me, stating that Neika and Stephanie wanted me in his room. I scramble to his door, concerned that something is wrong, but I'm greeted with genuine smiles. The lights are illuminating his room, and several nurses are surrounding his bed. I watch in stunned silence as they command Zack, "Close your eyes, keep them closed, now…open them." He follows all of their requests, repeating his performance several times. All of 5West shares in our excitement at this new development. Just yesterday, I felt as if he was trying to communicate with his eyes and now, we have irrefutable evidence.

Dave Stone and his daughter, Sadie, come by while Scott and I are still high off the experience. They listen intently as we take turns explaining all that has occurred over the last few days and pray with us, thanking God for His perfect timing. It seems bizarre to get such joy out of a simple act like closing and opening his eyes. It takes me back to when he was a tiny baby, and I remember how we delighted in each new talent. I imagine that's what it will be like in the weeks to come as we witness his recovery.

As night engulfs his room, and we are alone again, Zack and I experience a very touching moment. He is completely relaxed, with no tension in his arm. I take his left hand and touch it to his face. He stares at me intently and holds tightly to my hand. When I stop, he raises our hands towards his face, and I help him caress his cheek. It seems as if he is discovering who he is, and I consider what he must be thinking. Sitting in his dimly lit room and holding his hand, I am content, and I feel extremely blessed to be here. A peace seems to envelop the room, and my tears now come from joy, rather than pain. As I bow my head and begin to pray out loud, he closes his eyes, apparently praying with me. I whisper, asking God to intervene through morning rounds and prompt his doctor to sign the order to move to the Critical Care unit, smiling at the thought that 24 hours later, we will be transferring to Frazier Rehab. I pray that in our remaining days at University, we will have opportunities to spread hope to other families dealing with their own trauma. To be His testimony of how prayer got us through this life-threatening ordeal. I can't wait to see what tomorrow brings, how God will bless us and use this tragedy for His glory.

On my way to the parking garage, I walk slowly down the hall, glancing into other rooms. There are patients of all ages—most significantly older than Zack. This late, there are only a few visitors, and I can feel their desperation as they hover over critical loved ones. I pause, wanting to pray with them, but both rooms seem to be in heavy discussions with their nurses. I wonder if they know God, if they have claimed the saving grace of Jesus. Do they have the assurance that if their loved one died tonight, they would claim their reward of eternal life in heaven? I can't imagine what it would be like to be sequestered here, totally dependent on the skill of the doctors and not know the Great Physician. I walk to my car, and my heart is heavy as I pray for nameless strangers fighting horrendous battles.

*Dear God, may this be the tragedy that draws them to you, so they, too, can experience a peace that passes all understanding.* On my silent drive home, consumed in thought, I remember another promise from scripture. "Because of the Lord's great love, we are not consumed, for his compassions never fail." –Lamentations 3:22

## Third Saturday

Nurse Neika is checking the G-tube to ensure the extension is properly connected to the tubing when I arrive in Zack's room. This feeding tube will provide more required nourishment than the previous tube in his nose, but it is also a potential site for infection. Preoccupied with the task at hand, she doesn't notice how his eyes track me as I walk from the foot of his bed to his side. His head is slightly turned to the left, giving me full view of his face. I smile at my boy, bringing his left hand to my lips for a good morning kiss. No response, but my mood is not daunted. Zack is sporting a new black brace with Velcro wrapping around his right arm that runs from his shoulder to his wrist. He had been keeping this arm bent with his hand unnaturally drawn up to his shoulder, so this brace is meant to correct this posturing. Neika reports that he had a good night and excuses herself as more staff arrives.

Dr. Raff from Infectious Disease Control makes rounds with his residents and notes that Zack has been fever-free for 72 hours, and his white count has improved. He places his stethoscope on Zack's chest and listens to his lungs. As a matter of habit, he tells him to take a deep breath, and Zack inhales. Dr. Raff looks up, his eyebrows raised in surprise and asks him to do it again. Zack inhales deeply.

"Well, I wasn't expecting such a cooperative patient, and your lungs sound much better!" Dr. Raff chuckles. "Whatever you're doing, keep it up." He ushers his staff out the door as several comment on Zack's progress. It is obvious that Zack's response made the day for the ID staff. At this stage, taking a deep breath on command seems to be easier than other responses.

Dr. Densler and the Neuro Team complete morning rounds by confirming that the results from the last CAT scan showed no change, and Zack would be transferred to Frazier Rehab on Monday. Our relationship with the hospital staff has certainly evolved. That includes Dr. Densler. In the beginning, he had been taken aback when I had hugged him after a successful surgery, or when he delivered good news. Now, when I approach him, he opens his arms in anticipation. I think behind that cold, professional exterior, he secretly looks forward to my fond gestures of appreciation. The gravity of his chosen profession doesn't permit him to show emotion, but he absorbs my sentiments vicariously.

Throughout the morning, Zack's eyes are wide open, and he watches TV for several hours. I find this behavior bizarre, since he still is not considered "awake". Once he is moved to his therapy chair, the visitors start their daily parade, lining up at the door of ICU, waiting for their turn. He does not disappoint them. Because subjecting the other patients on 5West to a constant flow of teenagers can be disruptive, I instruct them to remain quiet. I usher four or five to his room and close the door. Each group is rewarded with a thumbs up and are delighted when he wiggles his toes at their request. He remains in his chair for four hours, the longest time since they started getting him out of bed.

Zack is exhausted when he returns to his bed and sleeps until he hears the voices of some friends in the room. He opens his eyes, interested in who is there. He starts getting very purposeful with his hand, which slowly creeps up to his trach tube. I redirect his fingers, but a moment later, he has his hands on his feeding tube. Again, he is redirected, but immediately grabs his respiratory monitor cable and yanks it off. Well, if he's not "awake", he certainly is more active.

Nieka reattaches the cable and cautions me to monitor him closely to prevent more serious damage. After repeated sessions of cat and mouse with his hands, she elects to put them back in the braces. Since these keep his hands in a rest position, they don't curl into a fist, so he can't grasp hold of anything. The braces on, she adjusts his bedding and asks him to move his legs. He responds. I'm encouraged that it seems as if he is back to where he was last week before the pneumonia and MRSA set in. He is so close. Wouldn't it be wonderful if he "woke up" on Sunday? What a great story for our pastors, Bob Russell or Dave Stone, to work into a sermon about how not everyone sleeps when they are preaching.

Visitors share with me about how Zack's story has touched so many people, and we hear teenagers talk about the consequences of their actions. God has taken something extremely traumatic and turned it into Zack's silent ministry. Although I have engaging conversations, I keep anxiously glancing at the door, expecting someone to announce a bed is prepared for us in the Critical Care unit. I recognize that we have to be transferred out of ICU by tomorrow if we are going to be released to Frazier Rehab on Monday. I have high expectations of the progress that will happen at Frazier. I've heard stories of patients who suffered serious spinal cord injuries and left Frazier walking, after doctors said it was impossible. Just waiting to get there is giving me a headache. You can't even get an aspirin in this hospital if you are not a patient. After 9 p.m., I realize I've not eaten all day. Maybe that's what has my temples pounding. The staff coaxes me into going home to get rested up for the real work that will begin when we start rehab. I feel guilty leaving Zack, until Stephanie reminds me that she's his favorite nurse, and they have a date tonight.

Lowering the bed rail, I prop myself on the edge of my chair and scoot it closer to him. I no longer notice the hum of machines or pay attention to every blinking number. The shadows in his room don't feel threatening. I take hold of Zack's hand and squeeze gently. His fingers curl around mine in response. His eyes are closed, and I lay my forehead on his arm as I silently pray that a bed is available tomorrow.

Then, I remember the anguished faces of the other families I saw on 5West last night. I ask God that as we move from the sanctity of our home in ICU, that we will have the opportunity to share the comfort of Christ with the brokenhearted. My stomach grumbles as I pray for strength to carry us through this next phase, which could prove more difficult than my imagination conjures up. I lift my head and finish with an audible, "Amen." Zack responds by squeezing my hand, which gives me the courage to leave him.

# Glorious Sunday

Arriving before dawn, I get a complete update from the night nurse before rounds begin. Since the doctors only spend about 10 minutes with each patient, I need to be prepared with questions when the Neuro Team arrives. Zack is sleeping when I slip into the room and greet Stephanie as she switches out his IV bag. Taking my usual position on his left, which is the direction he turns his head, allows me to get a good look at him. His brain has stopped swelling, so his head is no longer distended. Since he is missing the right bone flap, and the skull shapes your cranium, his head is no longer round. It is oddly shaped, and the right side is flat. Much of his hair has grown back, but you can still see the staples holding his scalp together at the incision, as well as the laceration on top. I wasn't fond of his engorged head, but this new shape is just as disturbing. Other than a hint of pink scar on his forehead, above his bushy eyebrows, all of the other superficial cuts have disappeared. He still retains his summer tan, and I trace my fingers down his arm to hold his hand, waiting for staff to arrive.

Dr. Han, attending neurosurgeon, makes rounds with Dr. Densler and another resident. I remain quiet, mentally preparing my inevitable questions, while they conduct a thorough examination. They discuss the laceration on his head and his impending transfer to Frazier Rehab. Concerned about potential infection, Dr. Han instructs me to request a wound care nurse once he leaves University Hospital. As a precaution, they elect not to remove the staples at his incision for another week. Any infection could cause his brain to swell and open the scalp at the incision, creating a dangerous situation that Frazier is not equipped to handle. The role of the wound care nurse is to keep the laceration clean and free of impurities.

After listening to their conversation, I timidly inquire when his bone flap might be replaced, reasoning that it would help to protect his brain from infection. Dr. Densler begins to speak, presumably to educate me on brain contagion, when Dr. Han raises his hand and interrupts. He patiently explains that after removing his bone flap during the initial operation, it was assigned to the Bone Bank for inspection, and the report indicated it was contaminated. During surgery, they discovered that the deep laceration on his head was full of glass and debris, caused by a guardrail crashing through the front windshield, striking Zack in the head, and ultimately resulting in the traumatic brain injury. The cultures taken at the Bone Bank will be examined to see if any bacteria or viruses develop, requiring his bone flap to be discarded. If that occurs, he will be measured for a custom-made, acrylic bone flap. Medically, his natural bone is preferable, since in theory, it will continue to grow with Zack.

Dr. Apfel, attending anesthesiologist, is the next to arrive with his residents. Each medical team requires an examination prior to his transfer, and Dr. Apfel uses this time to discuss the underlying brain injury with his residents. He is pleased that there are no respiratory issues currently causing distress and comments on the advantages of having the CDC monitoring his MRSA. Our conversation turns to Zack's accident, and the fact that no one in the car was wearing their seatbelt. Dr. Apfel holds an interesting point of view. He is from Germany, where only two percent of the population do not wear seatbelts. The U.S. has twice as many car fatalities, and he believes that Americans value freedom so much that individual freedom of choice overcomes rational thinking. We choose not to wear our seatbelts as a subconscious assertion of freedom. It is even more prevalent among American teenagers, because they are trying to pull away from their parents, struggling for independence and desire even more freedom.

Zack was not wearing a seatbelt at the time of the accident. I was diligent and always required my kids to put on their seatbelt before we pulled out of the driveway. In hindsight, perhaps Dr. Apfel is right. Zack didn't wear his seatbelt because he was 15, starting to pull away from us and wanting more freedom. It is alarming to consider that the freedom we hold so dear also causes us such tragedies.

Neika transfers Zack to his chair just as Scott strides in to relieve me, so I can go to church. With much fanfare, he declares that the personal trainer has come to really work him over. Scott has a big personality and takes a different approach to getting Zack to respond. Neika tosses me a sideways glance as he claps his hands announcing, "You ready, Zack!"

I whisper, "good luck" to Neika and slip out the door. Somewhat concerned that Scott might be a bit overzealous, I am still grateful for the opportunity to go to church. He has made arrangements with his mom to meet me in the atrium, and I am surprised to see my girls, as well. Dylan has joined his friends for middle school worship, but the girls had begged to go to big church with me.

Last night, I was home in time to cuddle with them before bed, but at a second glance, picking out appropriate church clothes should have been on the agenda. Logan looks part fairy, in leggings over some kind of tutu I had never seen before, and cowboy boots. Kyle tried hard to be stylish, but reminds me of Cindy Lauper—very colorful. Rita didn't seem to care, but is intent on splitting up the candy that Grandma always carries in her purse.

Sitting in the pew for the first time in weeks, I couldn't stop the flow of tears. I inhale each verse of every song, making them my personal prayer. Kyle strokes my arm to comfort me, and Logan's head rests on my other shoulder. Rita wipes black smudges from tears off her face and passes me butterscotch candy. I experience a communion of mercy and grace. Saturated in God's promise to rescue me from despair, I leave the sanctuary, restored. Rita volunteers to take the kids to lunch, and I head back to University Hospital.

When I return to 5West, Scott proudly announces that Zack managed to do 30 crunches with his legs and arms. This is not the same type of exercise you might see in the gym. Obviously, our idea of crunches has changed significantly over the last few weeks. Zack was able to tolerate another five hours in his chair before Neika transfers him back to bed. It doesn't seem difficult to just sit up in a chair, until you understand how much energy and muscle strength it requires for someone with a traumatic brain injury. We realize the effort he puts forth and literally have to wipe sweat from his brow when we remove his helmet. He is exhausted, but recovers after a short nap before visitors begin to arrive.

Zack has a plethora of friends—many of them female—who relish their time with him. In one visit, he squeezes Avery and Caroline's hands, and they excitedly return to the corridor to tell the other friends who are waiting for their 15 minutes. After some coaxing, he sticks out his tongue a few times for the staff. A flicker of his old personality surfaces, that willful teenager who chooses what verbal commands he will follow. I chastise him in a teasing tone, "Stop being stubborn, Zack." That's the correction he needs, and he cooperates with further commands.

It is late when Dr. Miller appears in our doorway for a visual inspection of the stoma. It has healed, and the stitches need to be removed before we transfer to Frazier. He explains that the skin, supported by the collar which wraps around Zack's neck, will now hold the trach in place, making the stitches no longer necessary. He snaps on sterile gloves, turns on the overhead light and disinfects the area. Zack is still as each suture is carefully removed. Dr. Miller reviews proper cleaning procedures with Stephanie and wishes us good luck in therapy, dimming the lights before heading out the door. After making notations in his chart and checking all his fluids, Stephanie returns to her duties at the nurse's station, leaving me alone with Zack.

He seems especially alert tonight and holds firmly to my hand. When I try to pull away to adjust my chair, he won't let go. He stares intently at my face, his eyes meeting mine in a magical connection. Scott had brought me a cassette player, and now, worship music softly fills our dimly lit room. I allow my mind to drift as I consider the events of the past few weeks and marvel at how God lovingly doles out discipline in perfect amounts. This trial we presently experience will change us, make us stronger. It teaches us that when we fear the future, God sends us reminders that He is in control. This life is but a whisper in God's ear. We do not know what he has planned for us, only that it will be perfect. My dear friend, Donna Jaha, explains that Zack is like a pebble thrown into a lake. You can see the ripples traveling out in all directions. He is the catalyst, but it's not about him. It's about the ripple that God created through one imperfect pebble. Waves that impact his friends, our family, the staff, and even strangers who hear our story or see us gathered in prayer.

Zack rests peacefully on 5West another night. We didn't get our orders to transfer out of ICU in preparation to go to Frazier Rehab. There wasn't an empty bed in the Critical Care unit suitable for him. Zack is a minor and can only be placed in a room with another minor. His MRSA, which is a highly contagious infection, further limits their options. Stephanie gives me a lopsided grin as she tapes a printed sign to our door. With no suitable room available, and the state insurance prerequisite that you can't move from an ICU into a rehab facility, a decision was made to treat his ICU room as a step-down unit. The staff theoretically aren't coming in our room every hour to check his vitals like before, but they still respond each time I call. So here we are, in our ICU cocoon, with the same dedicated nursing staff we have had from the beginning.

How ironic that only days ago, I had panicked in fear of being transferred to the floor and thought the answer was moving to Kosair Children's Hospital. God closed the door on that option and answered with our improbable acceptance into rehab. Then, He gives us more than we could ever hope or imagine. Filling up the beds in Critical Care, so we can remain right here, where I wanted to stay all along. The power of prayer provides in ways we never thought possible. I believe God has a reason for keeping us in the "miracle" room on 5West one extra day, and I can't wait for tomorrow to find out why.

Anticipating our move to Frazier Rehab, I'm beaming as I bounce into Zack's room. A simple wave from the nurses' station reminds me not to expect the usual morning update. However, being a "step-down" patient doesn't inhibit special attention from Dr. Raff, who arrives to report on Zack's infection. He explains that while Zack has been fever-free for over 72 hours, his white count is back up. He listens to Zack's lungs, nodding his head in agreement with whatever he hears. Rattling off a list, checking for symptoms, he decides he's not concerned. He looks at Zack quizzically, asks for a thumbs up, and Zack immediately complies. Dr. Raff chuckles, "Well, that's encouraging."

Karen arrives for physical therapy, and he continues impressing us with his responses. He grants her requests that he stick out his tongue and wiggle his toes. She leans him forward to put on his helmet, carefully buckling it under his chin and moves him to the chair. He has to sweat it out there for the next three hours.

Jennifer Gallaway, with Frazier Rehab, knocks on our door after Zack is returned to his bed. She informs me that the doctor has signed the order to move him. Frazier will accept him; however, she has to get approval from our insurance company. This will be a new battle. I remember my thoughts last night, wondering what God had in store for me today. I was expecting something different, more pleasant. But in His infinite wisdom, God knows what encounters make me stronger, and this day is devoted to maneuvering through insurance regulations. Traumatic brain injury patients are graded on the Ranchos Cognitive Scale on how they respond. Zack is currently a level three. Frazier's admittance policy requires patients to be level four, but Zack is young and has great potential, so Dr. Mook waived that requirement. However, the insurance company regulation for starting rehab is level five. Our policy only grants Zack 60 days of Acute Rehab benefits. Jennifer explains that they don't want the clock to start ticking, and our time run out, before he has sufficiently recovered to be treated as an outpatient. She will continue conversations with the insurance caseworker to get him released to Frazier at his present level.

A member of Westport Road Church of Christ arrives to encourage us through prayer. She focuses on Isaiah 43:10, "You are my witnesses, declares the Lord, and my servant whom I have chosen, so that you may know and believe me and understand that I am he." Believing that God chose Zack for a reason is a humbling concept. I eagerly await the day when Zack can feel honored that God knew he was strong enough for this mission, whatever it turns out to be. I pray, silently asking God to help me accept His perfect plan and to have patience with His timing. Our visitor is gifted with an angelic voice, and we are uplifted as she sings worship songs that focus on God's rescue.

Our occupational therapist leans in the doorway to hear the impromptu concert. She introduces herself, and our guest slips out the door, promising to keep us in prayer. The initial goal of occupational therapy is to help Zack recover his fine motor skills and identify any deficits. As she rotates his wrist, flexing each finger, she explains that it is critical for recovery that his brain is stimulated. This happens when he is awake. She stresses how important it is for visitors to talk to him and touch him. That's one area that won't be an issue. I recall a recent visit with one chatty high school girl, whose mom kept apologizing, saying her daughter could talk to a brick wall for an hour. She was just what Zack needed, relaying all the gossip at school, who was dating who and what teams were moving on to regionals. She even asked him if he liked her haircut, and I'm fairly confident Zack didn't even know who she was.

At 4:30, Dr. Mutchnick hands me a card and tells me that I need to call my insurance caseworker. He clarifies that my insurance provider is not in favor of the transfer to Frazier, stating our benefits would be better utilized at a nursing home, until he could be assessed at a level 5 on the Rancho scale. Vivid images of depressing nursing homes with withering patients cloud my mind. This is not where my son belongs, and I choke back the lump forming in my throat as I dial the number. A woman answers, cutting me off when I offer an explanation for the call and goes to locate his file. She confirms all the pertinent data and coolly suggests that we consider the brain injury unit at Pathways Nursing Home.

She continues to talk over me as I explain that we had already been accepted at Frazier Rehab. Finally, after a moment of silence, she lets me talk. I have to convince her that Zack was a healthy, driven 15-year-old before his accident, and he can't be evaluated with subjective numbers. Our conversation is difficult. My hands are shaking, and I see the nurses look up from their station just outside our room when I raise my voice. It feels like we have everything lined up with Frazier only to have some insurance bureaucrat dismiss our plans under the pretense this is better for Zack. I lean against the wall, fighting back tears as I look at my precious son, lying helpless in his hospital bed. I can't fathom him sitting in a nursing home, even if it is with other TBI survivors, knowing that he will get minimal therapy.

It seems like a death sentence to me. I try to concentrate as she explains how this process works. She has to be sure I understand the benefits before she will issue the order to release him to Frazier. That we have a fixed amount of Acute Rehab benefits, regardless of how he responds. I stare at the clock above Zack's bed, hating how time seems to be against us again. I cannot stifle my sobs, but I can sense a crack in her bureaucratic wall. After 20 minutes, we come to a mutual understanding that if my benefits run out, I will find a way to pay for therapy on my own. Finally, she agrees to make the call, authorizing his move to Frazier.

I am confident that God is in control, but it is still very difficult for me as I try to understand what the next best move should be for Zack. Learning the ropes is difficult while riding an emotional roller coaster. I hang up the phone and slump to the chair, my hands covering my face, so Zack won't see me crying. I don't even realize that Scott has entered the room, until he drops to his knees to hug me. I tell him the insurance company was signing the order for Zack to move to Frazier, as he pulls me to my feet.

"That's good news and no reason to cry." Before I can protest, explaining the battle I just went through, he smiles and says, "Watch what we can do." He starts coaching Zack through leg crunches, and I see, firsthand, how hard Zack tries when Scott pushes him. He presses his knees together and then releases them on command. As Scott counts, he is overcome with emotion and tears slip down his cheek. It is exhausting for all three of us, but it does make me focus on Zack again, and not my insurance adversary. Scott and I hold hands with Zack and thank God that when our strength runs out, He is always there to carry us.

After Scott finishes his coaching session with Zack, I walk him to the elevator, and the doors slide open. One of Zack's classmates greets us, and we walk arm-in-arm to his room. Randy Marshall has just returned from a mission trip to Honduras. She says the church in Honduras is praying for him. I tell her I know of a church in India and a monastery up north that is also praying for him. It provides such comfort to hear about the churches that lift him to God in prayer, so we can encourage Zack to be strong.

As darkness falls, I notice that Zack is intently looking out the window. He is moving his legs and turning his head to get in a better position. Something outside has had his undivided attention for the last hour. I scoot my chair closer to the bed and lean in to get the same view. One block over, there is an old church steeple with a cross on it. Bathed in moonlight, cast against a cloudless sky, it seems surreal. I wonder if that is what he sees. It's a comforting thought, as I imagine that there are angels guarding over him. I start to cry and slip to my knees. I whisper a prayer, pleading with God to guide our therapy, so Zack will not need more than 60 days at Frazier and our benefits won't run out. I ask for opportunities for Zack to glorify God through his complete recovery there. Sliding back into my chair, I take Zack's hand and tell him we won another battle. Then, I look at the clock over his bed and defiantly stick out my tongue in a little victory gesture. Feeling somewhat childish, I glance at the nurses' station, relieved that no one was watching. I bow my head with one last prayer request of gentle lessons in patience and head home.

Arriving slightly later than usual, I find that Zack has already had a shave, a bed bath, and a hair wash, although there isn't much there. He looks so good. He is holding the teddy bear that a friend's little sister sent. Nurse Stephanie smiles and says that he had slept most of the night, but at one point, he held her hand tightly and didn't want to let it go. Stephanie gives Zack lots of attention, but our current status prevents her from spending a lot of time in our room. She needs to tend to her other patients, so she put the bear in his hand. He held that little bear all night and still had it in his hand when I arrived. She moved to the opposite side of the bed and affectionately patted Zack's arm. Her gaze remains on Zack's face as she reports that he had no fever, but his latest white count had risen again.

She is explaining the significance of monitoring his white count for signs of infection when Jennifer Gallaway with Frazier arrives. She is also concerned, informing me that the arrangements for our transfer were complete, but Frazier requires verification that his elevated white count didn't indicate any new infection. She moves to the foot of the bed, where Zack watches as she casually examines the compression device that he wears on his lower legs to prevent clots. She focuses on Zack as she rattles off a list of items I need to take to Frazier. She explains that he will require shorts, t-shirts, socks, and tennis shoes, because he will be dressed every day for therapy.

Dr. Raff shows up with his residents in tow to discuss the latest elevated white count, but calmly says he is not concerned. He explains that many things could cause it to fluctuate, so he would check out a few possible sites for infection. He instructs his residents to pull the main line and draw a blood sample. They switch out the type of catheter to check for a urinary infection. They draw blood again. For the next two hours, Zack is a human pincushion. I have an unrealistic fear of needles and watching everything they do to Zack sometimes makes me queasy. Although nothing makes me more nauseated than when they suction his trach, which happens several times a day. Finally, they check his white count, and it is back down to an acceptable level, so Dr. Raff was right... no problems preventing us from moving to Frazier. Dr. Raff reinserts the PICC line, so they can continue with Linezolid, a 28-day antibiotic regiment that we only started on July 18th.

Late afternoon, Mr. Greener, Christian Academy High School principal, is directed to our room as I'm pouring over all the pamphlets from Frazier. Zack is asleep, and Mr. Greener laughingly comments that he is used to seeing him sleeping in study hall anyway. Fortunately, Zack didn't spend a lot of time in the principal's office. After the usual small talk, the conversation turns to the accident, the fact that Zack snuck out of the house in the middle of the night and went on a joyride with an older guy and three girls. We lament over the choices that everyone made that night and how the resulting consequences came down hardest for Zack. He reiterates the same opinion I have heard from so many others. The impact the accident and his life-altering injuries has had on an ever-increasing number of teenagers.

Zack was a popular, good-looking athlete on the honor roll at an academically challenging school. No one ever expected anything this tragic to happen to him. This poster boy now has all their attention. He is the perfect example of how a seemingly simple decision to sneak out after midnight can change your life forever. More significantly, he has become God's illustration of the power of prayer. Friends who visit see, firsthand, the devastating trauma Zack sustained. They pray with us and witness those prayers being answered. Zack can't talk, but his message is loud as thunder. Mr. Greener says goodbye, and a resident comes to take Zack to x-ray. He explains that they need to be sure his PICC line is situated properly, and he will return to the room in an hour.

Glancing at the clock, I discover that it's already 4:30, so I'm not surprised that my stomach is grumbling. My friend, Donna Jaha, convinces me to break for lunch while Zack is gone, so we head towards the cafeteria. We take the elevator to the basement, maneuvering through multiple corridors that tunnel under the pavement, to the medical building across the street. This give us plenty of time to discuss our move to Frazier. She shares in my excitement, but I confess of an uneasy sense about the timing. Checking the time on my phone, I reason that once Zack is finished in x-ray, it will be getting late, and I think it would be better to just wait and go to Frazier in the morning. Before we can even select our food, my cell phone rings.

Jennifer confirms that since it would be 6:00 p.m. before they could arrange transport to Frazier, they decided to postpone the transfer until tomorrow. I thank her, smiling to myself, acknowledging that God made that decision as we strolled the sterile hallways to the cafeteria. I consider what the reason might be for us to remain on 5West, and I remember our neighbor in ICU. Perhaps He wants us here one more night for Nia, the girl in the room next to Zack. She is 20 years old with a brain tumor. I've prayed with her mother, often in the hallway outside of our adjoining rooms. Nia had surgery today to remove the golf-ball-sized tumor, and Sharon tearfully told me that the cancer had spread to her spine. We embraced, and she invited me to her room to see Nia, who frequently asks about the boy next door. She hears the incessant commands of the doctors and nurses and wants to know what's wrong with Zack. Why are they always requesting a thumbs up or telling him to stick out his tongue? She knows him only through the wall they share, and yet, her concern is genuine. Her parents are strong Christians and over the last few days, we have been lifting each other up, each praying for the others' child. God knew we needed to be together one more night.

Zack is gone longer than expected, and when a resident finally wheels his bed back into the room, I notice the staples have been removed from his skull. Shaking my head, somewhat confused as I recall only two days earlier when Dr. Han said the staples would remain for another week. The resident explains that after examining the latest CAT scan, the Neuro Team agreed that the incision was sufficiently healed to warrant removing them. I won't complain, because without the staples, he doesn't have such a Frankenstein appearance. The resident continues to share that it will still require at least two months to ensure swelling won't return, and then, his bone flap can be replaced. He reminds me that whenever he is out of bed, he must wear a helmet to protect his fragile brain. Zack had been sedated for this procedure and was still sleeping off the tranquilizers, so I head downstairs in search of Scott.

I return to the second floor waiting room, excited to spend a little time with Kyle and Logan. A hospital waiting room is not exactly a fun place for little girls, but at least here they get plenty of attention from Zack's friends. They spend a lot of time at home with our neighbor,

Morgan Getz. It would never work if Dylan was in charge, so Morgan is our saving grace right now. I enjoy listening to the girls describe their shopping trip, picking out school supplies with the Christian Academy cheerleaders and showing off their new sneakers. I hadn't noticed that Scott had disappeared. Returning to the room an hour later, I find him sitting on the side of the bed.

I stood in the doorway watching as Zack lifted his head off his pillow about a foot. His hand inched up to Scott's chest, and he began fingering his chest hair between the buttons on his shirt. Normally, he would have found this irritating, but Scott was beside himself with joy. His son was showing him a tender affection, like he hadn't experienced since Zack was a baby. Tears trailed down his face as he kept perfectly still, relishing the moment.

It seems as if we are always crying, but our emotions are raw. Most of the time, we are physically exhausted, just trying to keep it all together while our world seems to be falling apart. It was difficult to convince Scott to leave. Friends had taken the girls out to eat, but he still needed to pick up Dylan. I usher him to the lobby, understanding how painful our situation is for him. Our arms are draped around each other's waists, lost in our own thoughts as we silently wait for the elevator. Kissing his cheek, I nudge him into the cab and notice his solemn expression as the doors slide shut. I make my way back to our room and take my place beside Zack's bed.

A short time later, the phone interrupts my thoughts. I'm surprised to hear Scott's voice, full of emotion as he describes the last 10 minutes, explaining that he was sobbing as he pulled out of the parking garage and was so overcome that he pulled his truck to the curb. He fell to his bare knees on the sidewalk, wanting the concrete to hurt, so the physical pain would mirror his emotions. He cried out to God, pleading for Zack's recovery, and thanking Him for saving his life. He climbed back into his truck with a strange awareness that he was not alone. He felt the seat next to him in search of the heavenly passenger that had rescued him from his grief. His emotions are fragile, but his faith has grown so strong. He tells me that that when you walk through the valley of death, you can cry out to God, knowing He hears you.

It is late as we move Zack from his chair, and I play the CD from the Vine that a Southeast Christian Church volunteer had delivered earlier in the day. The music echoes through the corridor and brings Sharon out of Nia's room to stand quietly in our doorway. I move towards her, and we greet each other with a silent hug, our foreheads touching, as if bowed in prayer. Our rooms are directly across from the nurses' station, and this touching moment doesn't go unnoticed.

There is a somber mood among the staff, knowing this is our last night on the floor. I feel so blessed to see Zack staring at the steeple outside his window again, the cross vivid against the sky as we listen to worship music. Fatima, our nurse's aide since we have been here, comes to say goodbye. She knows tomorrow, when she begins her night shift, we will be gone, and she is sentimental as she talks with Zack. She hugs us both and tearfully promises to come to Frazier to see his progress.

It will be bittersweet to leave here. I think of all the staff we leave behind and pray that those who don't know Jesus will see a glimpse of Him in our hope for Zack. Nurse Yolanda hears the worship music and drifts into the room. In the midst of our farewell, she asks for information on Southeast Christian Church service times. She's inspired by the melody and wants to check out the Vine, our college-age ministry. God is using our situation to draw others to Him. I have an overwhelming sense of peace tonight. A renewed confidence that Zack will be healed, and God will be glorified. I lean back in my chair and listen to a song describe how heaven came to rescue me. I close my eyes, feel His presence, and just breathe.

I arrived later than usual to the hospital, because I was packing clothes for Zack to take to Frazier Rehab. As I was selecting t-shirts, shorts, and sweatpants, I couldn't stop from smiling, even though this task was putting me way behind schedule. It didn't matter. We would finally see Zack in his own clothes, instead of a hospital gown. And he was going to Frazier, not a nursing home, as many had predicted. Zack was lying in bed with his legs crossed when I slipped into his room. If not for his oddly shaped, shaved head and the cables leading to his monitor, he could have been any teenager relaxing in bed. I was driven back to reality as I noticed both hands fingering his trach.

I stood silently in the doorway and watched as he moved his left hand up to touch his face. It is almost as though he is trying to figure out who he is. Like Rip Van Winkle, awakened from a deep sleep, trying to remember who he was. His fingers crept from the trach to his lips, touched his nose, and slowly inched back to rest on the hose connected to his trach.

Dr. Raff with Infectious Disease makes his final assessment and comments that the "storming" Zack exhibits is common with all critically brain injured patients. Despite the profuse sweating and his slightly elevated white count, Dr. Raff is not concerned. He looks at Zack and says, "Go to rehab," as I excitedly clap my hands like a child at a circus. Dr. Apfel listens to Zack's lungs with a stethoscope and nods his head in approval. To my surprise, he asks for the address of the blog, so he can keep up with our progress and says he has a good feeling that Zack will be a star patient in rehab. We wait with eager anticipation for the ambulance that will take us to Frazier. Karen manages to work us into her morning, even though we are not scheduled for physical therapy. She couldn't miss saying goodbye and promises to visit, commenting that P.T. in therapy will be much tougher than what we've experienced in ICU. Our chariot finally arrives at noon for the short ride to Frazier Rehab. As we pull up to the curb, I glance back through the buildings looking for University Hospital, as though I'm leaving family behind.

As we enter the main lobby, I immediately notice that it seems calmer than the one we left behind. The elevator whisks us to the eighth floor, where a smaller lobby leads to a secure hallway, accessed by pushing a button to open automatic doors. I am naturally curious as I walk down the hall, glancing into rooms, hoping to see patients doing miraculous things. We are settled into a private room with sunlight emanating from large double windows. There is another bed for me and our own bathroom.

Zack is transferred to his bed, and our day nurse introduces herself while comparing his wristband to our paperwork. Courtney begins the required medical appraisal, checking blood pressure and noting the precautions necessary for MRSA in his chart. She takes him to be weighed, and I discover he has lost over 10 pounds, now down to 139 pounds. Dr. Miller, the resident specialist in physical medicine comes in. I instantly like him.

We talk for a while, and I tell him that we also had a Dr. Miller at University Hospital, who was the resident anesthetist. Ironically, both of their first names are Jason, and it turns out, they went to medical school together. Small world...or perfectly planned. Dr. Stevens, attending physiatrist, is next on staff to introduce himself. He explains that they may use trazodone, a drug for anxiety and a sleep aid, if they feel it's necessary. Their philosophy at Frazier doesn't include a lot of medication, but they want him well-rested and at his best for therapy. The staff is kind and welcoming, making sure that I have everything I need.

At 5:00, I meet part of the team who will be instrumental in Zack's recovery. His physical therapist, Amy Raque, along with an aide, move him to a sitting position on the side of his bed. Coaxing him to hold his head up while they support his body, they pull him to his feet. Amy explains that they want him to feel the weight of his body and the floor beneath his feet. His legs are weak and trembling, but they support him one on each side, with Russell's arm around his back. I am struck at how tall he appears and notice that his clothes seem way too big. My previously muscular athlete looks puny, like a skinny scarecrow. Although he only stands for a brief minute, this simple task takes a lot out of him.

When they get him back to bed, he is exhausted. I expect him to recover with a nap, but soon, that hand goes up to feel his face. His left index finger traces his eyebrows and feels his lips. I watch as he glides his hand over the bridge of his nose, finds a hole, and sticks his finger in his nostril. He moves his legs, his left foot crossing at the ankle, and then back across the bed. He seems a bit restless, but after lying still for so long, I am thrilled to see him moving around again. His fine motor skills are intact, and he uses the tips of his fingers to find some tube to pull on. Recognizing the danger, I hold his hand, gaze into those big brown eyes, and talk to him, so he's distracted.

Even after all his surgeries, he is still so handsome, and the nurses fuss over him. I was afraid to leave the nurses in the ICU and had grown fond of many of our doctors at University Hospital, but this place already feels like home. They know what they are doing, but they are gentle and explain everything to me. They make me feel as though I am part of the team that will insure Zack's successful recovery. They bring me dinner and encourage me to ask for anything we may need.

As evening approaches, Scott's parents, Rita and Louie, bring Kyle and Logan to see him. Kyle immediately puts sterile gloves on and holds Zack's hand. Not disturbed by his appearance, she strokes his arm. Dissatisfied with this passive attention, she spies the lotion on his bedside table and asks if she can rub it on his feet. As she uncovers his legs and removes his socks, Logan becomes overwhelmed, climbs on my lap, and begins to cry. She is scared of this patient who looks like her brother, but doesn't act like he's supposed to. We take a walk down the hall. Wiping her tears, I promise her Zack will get better. I am confident he will. I trust that God has a plan that is better than anything I can dream up. As we approach the nurses' station, Kendra, our night nurse, sees Logan crying and offers her ice cream. Returning with the treat, she offers her some paper and markers to make Zack a picture for his room. It is obvious that the staff here understands and cares how this situation impacts our whole family. Caught up in the chaos and medical drama, I sometimes forget how hard this is on Zack's siblings. Friends and family have stepped up, taken them places, and at times, it seems like a big slumber party, but their life is dramatically different, and they worry about their brother.

When visiting hours are over, I settle in with Zack. I check the clock and decide it's not too late to call Scott with an update. Kendra busies herself, checking the tubing that runs to his I.V. bag and adjusting his bed. She leans down and asks Zack if he is okay. He nods his head and mouths yes! My back is turned, and she waits as I finish my call with Scott. She asked me if he has been nodding in response to questions, and then reveals his silent reply. As tears well up in my eyes, she attempts to persuade another response, but he refuses to repeat himself.

I'm encouraged by this new development, but dismayed that after waiting by his bedside for weeks, he chooses to speak first to a stranger. She senses my disappointment, offers a sympathetic hug, and promises there is more to come. Noting the response in his chart, she slips out, closing the door behind her. I move to his bed and gaze at my scrawny son, pondering what therapy may look like tomorrow. We know it will be tough ahead, and he will go through phases of recovery that won't be pleasant. The Zack we knew may not come back, but he will be a new creation that God will use for His glory. It dawns on me that the "storming" he does is the furnace God is using to mold him into His servant as scripture describes—"Behold, I have refined you, but not as silver; I have tried you in the furnace of affliction." Isaiah 48:10. Zack is settled, and I retire to my chair, open my laptop, and update our followers on the move to Frazier. I have so many emotions right now that tears unconsciously slip from my eyes. I am tired, grateful, encouraged, and anxious all at once. I glance over at Zack in his own clothes, sleeping peacefully, and wonder what I am supposed to say. Then, I notice that I have received a message from one of his friends.

"Hornback Family. I just got an email back from Honduras. Zack has a whole town (La Paz) in Honduras praying for him. I sent news of Zack's accident to Honduras, and their church has been praying daily. They asked how he was doing and if their prayers were being heard, and I thank God that I could tell them that Zack is going to be alright. That by God's will, he will probably make a full recovery. I mean, God is so big. Even a town from another country at least 3,000 miles away is praying for Zack. Who knows who else is praying for him? I can ensure one thing: God is definitely hearing the thousands of prayers that we lift to Him for Zack every day. I know that when Zack makes a full recovery, God will allow him to pursue his dreams. For all we know, God may plan Zack to be recovered enough to come back his junior year and play varsity baseball for CAL and go on to play at a college. God is awesome, and he can make miracles from seemingly nothing. At the baseball retreat in April, we watched *Miracle*. And we all knew that this movie was going to pertain somehow to this year's team. It didn't happen in our record, but I can now see that Zack's recovery was the theme that we believed in for the entire season—"DO YOU BELIEVE IN MIRACLES?" My answer to that is YES, because Zack will complete a full recovery, even when most of the doctors doubted him at first. You keep talking about the Miracle Room that Zack is staying in, and we have already seen many amazing miracles and we will continue to see them, and we do believe in miracles. I also pray that God will use you after everything settles down to be a witness to those around you who need it the most."

Tears stream down my face and soak the keyboard. I needed to hear this message and be encouraged by how far we have come. I bow my head and am thankful for the prayers that have already been answered and feel emboldened to believe God's plan is complete recovery. I wipe my eyes on my sleeve, and before long, I drift off to sleep, imagining Zack at a podium, speaking in front of an auditorium of teenagers. They are applauding, then stomping their feet. My subconscious nudges me awake, and I realize it's Zack over there making so much noise. He constantly moves his legs, like he's doing some kind of river dance. He is all over the place, and half the time, both feet are hanging off the bed. I keep getting up to put his feet back in bed and cover him up.

I remember at University Hospital, when he wasn't moving his legs at all, I would pray for any sign of life. The nurses told me that there would come a time when I wish he would just hold still. Well, at 2:30 a.m., that time has come. It seemed like I had just drifted back to sleep, when Dr. Stevens and his resident, Heidi, stomp into the room and turned on the bright overhead light, waking us both up at 5:30 a.m. It seems comical that they start asking me questions after only three hours of sleep, and my brain wasn't functioning much better than Zack's. Since they are filling in for Dr. Mook and have other patients to see, rounds start early. I may have to reconsider sleeping here, even though there is a bed for me. Between Zack's dance show last night and the early doctor visit, I won't have the stamina to make it through a day of therapy.

Our nurse for today is Jennifer, a five-year veteran at Frazier. She introduces herself and notices how frazzled I am. She assures me that Zack will be well taken care of, stating she has witnessed many family members crash in exhaustion and suggests that I would be better off sleeping at home.

Dr. Skolnick, our pulmonary expert, discusses changing Zack's trach to one that can be plugged, so he can talk when he's ready. Oh, to hear my sweet boy's voice again. As they leave, Zack is reaching up and feeling his face. His fingers roam all over his head, feeling his eyebrows and over to his ear. Finally, his left hand touches his lips. I love watching him, but today, I am very emotional. I guess fatigue gets the best of me, and the floodgates open. Zack seems to handle this whole ordeal with such dignity and grace that I am ashamed of myself. I feel a desperate battle within me, between God's will and my fear.

I attempt to read my Bible, but can't focus, thoughts swirling around in my head. I get out my journal and pour my feelings into it. I hadn't noticed that another resident had entered the room to check on Zack. Dr. Borhan can see I'm upset and sits down to talk with me. He explains that he had heard what a serious accident Zack was in and knew his injuries would be severe, but he is heartened by his progress in such a short time. I am struck by the different approach the staff here takes: intentionally encouraging, instead of the foreboding doom of ICU. Each person we have encountered has shown such empathy, not just for Zack, but also for our family.

A nutritionist comes by and explains that Zack has been getting 1,800 calories a day through his G-tube, and they want to start beefing that up to 2,100 to build up his strength, so he can fully participate in therapy. When she leaves, I notice some blood on his pillow and realize that while we were talking, Zack reached up, scratched his head wound, and now it is bleeding.

I call out for Jennifer, who rushes into the room. She looks at Zack's head and bloody fingernails, emphasizing that we must pay close attention, because stitches itch, and his hands are roaming everywhere. Then, I remember Dr. Han's instructions to request a consult with a wound care nurse to review the orders on how to care for it. Before lunch, Amy arrives to provide some bedside physical therapy, which mostly consists of just getting Zack dressed. Then, he is introduced to his wheelchair, and we go to the gym for the first time.

Rehab therapy is hard work, and at times, Zack resists, even appearing to get a little angry. Amy tells me that's a good sign. They bring out a full-size mirror, and Zack sees himself for the first time. He stares intently, and I get the impression that he doesn't believe it is him. Mary Beth, his occupational therapist, demonstrates several moves I can continue to work on with Zack in his room, to improve tone in his right arm and shoulder. They explain that he is neglecting his right side, rarely using that arm. It's like the world on his right doesn't exist, so he will not look at anyone to his right.

Apparently, right-side neglect is a common reaction with a brain injury on the left, so we need to stand on the right to encourage him to look in that direction. This is hard in practice, since you naturally want to stand where he will look at you with those big, brown eyes.

Our time in the gym complete, we move to speech therapy and meet Kathy Pfeiffer. She turns out the lights and uses a small flashlight, tempting him to track to the right. She reiterates that our biggest battle right now is getting Zack to recognize that side of the world. She uses ice cubes on his cheeks to stimulate him and rubs them on his lips to encourage him to lick them. He salivates, but doesn't swallow. Breathing on his own, he will now have to learn to swallow. So much of these actions come naturally, but they must be relearned after traumatic brain injury.

Zack is visibly tired after therapy, but several friends are waiting when we return to his room. One of the nurses suggests that we take him outside, since it was such a pretty day. Embracing the idea, I was practically skipping down the hall as we pushed him towards the elevator. Zack has not felt the sun in nearly a month, and we were all excited to spend the allotted 15 minutes outdoors. It proved to be a bit overwhelming for him, with the bright sunlight and traffic noises. I could tell after only a few minutes it was too much stimulation, so we return to his room and his friends say their goodbyes.

Zack is moved to the bed ready for a nap, falling asleep almost instantly. I'm quietly reading, my eyelids getting heavy, when we receive a visit from Larry, a 21-year-old who survived a brain injury after a motorcycle accident, and his mom. Zack is still asleep, worn out from therapy, and I need to be asleep. We talk about Larry's recovery, and again, I am overcome with emotion. I want so badly to see Zack in the same condition as Larry. Walking, talking, going to school, and having fun with his friends. It must be awful for Larry as his mom tries to comfort me, but all I can do is look at him and cry. He appears uncomfortable, but I assure him that I am glad he came, that it is encouraging to acknowledge him and envision Zack in the future. Larry seems more than ready to leave as his Mom hugs me, whispering that things will get better, and they hurry down the hall.

Dr. Miller has read the nurses' report of our short trip outside and comes to speak with me. He explains that we must be aware of over-stimulating Zack at this point in his recovery, or he can become agitated and stop responding. He instructs the staff to put a "quiet zone" sign on our door and decides to limit how many people are in his room at one time, stating that multiple conversations could be distressing. I tell him that we need visitors, justifying that his friends are an important part of his recovery, so he agrees, as long as we are sensitive to Zack's responses. Dr. Miller describes anticipated reactions as he moves through phases of recovery, reiterating that we have to be flexible, especially after a big day of therapy, when he will need rest.

Donna was waiting for the elevator when Scott arrived, so they enter Zack's room together. She immediately sees my tear-stained cheeks and hugs me as I explain my reaction to Larry's visit. Scott turns his attention away from Zack and gently puts his hands on my shoulders, looking me in the eye. Both proceed to lecture me about how I will be of no help to Zack if I don't get rest myself. It doesn't take much for Scott and Donna to convince me that I need to go home and get a good night's sleep. I know that is what I should do. Being with him all the time prevents me from recognizing how far he has come; how much more alert he seems. I realize if I am stressed out and emotional, it is not good for Zack, so as much as I want to be at his side, I agree to go home.

Scott will stay until it is time for Zack's bath, knowing that afterward, he will sleep for the night. As I drive home, I ask God for patience with His timing and wisdom to know when it is better for me to leave him in the excellent care of the staff. I pray that when his friends visit, they will leave believing in the power of prayer and that we send out of Zack's room many witnesses for Christ, encouraged to speak of their faith. When I pull in the driveway, I see trash cans overturned and remember Scott telling me about our skunk problem. Oh, please don't let me find that they have attacked our dog again. I am very tired, and it is hard to sleep with your fingers holding your nose.

Three weeks since the accident and day two at Frazier, I arrive to find Zack chilling in his bed with the lights out, watching TV. He has his left leg swung over the side rail and looks completely relaxed and at home. As I walk across the room, he tracks me all the way to the right. Kendra has left a note on his door, informing me that he had a peaceful night and nodded twice.

I grin at Zack, wondering when I will get to witness that response. Dr. Skolnick and Dr. Borhan make rounds at 7:30 a.m. to change out his trach with a number-six, Jackson metal one that has a plug. This trach is smaller, much easier to clean, and the plug enables him to speak when he's ready. After his trach was changed, I watched as he stretched his left arm over his head. He noticed me watching him, so I asked him to raise his hand. He held it over his head until I instructed him to put it down. I smiled and moved to the bed to kiss his cheek, pleased that he was following commands.

Our morning session with Amy and Mary Beth takes place in his room. They take pictures of him in different positions, so I will understand the correct posture to correct the tone in his right arm and shoulder. Mary Beth cancelled the dynamic arm splint that Dr. Mook ordered, stating she would make a custom one that will be more suitable and less expensive. When they are ready to leave, Mary Beth asks him to squeeze her hand if he wants her to leave him alone. Zack just stares at her. She tries again, *"Do you want me to leave you alone?"* He pauses, and then slowly shakes his head "no". Squeezing his hand, her lip quivers as she explains that most patients offer an enthusiastic yes when asked this question. I think we will get lots of extra attention now that Mary Beth has fallen under Zack's spell.

Zack napped until it was time to get dressed for the gym. When he was moved to a sitting position on the side of the bed, he began to cough, and I noted the grimace on his face as though he was about to cry. I ask him what is wrong, and he shakes his head and says, "No". He finally speaks, and I hear it. There are several visitors present as we move him to his wheelchair. I bend down to eye level and ask if he wants to go to the gym and again, he says, "No". Surprised, I reply, "Mary Beth is at the gym. Don't you want to see her?" Zack mumbles three or four words that we can't understand.

During physical therapy, they use beanbags of different colors, asking him to take one and give it to me. He reaches for the first one and releases it into my hand. Smiling, Mary Beth and Amy both agree that he has reached an impressive milestone, since it is more difficult to release than to hold something. After the first beanbag, he isn't ready to give the next one up, preferring to hold it and finger it like a baseball. When therapy is complete, they request a high-five, and he quickly raises his hand, encouraging us all. The therapists update his file, noting his progress, and my spirits are lifted as I wheel him up to our room.

It is after to 5:00 p.m. when we return to the room. Zack is very tired, and I remove his sneakers while an aide helps get him into bed. He rests peacefully for an hour until Scott arrives with his hairdresser in tow. Julie has been following Zack's progress through the blog and has offered to cut his hair. The side that wasn't shaved off for surgery has grown quite scruffy, so she is going to clean him up a bit. Zack sits up in his wheelchair, and Scott gently cradles his face as Julie carefully trims around his ears. She has been cutting men's hair for years, but this is a very different situation, and I notice her hands shaking ever so slightly. It only took a few minutes before we were brushing him off and returning him to his bed. Julie packs up her shears and hugs me goodbye, and Scott walks her to the elevator.

I look at my son, with his hair neatly trimmed, accentuating his misshapen head. I reflect on the grace and love of God, that He would give me such a fantastic day after the emotional one I had yesterday. He gave Zack back his voice and grants us an encouraging day in the gym. He always sends the right person or post on the website at just the right time. God heard my cries yesterday, and He blessed me with so many positive things today. When I left here last night, I commented that I wish I could just go to sleep and wake up months from now, when Zack was well. After today, I don't want to miss a moment. Memories flash across my mind of my toddler taking his first steps, and I relish in the thought of experiencing that delight again.

I close my eyes, take Zack's hand, and voice my prayers. I want Zack to hear that we need only to put our trust in God, to let go and let Him perform miracles. We are blessed to have God carry us through an experience that not many others can fathom. At times, it has been terrifying—our future unsure—but today, I am emboldened by the promises of scripture in Romans 8:18— "I consider our present sufferings are not worth comparing with the glory that will be revealed in us."

Arriving a little later than usual, I hurry through the lobby and catch the first elevator. Zack is awake and mumbling, although we can't understand a word, almost as if he is speaking another language. It is still fairly early when our first visitors arrive. Jude Thompson, Sr. and his son, Jude—who is a classmate of Zack's—drop by to check on his progress and offer encouragement. His dad explains that Jude had played a bad game of golf the day before and normally would have been really upset about it, but he realized how fortunate he was to be able to play at all. He thought about Zack, trapped in a hospital room, not able to enjoy the summer, not able to play baseball, nor even walk outside, and he was humbled. Jude signed his golf glove and gave it to Zack, telling him that he is praying for his swift recovery. As they leave, his dad hands me his business card and offers to help with any insurance issues. They politely walk out the door, and I turn the card over in my hand to examine it. I'm quite surprised to read "Jude Thompson President Anthem BlueCross BlueShield KY". That's my insurance company. All these years, we had sat in the bleachers, cheering as our boys played basketball together at Christian Academy, and I had never known what Jude did for a living. Another dot connected. I put the card in my pocket and think about what young Jude had said to Zack. This is a humbling lesson for many of Zack's friends. Reflecting on Zack's situation makes them appreciate activities that they previously had taken for granted.

Noticing the time, I help an aide get Zack dressed for therapy, and Mary Beth arrives in time to get him into his wheelchair. He mumbles something, but the only word we can make out is, "Head." As we finish putting on his sneakers, Andrew, Taylor, and Blake stride in, excited to see him in a wheelchair and wearing familiar clothes. Zack hardly acknowledges his friends, and just stares longingly at his bed. He obviously does not want to be in his chair, fidgets restlessly, and says, "I don't want get up." We all just stood there, astonished. They talk to him, trying to elicit other responses, but Zack is too busy attempting to break free of the seatbelt that keeps him restrained in his chair. Covering my mouth to stifle a giggle, I bend down to eye level and explain that he can't go back to bed. As we make our way to the gym, a nurse chases after us, stating that Zack needs to be weighed before therapy.

His friends agree to come back later, and as the boys leave, he finally acknowledges Andrew and Blake with a high-five. We follow them down the hall, and they disappear in the elevator as we wheel Zack into another room. Placed on the scale, we learn he has lost more weight, down to 135 pounds. His body burns a lot of calories, just healing his brain, and then, there are those late-night river dances in bed. The nutritionist decides to increase his tube feedings to 2,160 calories. As we are hanging around the nurses' station, I notice Zack keeps putting his foot on the floor, like he's getting ready to bolt. I ask him to put his foot back on the footrest, and he complies. He is following more commands, and we no longer ask for a thumbs-up. We wore that request out at University Hospital. I wheel him towards the elevator, and as we wait for the cab, I see Zack intentionally scoot himself back in his chair. He is gaining more control over his body.

Saturday schedules are limited, so it is already 4:00 p.m. when we arrive for our first gym session. Scott walks in just as the weekend occupational therapist is explaining that Mary Beth was scheduled at Jewish Hospital today. Ann had barely finished with introductions, when Mary Beth races in, announcing that her schedule had changed, making her available for Zack's session. I smile, thinking to myself that Zack has her under his spell. With two therapists, Zack is much more aggressive in his responses. After 15 minutes of working him in a sitting position, they decide to lay him back on the mat. He immediately throws up. Scott and I are both freaked out, but they assure us that it is not uncommon. They pull Zack to a standing position, bracing his upper body while he supports his weight on his own. We can see him flexing his thigh and stomach muscles through his thin t-shirt, his face determined as he focuses on trying to stand. We notice, for the first time in 23 days, that he has grown taller.

He is now taller than Scott and looks to be over six feet, even though his wobbly legs make it difficult to stand up straight. They place him in front of a full-length mirror, so he can see himself standing, but I think he is more focused on Scott celebrating behind him. While I'm able to go with Zack to therapy every day, Scott is only able to witness his progress on the weekends. Ann and Mary Beth discuss Zack's development and place him at a four on the Cognitive Scale, but, ultimately, his speech therapist will have the final word—no pun intended. They explain that Zack will move into the next phase, which is a step forward, but not necessarily pleasant. He will become increasingly more agitated and aggressive. He will talk a lot more, but only to express negative thoughts and emotions: "I don't want to," "I can't," "You're mean to me." They warn that he is also likely to get foulmouthed, a common reaction in patients with traumatic brain injury. Let the cussing begin, if that's a sign of recovery.

Scott hurried home to pick Dylan up from football practice and relieve Morgan. I don't know how we would manage without our neighbor stepping in to help with Kyle and Logan. It's impressive that a 13-year-old can calm the nerves of two little girls living through a family tragedy, but they adore her. Morgan folds our laundry, helps with dishes, reads them the updates on their brother and wipes away tears as she prays with them. Thankfully, we are blessed daily with food delivered by friends from Southeast Christian Church and Christian Academy. This enables Scott to work, while I remain with Zack.

When we return to our room, Zack is eager to be back in bed. He is physically weary from therapy and weak from throwing up. Fussing over him as she connects his G-tube to the feeding bag, Kendra listens to me recap our gym fiasco. Suddenly, Zack coughs and his trach comes out, spilling mucus down his neck. She calmly reinserts it, adjusts his collar, and cleans him up again. She puts a call into Dr. Skolnick in pulmonary and updates her report.

We have plenty of visitors to keep me occupied until Kendra returns with a message from Dr. Skolnick. He ordered that his trach be plugged at night, as well as during the day. If Zack handles it as well as they expect, oxygen levels close to 100 percent and able to cough up secretions, they will remove his trach next week. I breathe a big sigh of relief, recognizing that would be one less aggravation. If only we can keep his hands off his head wound. It itches, so he frequently scratches it, often drawing blood. With our guest departing, the staff encourages me to go home early tonight, so they can get Zack settled. I putter around, making excuses, not wanting to leave, when my phone rings.

Scott promised the kids that I would be home before they went to bed, and his call was my reminder. Kendra chuckles and points at the door. As I drag myself to the elevator, I suddenly realize how fatigued I am. I lean up against the wall on the ride down to the lobby, and my mind drifts back to University Hospital. Only four days ago, he was in ICU, and I was worried about some infection killing him. The power of prayer is undeniable.

God gave me a special gift today. Not silver or gold, but just as priceless. The sun was already promising a beautiful day, and I was still humming the worship music that I had been playing in my car when I entered the lobby. The melody resonated through my mind, putting a bounce in my step, as I skipped into Zack's room. He was awake, lying in bed. "Good morning, sunshine." His eyes light up, and he smiles at me. Not a toothy grin, but a sweet, angelic smile. Thank you, Jesus! I park myself in my chair, and without moving it next to the bed, I watch him. He lifts his left hand in the air and wiggles his fingers. He seems mesmerized, twisting his hand around and brings his fingers together. I feel almost as if I'm intruding, but I can't take my eyes off watching him discover that he controls those dancing digits. It again reminds me of when he was a baby.

It was still early when Jim Whitworth, a high school teacher from Christian Academy, finds his way to our room. We talk at length about the impact Zack has made on a lot of his friends and even teens who don't know him. Students from other communities have reached out, not only with prayers, but to express how our situation is changing the way they respond when facing adversity. We hear things like, "God can help us through anything," "God created us to glorify Him in every situation," and "Zack is a witness to God's healing power." The website is passed around churches, youth groups, and business offices, bouncing from state to state and beyond to other countries. God is working through Zack to touch so many lives. Jim reminds me that we are told to preach the Word daily, and if necessary, use words. Totally appropriate now that Zack doesn't have many words to say.

Jim makes his exit as a resident arrives to take a culture of Zack's head wound. Apparently, their lab didn't have a record of the culture taken at University Hospital, and they need to be prepared to treat any infection. His head is bleeding again, so I give Zack the golf glove to hold, keeping his roaming hand busy, so he won't be tempted to scratch his wound. I'm watching the clock, so I won't be late for church, and I see Zack holding the glove up in the air and shaking it. My attention is diverted when my friend Donna waltzes in, ready to relieve me, so I can make it to the service on time. In an instant, Zack somehow manages to get the glove onto his left hand by himself. Donna is so delighted that she kisses his forehead and asks if he wants to kiss her in return. She was holding his hand, and he pulls her towards his face and kisses her cheek. My sweet boy.

The 20-mile drive to church seemed to take only a few minutes with my mind replaying our morning blessings. How a simple smile can bring such hope. Overcome with emotion, I can't stop crying as I sit in church, thanking God for saving my son and praying for complete recovery. I find personal meaning in every worship song, and Scott doesn't even bother to wipe the tears from his face. When we return to Frazier, I notice that Zack is very active, pulling at everything, his feet hanging off the side of his bed. As instructed, I pay close attention to his roving hands, so that he doesn't cause any more damage to his head. Dr. Gormerly makes his rounds and reports that the culture they took of his sputum was negative for MRSA, however, there was an infection of *E. coli* present. He doesn't seem concerned. I am learning to let things go easily, especially if the doctors aren't alarmed, since we have plenty of other issues to resolve.

We move Zack to his chair, and he struggles with the weight of his helmet to hold his head up. This chair is not the modified stretcher version he used at the hospital, but more like a stiff recliner. Several times, his head bobs forward, and I gently push it back onto the headrest. He doesn't like it, and finally gets mad enough that he throws a washcloth across the room. He frowns and says, "Head hurt," in the midst of other mumbling. I don't know if it's the helmet or his brain injury triggering his headache, but I acknowledge how frustrating it is for him not being able to communicate. Since this is considered therapy, and we get no formal sessions on Sunday, we manage to keep him in his chair for several hours. He is resting in bed when Dr. Borhan comes in with news that Zack has a urinary tract infection, most likely from having a catheter for so long, so they are starting him on another antibiotic. I'm sure this won't be the last of medical issues we will face.

It is early evening, and Zack is sitting up in bed when several of his friends arrive. He is holding his baseball, rolling it around in his fingers. He holds it up in the air, and when Rick asks for it, he releases it into Rick's hand, an important indicator of progress. When Rick returns the ball, Zack automatically throws it about a foot to Trey. For the next two hours, he plays this simple ballgame with his friends. Hearing their occasional roar, our nurse drifts in to catch the excitement. Before long, Dr. Borhan comes back to check out their game and is actually impressed. Of course, his friends are delighted, recognizing that this game is great therapy. And since this is the ball that Scott brought to Zack at University, it holds a special meaning. The homerun God had sent as a symbol of hope for Scott, is now an encouragement to all of us.

Arriving this morning, even with the sun beckoning a new day, I didn't expect much, since no therapy is scheduled. But as I learn to wait on God's timing, I receive unexpected blessings. We say goodbye to his beaming friends, promising more games on their next visit. I consider Kyle Idleman's sermon on suffering today and the final message to just hold onto God. I can't imagine going through this trial without clinging to our Savior. To be able to approach the throne of God and know He feels our pain is a great comfort. I sit back in my chair and close my eyes. I picture myself sitting at the feet of my Heavenly Father, His hand resting tenderly on my shoulder, His face full of compassion as He listens to my requests. I ask for healing, for Him to show us new ways to reach Zack in therapy. I ask that we will be satisfied with the little blessings that He decides to give us, so that we can experience greater joy on days like today. When I finally open my eyes, Zack is sound asleep, still clutching his baseball.

Starting off a new week, with new challenges, I swing into Zack's room before 8:00 a.m. to find Nurse Jennifer changing the bedsheets, while he sits patiently in his wheelchair. She reports that Zack had disconnected his feeding tube four or five times during the night, making a mess of himself and his linens. His roaming fingers curiously explore every cable and tube, requiring almost constant attention. He will have one less temptation when his trach is removed, hopefully in the next few days. Tackling physical and occupational therapy in his room, Amy asks Zack if he wants to stand up and he emphatically responds *"Yes!"* Once he is standing, he immediately tries to take a step. Amy and Mary Beth prevent him from moving forward, explaining that you must support your upper body in order to walk, and Zack can barely hold his head up. Complicating his effort to walk is his observable right-side neglect, which sends incorrect messages to his brain. He considers "center" as down and to the left, so that is his focus when trying to take a step. Obviously, it is difficult to walk straight when you don't know where your center really is. This reinforces our goal to get him to recognize the world to his right, because that impacts everything.

Mary Beth selects one of the posters his friends delivered to decorate his room and asks him where Andrew is in the photograph. Zack points to Andrew. This is a positive sign that at least parts of his memory are intact. She introduces a toothbrush and asks how to use it. He brings it to his mouth and attempts to brush his teeth. This will require more attention, since he kept biting down on it, rather than moving it across his teeth. Zack was always meticulous in his grooming habits, so I feel confident that he will master this task fairly quickly.

Early afternoon, we wheel to speech therapy, and Zack gives us all sorts of surprises. Staring at himself in the mirror as his therapist puts applesauce on his lips, he quickly licks it off. Kathy decides to try a spoon, and before she can react, Zack grabs the spoon and begins feeding himself. He was quite messy and only able to scoop up very small bites, but he was doing it on his own. We were interrupted by her office phone. She moved across the room to answer it, with the spoon in her hand, Zack looks at her walking away and wistfully says, "Applesauce." It was marvelous to hear him talk, but my poor boy has had no food by mouth for over three weeks and is famished. She returns with a cup of water and puts it to his lips to take a sip, but he isn't having any of that. He takes the cup and begins drinking from it, pushing her hand away when she tries to take control. Stifling a laugh, Kathy corrects me with an incredulous look, stating that he has to pass a swallow test before he will be allowed to eat or drink anything. It is difficult not to acknowledge his eagerness to eat. I have watched my son shrink to skin and bones over the last few weeks, and it's only natural to want to feed him. We end our hour of speech therapy and make our way to the gym.

Combining physical and occupational therapy allows them to work towards the same goal, while utilizing our rehab hours more efficiently. They intentionally focus his head back to center, and as I watch the various exercises, I think to myself if they only had applesauce, I bet he would follow that spoon wherever they wanted him to look. Food could be a real incentive for him, but only speech therapy is allowed to use it. After some strenuous work in a seated position, they lay him on his back, and he immediately vomits. They don't seem concerned, nonchalantly cleaning off the mat, but I make a mental note to discover why this is happening. Each time he regurgitates, Zack is visibly upset. They turn him onto his stomach, and Amy helps him support his upper body with his arms while Mary Beth holds his head up and center. Once he has mastered that position, it's time to play horsey. They place him on his hands and knees, a difficult position for him, since he has to support his body weight evenly. It appears to be a simple exercise; however, his brain labors to send the correct messages to his body on what to do. Like a champ, he is able to remain in this position, until both his therapists are sweating from assisting him. As he is relaxing on the mat, they praise him, congratulating him on a great job, and Zack picks up a towel to wipe the sweat from his forehead. Mary Beth raises her eyebrow, smiles, and grabs his chart. She points out that his speech therapist has moved him to a four on the Cognitive Scale. Encouraged, she makes the same remark in his OT/PT report. There is a joyful skip in my step as I wheel him back to his room. He has made definitive progress in a few short days.

Once he is back in his bed, he is asleep within minutes. He has been diligent, pushing himself to work hard. Every physical movement is also mental gymnastics, so he is just worn out. Nurse Jennifer says that we need to let him sleep, so his brain can heal, and I decide to go home early. I missed several calls from Scott while in therapy, and I can tell from his messages that he had a rough day, too. When I pull in the driveway, I expect to find him sitting in silence on the deck, where he spends most of his nights. He no longer watches TV and stays up much later. He works construction, so he is usually worn out at the end of the day and ready for bed by 10:00 p.m.

Since Zack's accident, he sits in the dark on the deck until after midnight, deep in thought and prayer, waiting for me to come home. I report on the positive progress of Zack's day, but he ends up in tears, frustrated that he can't be with him, and not sure if he can keep managing things at home. I kneel beside him and take both of his hands, placing them together in prayer. I speak softly, asking God to give him strength to handle the additional pressure at home and allow him to find special time to be with Zack. I pray for the Rivards, that they will find comfort in their faith as they support Matt through the legal ramifications of driving intoxicated, which resulted in the accident that caused Zack's traumatic brain injury. As difficult as it is for us to watch our son deal with TBI, we still recognize how heart breaking it is for the Rivards. As I hug Scott and urge him to go to bed, I can still sense his despair, and a scripture verse comes to mind. I tell him to remember the promise in Revelations 21:3, that the Lord will make "everything new" and to see the journey that Zack is on now as a glimpse of what the future holds for all who believe.

# First Tuesday

It was inevitable, so I wasn't all that surprised, when his nurse explains that they had to restrain Zack's left arm throughout the night to keep him from picking at his head wound and messing with his feeding tube. His right-side neglect prevents him from using his right hand, so thankfully, he won't have to be in a straitjacket all night, just restrained on one side. Joan Hardin, our wound care nurse, comes for a consult and instructs the staff to clean his head wound three times a day with saline. She explains that this process should dry it out, so that the stitches can be removed, and the itching stopped. When we move Zack to his wheelchair for his morning trip to the gym, I am encouraged with how well he is holding his head up. *This is going to be a good day*, I think to myself as we ride the elevator downstairs.

Then, suddenly, he starts to vomit. Not just once, but several times. We are alone on the elevator, and puke is coming out around his trach every time he heaves. Both of us are terrified, not knowing what to do, and when the elevator doors open, I start screaming for help. Zack is mortified that he has puke on his hand, his baseball, and all over his lap. Mary Beth and Amy calm me down and clean Zack's hands off. They wash his baseball, instructing me to take him back to his room for clean clothes, and they would come upstairs for therapy. I'm scared to even get on the elevator with him by myself, so an aide rides up with us. The nursing staff is surprised to see us return so quickly, and tears slip from the corner of my eyes as I explain why Zack is such a mess. They fuss over him, get him in a clean shirt and shorts, and assure me that Dr. Mook will figure out why this keeps happening.

Mary Beth and Amy take him down the hall from his room to where they have placed a mat. They position him on his knees, holding onto the windowsill. He maintains this position, shifting his weight to balance his upper body for several minutes, and then he starts puking again. He has a pitiful expression on his face, his brows twisted in confusion while his eyes plead for help. Fortunately, Amy has a clean towel to wipe his mouth, while Mary Beth soothingly suggests that we return to his room for another change of clothes. They discuss a variety of options that might cause this reaction and instruct the nurse to page the doctor on call. With therapy cancelled, they return to the gym, and I am left alone to wait.

Sitting in his wheelchair, Zack starts throwing up again before the doctor arrives. I'm trying to catch puke in my hands, to avoid it getting on his lap, telling him it's going to be alright with tears streaming down my face. I can't even convince myself, so I'm sure Zack wasn't consoled. Nurse Jennifer rushes into the room with his chart and thinks she has it figured out. He was started on a new antibiotic, Bactrim, yesterday for his urinary tract infection. Bactrim frequently makes people nauseous. She explains that all of his cultures have come back, and his white count is under 10. They conclude that Zack only has a mild urinary infection that his body can fight on its own, so the order for Bactrim is cancelled.

She gives him Phenergan to stop him from puking. He looks solemn, almost resigned that this is his fate. Having watched how hard he fought to do the simplest gesture like giving a thumbs up, I have a new appreciation of his determination. I feel like he can handle almost anything, except puke on his hands. He doesn't like that at all.

After consulting with the doctor and nutritionist, Jennifer describes how they will introduce Bolus feedings, a method of feeding him through a syringe directly into his G-tube three times a day. This will create a more natural digestive rhythm. Fill the belly up, digest, stomach is empty, fill it up again. Not very appetizing, but it will prevent him from vomiting and should start to put the weight back on him. Relieved that we have a plan, I adjust Zack's pillow, patting his hand as I tell him he is going to be fine now. I try to sound more confident than I actually feel, but I don't want him to be scared.

At noon, we get an unexpected visit from Dr. Kraft, Director of the Spinal Cord and Brain Injury Program for Frazier Rehab. He had reviewed Zack's case file and wanted to know if I had any questions. Ironically, his son dates Lyndsey, a good friend of Zack's. They had been praying for him, and once they learned he was transferred to Frazier, Dr. Kraft agreed to check in on Zack. Just another instrumental person God placed in our path to guide us along the way. Instantly, I whip out my little notebook that is always in my back pocket, rattling off a list of questions as I flip through the pages. Taken aback, Dr. Kraft says he wasn't expecting me to be so thorough and suggests we take a walk down the hall, where we can talk privately. The staff watches curiously as he guides me into a small conference room and directs me to take a seat.

Dr. Kraft patiently describes in an overly simplistic way that when you have a brain injury, it's like a two-liter bottle of soda, getting shaken until there is nothing but fizz. The messages the brain needs to relay to various parts of the body—to the lungs to breathe, the arms to raise, the eyes to blink—have to make their way through all that fizz. He explains that as you recover from a traumatic injury, your brain develops new neuropathways around the damaged parts, which is why you have to learn to walk, talk, and do everything all over again. He also clarifies that "working memory" begins at Rancho level six. This is when Zack will have an awareness of time. Right now, at a level four, when someone walks into the room, no matter how many times he has seen them that day, to him it seems like the first time. He lives only in the moment. Dr. Kraft gets quiet for a moment and then leans in as if to tell me something really important that he doesn't want me to miss. He reveals that they know a lot about brain injuries, but only recently discovered why some people recover more completely than others.

He compares two 15-year-old, athletic, intelligent males, with the same part of the brain injured, yet they will recover differently. He describes how, in the last few years, they have discovered that the difference is the level and type of "family support". Patients who have a family member involved in their therapy are the greatest assets to recovery. Speed of recovery is not the issue. It doesn't matter how fast he is getting through a particular phase, but rather how "complete" his recovery is. Whether it takes six months or two years is irrelevant. What is important is complete recovery. Dr. Kraft sits back in his chair and looks at me intently. He cautions me that Zack will likely be left with some deficits, but then he puts that potential into perspective with a story. He tells me of a patient of his with a spinal cord injury and is a paraplegic. He says that although he is severely physically limited, he has written a book, goes on speaking engagements, enjoys dinner with friends, and travels. By contrast, he describes his neighbor, who has no physical limitations but comes home from work, sits in his garage, and drinks himself into a stupor every day. Dr. Kraft crosses his arms, leans back in his chair, and asks me "Who has the more fulfilling life, my patient who will never walk again or my *neighbor?"* He reveals that it is very unlikely to suffer such a traumatic injury to the brain and not be left with some deficits, but no matter what issues Zack may have to deal with, he can still have a fulfilling life. This wise, compassionate man smiles, checks his watch, and stands up to leave. I could have talked with him for hours, but was lucky to have his undivided attention for 20 minutes. As I walk back to the room and he hurries off in the other direction, I am reassured that Zack will recover knowing that he has mountains of family support.

When I return to the room, my demeanor has changed. I am reenergized as I wheel Zack to speech therapy, but he is not. Phenergan prevents vomiting, but it also makes you sleepy. We discuss how Zack's midline is improving, that he is keeping his head and eyes straight forward, but we get very little effort out of him. We give him a sip of water, which he accepts without even trying to hold the glass. We move to the gym and PT/OT is not much better, since he can hardly stay awake. His therapists stretch his leg muscles and show me some exercises I can do with him in his room. They agree that he has very little energy, so we are dismissed early, and we head back upstairs. Jennifer helps to get him in bed, where he sleeps until 6:00 p.m. When he wakes up, he is very relaxed, and I notice as he turns his head and eyes to the right. This is decisive progress, considering his right-side neglect.

When his friends arrive later, I remind them to talk with him as if he will answer. Tell him the latest gossip and assume that he is interested. They readily agree, babbling on about school preparations, and their passing recent driver's license tests. He looks at them intently, appearing to understand the conversation. As we approach the end of visiting hours, we get a delightful gift. Andrew, Taylor, Trey, and Allie are chattering away, when suddenly, we get the biggest smile…full teeth. We are exuberant, celebrating with high-fives. Several nurses hear the commotion and run into the room. I grab my camera to capture the remnants of his smile. God is so good. Knowing what a stressful day we experienced, he gave me what I have longed for…that beautiful, full smile. What a blessing! His friends are reluctant to leave, and I hear them continue to rejoice as they gallop down the hallway towards the elevator. Kendra pokes her head in the room to announce she will be in shortly to check on us. I move to the bed and gaze into my son's eyes, taking his hand. He curls his fingers around mine. Slowly, his lids get heavy, his lashes flutter, and he takes a deep breath. I smile and as if to remind myself, I whisper, "Take each day as it comes, and find God in the midst of all of it."

## First Wednesday

Arriving early this morning, I waltz into Zack's room to find him awake and relaxed, with his left arm up over his head. I approach his bed and tickle him under the arm. Not eliciting much of a response, I teasingly inquire if he likes it. Slowly, he shakes his head, glaring at me with an annoyed expression. Feeling chastised, I push my chair back and discover his bear on the floor. Holding it up, I ask him if he wants it, and he responds by nodding his head. He nods to several other questions, and it's like déjà vu, taking me back to conversations we had before the accident. Trying to be diligent parents, we were constantly asking, "Where are you going, who is going with you, and when will you be home?"

As a teenager exerting his independence, his answers were short and somewhat annoyed. Zack was an excellent student taking honors classes in a private, award-winning school. Most of his courses came easy for him and didn't require much time studying. An athlete focused on baseball, he also played football, basketball, and track. He was a handsome guy, especially popular with the ladies. Until our recent arguments over his curfew, he never really gave us reasons to be concerned. Then again, I may have been oblivious to what was really going on when he was out with his friends, but Scott had always been suspicious. I believed if

Zack was performing well in school and active in sports, he should be rewarded with more freedom during the summer.

Scott didn't trust him. He wanted to know where Zack was at all times and interrogated him when he came home. It frequently led to them yelling, with me trying to mediate the dispute. It would be peaceful for a few days, and then, Zack would push the curfew to its limit, and the battle would start all over again. Perhaps that's why we were both surprised when Zack came home well before curfew the night of his accident. I remember smiling smugly at Scott while I commended my good boy for coming home early. Boy, did he have me snookered. Zack knew he would only have to wait a few hours, ensuring we were asleep, before climbing out his basement bedroom window to sneak off with an 18-year-old troubled kid and three teenage girls.

Reflecting on that dreaded phone call, I remember it was difficult to believe what the officer was saying. How could my son be in an accident, when I felt certain he was asleep in bed? That was 26 days ago. Zack had a full head of hair, was 20 pounds heavier, and was not dependent on others to get him dressed. Those are the thoughts clouding up my mind as I bring his toiletries to the bed and begin to brush his teeth. He puts his hand over mine and slowly pulls away. There is a tinge of triumph in his eyes as he starts to brush his teeth by himself. He looks so scrawny at six feet and only 135 pounds, but I am pleased that he is attempting to do things for himself.

Dr. Mook comes in with his chart and reports his chest x-ray was clear of fluid, so they will schedule to remove his trach tomorrow. Jennifer helps get him dressed, and I wheel him down to the gym for our morning PT/OT therapy. After some initial exercises to stretch his muscles, Zack is sitting up on the edge of the elevated mat, supporting himself with his hands. He is very nosey and constantly tries to see what's going on outside of our curtained therapy area. Mary Beth distracts him with his baseball and comments that perhaps he wants to read what is written on it. He gently fingers the ball, turning it over in his hand to examine the writing. He loves this baseball. She reads out loud what is written on it: "Home run hit out of the park for you. I love you, your dad, Scott." Zack always has this ball with him, rolling it around between his fingers of his left hand. It was just the distraction we need to refocus his attention to our area of the gym.

Amy kneels behind him on the mat, reaching around to hold his chin, preventing him from turning his head to the left. Mary Beth stands in front of him with a plastic disk, raised at eye level to the right. Instructed to touch the disk, he begins to raise his left hand and is quickly corrected. "Use your right hand, Zack." Mary Beth pats his right hand and places his left hand on his knee. Amy nudges his elbow from behind, and Zack's right arm shakes as he tries to lift it. It is almost as if this arm is injured. His brow is furrowed as he grimaces and struggles to move his right arm. His shoulders slump, and he lets out a big sigh, "No." Mary Beth lowers the disk, and Amy rubs both arms and softly encourages him. Zack was a pitcher, and this right arm could throw a mean curveball before his brain injury. Frustrated with this exercise, he turns his attention back to his baseball lying on the mat. He swats it with his left hand, and it rolls across the floor. His eyes dart from me to the ball, as if willing me to retrieve it. I hand him the ball and comment to his therapist, "At least he didn't puke."

Back in our room, we get an unexpected visit from Yolanda, one of his nurses at University Hospital Neuro ICU. She is excited to see Zack in his own clothes, sitting up in his wheelchair, and she listens attentively as I report on the progress he has made in the first week at Frazier. She smiles sheepishly and says that Zack was the first patient she had ever visited after they left the hospital. Zack had made a big impact on her. She was uniquely touched by how God answered our prayers throughout Zack's recovery. Yolanda is now having conversations about faith and is sincerely interested in attending the Sunday night service at Southeast Christian Church. She would have never even known about this contemporary service, offered on her night off on the other side of town, had Zack not been her patient. God sure works in mysterious ways.

Donna arrives as we head to the gym for our afternoon session and decides to accompany us. Zack stands up in front of the mirror, assisted by Mary Beth and Amy on each side. He is so tall, and he eyes himself curiously, from head to toe, a quizzical look on his face. I ask them to explain the complications caused by his right-side neglect. Amy describes that the tone in his right arm is the result of his brain sending wrong messages of abnormal tone to his body. This causes contracture. In Zack's case, he holds his right arm near his shoulder because his brain tells him that is normal. Mary Beth made a brace that straightens his arm and stretches the muscle fibers that send the brain a message of correct position. She claims that, eventually, the brain and muscle will work together, and Zack will hold his arm correctly. They move Zack over to the mat and sit him on the edge of the elevated platform. He sits, totally unsupported, with his hands on the mat beside him. He sways slightly back and forth, shifting his weight. Suddenly, he stands up all by himself, fixes a wedgie, and sits back down. We are flabbergasted! Mary Beth laughs, "Sometimes, they just need their own, personal incentive." Apparently for Zack, it's a wedgie. She mentions that a soft neck brace would help him keep his head up, although he would still be able to ignore his right side. We have been using a hand towel wrapped around his neck to support his head, and he doesn't like it. When asked if he wants to remove the towel, he nods, but still keeps his head turned to the left, neglecting the world to the right. They ring a bell, trying to get his attention, but he ignores it. As we ponder our options, Donna gets a brilliant idea to use her cell phone. She makes it ring, and Zack immediately turns to take the phone and put it up to his ear. Teenagers... what else but a cell phone could capture his attention?

Feeling encouraged that we discovered a way to get Zack's attention, I'm considering all the gadgets we have at home that may be useful in therapy. I'm making a list of possibilities when Dr. Miller strides in to discuss Zack's progress. He has seen the notations from speech, PT, and OT in his chart. Then explains that he will not be officially moved to a four on the Cognitive Scale until he is consistent with his responses. Zack never wants to perform when the doctors are around. Of course, now my phone is charging, so we can't demonstrate his latest response. Dr. Miller listens, glancing down, and tapping his pen on the chart, but still confirms that he can't move him up on the scale until he is consistent. He agrees to attend therapy to confirm the reports. After he leaves, I tell Zack I don't think the good doctor was impressed. I ask him several questions, getting nods in response. I chuckle and shake my head, wondering why he doesn't answer Dr. Miller's questions.

Grandma Rita shuffles in, and I describe how his obsession with cell phones is paying off in therapy. Wanting a demonstration, she hands him her phone, and he is immediately in his own element. We call the phone, he flips it open, puts it to his ear and listens. When we say goodbye, he hangs up. We are amused as he goes through the menu and changes her ringtone. A large group of his friends arrive, and we have a cell phone party. They take turns calling him and sharing their phones until he has tried each one. For two-and-a-half hours, he is entertained with mobile devices. It is so heart-warming to see him act like a normal teenager. Watching from my corner of the room, I am bathed in gratitude. I silently lift up praises, thanking God for the creative people He has placed around us, seeking to find new ways to reach Zack. This is what "family support" looks like, and why it makes a difference in recovery. As visiting hours come to a close, I gather his friends in a circle to pray. I ask God to help us find the right method to teach Zack's brain where midline is, so we can welcome him into the world to his right. I remind them to worship the God who is carrying us when we are too weak to go on. I pray for God to keep whispering to Zack and to make him whole again. I close my eyes and imagine hundreds of cell phones ringing in heaven.

Several people occupy Zack's room when I arrive a little later than usual. Dr. Skolnick had removed his trach and was reviewing the stoma care procedures with our nurse. Dr. Mook and his resident were discussing changing his catheter, because there was blood in his urine. Apparently, he had been pulling on his catheter throughout the night and didn't sleep much after 3:00 a.m. Not a good way to start the morning. Dr. Mook ordered another CAT scan to check the hematoma beneath his head wound, with the intention of removing his stitches if the scan indicates there is no infection. Removing the stitches will alleviate some of the itching, and hopefully, keep him from scratching. Carla Herman, a nurse and friend of the family, was our first visitor, and she holds Zack's hand while Dr. Mook was explaining his decision process. Zack was watching Carla intently and suddenly winked at her. Very deliberately. It was delightful and amusing. Carla is a petite blonde, with an engaging smile, and was quite flattered that she had elicited a response that no one else had yet to see. Dr. Mook hurried off to his next patient, and Zack reluctantly released her hand in order to get dressed for morning therapy.

As I wheel him to the elevator on our way to the gym, I notice he doesn't seem quite right. It's odd to consider that I have a new benchmark for what "right" is with Zack now. I voice my concerns, and Mary Beth says that he is showing signs of "apraxia", a common side effect to brain injury. Amy explains that when given a command, you can see him trying very hard to oblige. He understands what you want him to do, but his brain just can't make his body do it. This is just another phase, in addition to right-side neglect, that we will have to work through in therapy. Zack sits on the edge of the mat, elevated on a platform, and he sways back and forth as they prepare him to stand. Abruptly, he projectile vomits all over both his therapists, as well as himself. I am spared, only because I was standing on the mat behind him. Amy ask him if his stomach hurts, and he nods. He looks nauseated, so they clean him up, and we head back to his room. As we ride up in the elevator, I keep hearing that bureaucrat from the insurance company reminding me that our clock is ticking, and I'm concerned that he just lost out on valuable therapy time. As an aide transfers Zack into his bed, I can tell from his expression he really doesn't feel well.

Now, I'm flooded with guilt for being more concerned with his therapy hours than his physical well-being. Dr. Miller is paged to our room and hearing of the projectile vomiting, orders the next Bolus feeding to be hung, letting gravity put it into his stomach, instead of injecting it. Zack has not had his stomach full for nearly a month, so he just can't ingest a lot of food right now. It's a catch-22, Dr. Miller explains; we need to increase his calories in order to get his strength up to participate fully in therapy, and the only way to do that is with volume. I nod my head in agreement, but stare at that bag they call food, thinking that Zack will have to consume gallons of it to feel full. My skinny boy needs pizza, fries, and those pasta-rich dishes they fed the football team before a game.

Zack recovers in bed until it's time to go to speech therapy. As we wheel our way to Kathy's office, we are delighted when Scott and Kyle meet us in the hall. Kyle is excited to present her big brother with a special surprise: key lime pie! Kathy told me to bring something in that Zack really likes, so we can work on his swallowing, and he loves key lime pie. Of course, he only gets tiny bites of filling, but it must have felt like a party of tangy goodness on his tongue. He is clearly enjoying this new sensation and is kind of making a mess, like when you feed a toddler baby food. Kathy gives him a hand mirror, and he can see pie filling on his lips. He studies his reflection and finally licks it off. We all clapped and licked our lips in unison. It sounds so simple, but the tongue coming out of the mouth, particularly to lick something off his lips, is a positive sign of recovery.

We are in high spirits as we head to PT/OT for the afternoon session. Mary Beth and Amy decide to try something different and see if Zack will use an answer board. They printed a question on a piece of paper with Yes and No printed separately on other pieces. They asked, "Is your name, Zack?" It took a little while, with him glancing back and forth, but he finally moved his hand to the "Yes" paper. They asked, "Is your dad taller than you?" and again, he gestures towards "Yes". Scott and Zack were very close in height before his accident, but with his recent growth spurt, I'm confident he could have honestly answered no. He tires of the game pretty quickly. He has the attention span of a two-year-old, except when it comes to cell phones. They proceed to the mat to stretch his muscles. He is in a seated position, his feet straight forward to stretch his hamstrings. Zack has an agonized look on his face and begins to cry. He is moaning loudly, and I think he might talk.

This was the first true sign that he was in any kind of physical pain during therapy. They move away from the stretching exercises to an activity that Zack seems to enjoy. With them supporting him on each side, they stand him up and squirt foam soap all over the mirror that covers one wall in our therapy area. They give him a washcloth and show him how to wipe the soap off the mirror. He catches on immediately. He cleans every speck of soap, even reaching far above his head, off of the left side, but entirely ignores the right side of the mirror. They write in the soap to his right and encourage him to remove their letters, but it is clear that world to the right just doesn't exist for him. We were so enamored with his efforts on the mirror, that it was 10 minutes before Amy mentions that he stood the entire time, with very little support.

Returning to his room, the nutritionist starts his Bolus on a two-hour slow feed, and they take him for his CAT scan. As I wait for him to return, I call Scott and tell him to thank Kyle for bringing the key lime pie. I talk with her for a while, and she asks a dozen questions, wanting to know what she can do next to help her brother. I hear Logan whining in the background, and Scott puts her on the phone. She is crying, and I finally understand that she wants to help her brother as she sobs, "But everyone ate all the key lime pie." She was heartbroken. I pacify her by suggesting she make a picture to hang in Zack's room. Logan has seen his wall at Frazier is covered with pictures, cards, and posters of his friends. They are always trying to outdo one another, creating artwork with photos of themselves with Zack. I promise Logan that her picture will be Zack's favorite, and we hang up just as they are wheeling Zack into the room.

The aide gets him settled back in bed, but I notice that he keeps trying to sit up. He seems very agitated and then begins vomiting. I call out for our nurse, and together, we change him into clean clothes while I express my frustration. When will we achieve the right rhythm of feeding, at a level that gives him enough calories, but not enough to make him puke? We had to turn away a few friends so he could get enough rest to participate in therapy tomorrow. I promise them their visit is appreciated, explain that he had a rough day, and beg them to come back again. As I tuck the covers around Zack, fussing over him like I did when he was a sick toddler, I see a card on the table that I hadn't noticed before. I sit in my chair next to his bed and open the envelope addressed to me from a coworker. A tender sentiment is printed inside, reminding me that we are part of a perfect plan designed by God, who loves us completely. We are in His thoughts every minute, and they are filled with a desire to bless us. I close the card, place my hands in my lap, and gaze at Zack as he's sleeping.

Reaching for my journal, I fill a whole page with one sentence as I write, "I can't wait for tomorrow to see how God will fulfill the promise in Romans 8:28—'And we know that in all things God works for the good of those who are called according to His purpose.'" This difficult journey has taught me that faith is willing to engage in the unknown. Faith doesn't mean the absence of fear, for I have plenty of that, but, rather, having the energy to go ahead, right alongside of the fear, knowing that we are not alone. I know God is always with us.

D eciding to spend the night at Frazier, being too sleepy to safely drive home, I am awakened at the crack of dawn. It takes me a while to shake the cobwebs from my mind and recognize Dr. Skolnick when he arrives to check on Zack. He reports that his stoma is healing nicely and should be completely closed up in a few days. That leaves one less potential site for infection. Before he has a chance to leave, Dr. Miller arrives to evaluate Zack's head wound. Deciding to wait until Monday to remove his stitches, he comments that it is only a precaution, the CAT scan results were positive. My attention is drawn to Zack. I notice that he is sitting up in bed, his foot on the floor like he's trying to get up. I glance at the clock and realize it's time to make our way to therapy. Dr. Miller helps transfer Zack to his chair, and we head down to the gym for PT/OT.

This morning, he is prompted to stand, holding onto a walker. He manages the walker really well, but still has difficulty holding his head up. I stand against the wall, scratching my head, wondering what his brain perceived so interesting on the floor to his left. When they sit him down on the mat, he starts to vomit. Mary Beth reaches for a towel just in time to avoid another clothing change. Amy looks thoughtfully at Zack and admits that he might just be dizzy.

It would not be uncommon for him to have some vision problems with the severity of his brain injury, and he could be seeing double. They express frustration and write in his chart that he needs to have his vision tested. We are all anxious for answers, since this nausea interferes with his therapy, and that's why we are here. Our gym time cut short, I wheel Zack to his room and put him back in bed to rest. Within 15 minutes, he is throwing up in bed. Shrieking for our nurse, I start grabbing towels to wipe puke off his chest. She responds, an aide following quickly behind her, and they take over cleaning up his bed. The nurse contacts Dr. Miller, and he orders Raglan, a motility agent that helps move food through the digestive system, hoping this will stop the vomiting. He had been holding off on the Raglan because one of the side effects is confusion— the last thing a person with a brain injury needs. He writes a new order, decreasing the amount of Bolus feedings during the day and increasing his tube feeds at night. Dr. Miller is looking for that perfect balance of the proper number of calories that his digestive system can handle. Zack gets his first dose of Raglan right before we head to speech therapy.

Zack is obviously peevish and does very little in speech therapy, except to rub his head. He gives signals like he has a headache, but won't respond when asked if his head hurts. Kathy is reluctant to give him anything to swallow, for fear he will throw up again, so we end our session. She pats Zack on the knee and comments that I should inform our nurse of his headache. We are glum as we head to the gym for afternoon PT/OT. I stop in the hallway, get on my knees to be at eye level and ask him if his head hurts. No response. I look at Zack with mixed feelings of compassion and anxiety. I had anticipated a good therapy day, since he was sick yesterday, and here he is sick again. Before we can get into the gym, Mary Beth approaches me and asks if I would sit this session out, so they can work with him in a private room with some sensory therapy.

Another blessing from God, since I was just thinking I couldn't handle watching another therapy session where he did nothing. I return to his room alone to wait, but my mind is racing as I review my little notebook, looking for answers. I have Dr. Miller paged to ask if Zack could have Tylenol for his headache. I'm still waiting for an answer when Mary Beth returns with Zack. She explains that he did very well, that they used a 12-inch kickball, and he made several baskets with it. He also caught the ball at least 10 times and used his right hand, which he has been neglecting. They introduced several smells, and he responded to lemon, even trying to bring it to his mouth. I smile at Zack and squeeze his hand, expressing satisfaction that he used his time well in sensory therapy. Mary Beth looks at Zack curiously, commenting that we need to have his vision evaluated, reminding me that it could be contributing to his nausea. I scribble another message in my notebook, and she promises her report will have the same notation.

While Zack is napping, we get another visit from Dr. Kraft, Director of the Brain Injury and Spinal Cord Injury Program at Frazier. I tell him that I still have a few questions, so we take a walk to the conference room down the hall and talk for nearly an hour. He is a brilliant man, and he appreciates my desire to learn as much as I can about brain injury. He patiently explains to me how neurons in the brain send messages, passed from one neuron to the next using chemicals. When an injury occurs, the brain experiences excitotoxicity; the neurons get excited and all start sending out messages at the same time, releasing so many chemicals at once, that they become toxic to the brain.

When an injury to the brain occurs, some of these neurons are damaged, some recover, and some do not. The human brain has 100 billion neurons. Some are specialized, designed to control a specific part of the body, like the leg, and some can do many different things. As you recover from a brain injury, the neurons that aren't specialized take over functions for the neurons that are damaged. Initial recovery takes about six months but continues for years, improving over time. As Dr. Kraft talks, I write furiously in my little notebook, trying to keep up with his lecture. He seems to be in his element, and I feel like a favorite pupil. Rubbing his chin thoughtfully, he continues to describe how the frontal lobe of the brain, which is responsible for reasoning and logic, is the last part of the brain to develop. It is not fully developed until about age 23, reasoning that teenagers with an underdeveloped frontal lobe don't always make good decisions.

I nod, thinking that Zack is the perfect example. Dr. Kraft finishes speaking, sits back in his chair and exhales sharply. He confesses that he way oversimplified the process, but reiterates that the brain is very complex, containing many neurons that can be trained to take over new tasks. He states that there are 5.3 million Americans with brain injuries and extensive research continues to find ways to enhance recovery. Then, he clarifies that brain injury is an inconvenience, but it doesn't have to be devastating. His tone softening, he says that we will never have the son back that we knew before the accident, but he will have depth as a teenager that you don't see in people much older.

"You don't have to accept limits on what he can do, but understand that it may be harder for him than most other people. This will make him stronger, with a deeper appreciation for life. We can be proud of the person he will become." Dr. Kraft smiles as I brush away a tear. He gives advice for the stage Zack is currently going through. He recommends a quieter environment, less visitors at a time. I cringe, realizing that the staff must have tattled on us with our constant flow of friends.

As if reading my thoughts, he agrees that his friends are a crucial part of his recovery, but too many conversations going on at one time could overstimulate him. He approves of their visits, but clarifies that they should talk directly to Zack about normal stuff; what's going on at school, who is dating who, that annoying dog down the street… gossip. We should talk to him honestly, tell him the good and the bad. He doesn't need to be told that he is "going to be fine", because he doesn't think anything is "not fine". He reminds me at this stage of recovery, time is irrelevant to him. To Zack, a minute is like a day, is like an hour. He doesn't need a cheerleader, but rather, someone to hold his hand and talk to him about ordinary, everyday events.

The support of his family and friends will contribute immensely to his recovery. Dr. Kraft checks his watch and stands up, signaling our conversation is over. I thank him profusely for his time and follow him out the door. I am energized to the point of skipping down the hall. I am not depressed about Zack throwing up or giving halfhearted effort in therapy. I am again blessed by God for sending just the right person to talk with me. I am eager to share what I have learned with Scott and the rest of our family and friends.

Ironically, many of Zack's friends come to visit this evening, content to spend their Friday night with him. Aware that summer offers them many other activities, I am humbled by their devotion. I explain my conversation with Dr. Kraft and ask them not to have side bar chats that could be distracting. I notice that Zack is more alert than at any other time today. He is engaged, looking to the right with very little tone in his right arm. He seems very relaxed, content, with a grin just beneath the surface. He glances around the room and then winks at Brittney Garr, reminding us that he still has the lady's attention.

If you look past the helmet, you see a teenager with a cell phone. He is a person who just happens to have a brain injury, that one day soon will amaze us all. I blend into the wall, just watching as his friends catch him up on their latest shenanigans. My mind wanders back to the conference room and Dr. Kraft's prediction. Zack will face challenges, but eventually, he will overcome them and be stronger than before. He will come through the fire with the knowledge that he was never alone. I close my eyes and whisper to myself. I believe that when his friends are gone and I leave to go home, there is one who never leaves him. He is held in the palm of God's hand while the healing continues.

When I arrive this morning, I walk into the room to find both Dr. Mook and Dr. Miller reviewing Zack's chart. They involve me in discussions about his vomiting, admitting their concern led them to order a portable stomach x-ray. This will confirm their suspicion that he is impacted and justify why the Bolus feedings haven't been working. Both feel confident that if we eliminate the impaction and adjust the Bolus feedings, he won't continue vomiting. Once they conclude that he can move the food through his digestive system, they will cut back on the Raglan, and that should help alleviate some of his confusion.

After the x-ray, it only took a few hours to recognize that they finally had it figured out. Zack was started on medication and seemed to be a different guy. I'm encouraged as we move to speech therapy. Kathy starts off by asking if he wants ice, and he immediately nods his head. He takes the cup, turning it up to allow the ice to fall in his mouth, chews, and swallows quickly. Kathy smiles and notes it in his chart. He nods a quick response to nearly all of her questions. Returning to our floor, we are greeted by an aide who takes him to be weighed. I'm not surprised to learn he has dropped weight again, down to 133 pounds, considering he has thrown up every meal in the last few days.

Back in his room, we find Scott's brother, Tony, and his wife, Jill, waiting for us. They had not seen Zack since his transfer to Frazier and were amazed at how he had progressed. Zack remains in his wheelchair, alert for their entire visit. When it's time to go to the gym, I ask him if he wants to brush his teeth. He replies, "Yes." It's barely a whisper, but still uplifting that he's talking again. They walk with us to the elevator, and I ask Zack to push the button for me. This is a new command. Without looking up, he pushes the down button. Do you remember how excited your toddler was when you got on an elevator and they pushed every button? That is how I felt when I saw Zack respond to my request so naturally. Tony and Jill exit the elevator at the lobby level, and we continue down to the gym.

It's Saturday, so we are met by the weekend therapists, Kristi (PT) and Angela (OT). Starting out in a sitting position on the side of the platform, they coax him to stand, and he rises with only light support on each side. Kristi asks him to sit down, and he complies. I notice that he has improved, holding his head up at midline. Angela shows me the neck collar that had been ordered, but decides to wait until Monday to try it out. The weekend therapy staff are agreeable and competent, but it's not like having Mary Beth and Amy. They have seen Zack every day since his arrival at Frazier and have a vested interest in each of his accomplishments.

Once we complete therapy and Zack is revived with a short nap, an aide comes to give him a bath. She prepares his toothbrush and hands it to him, and he brushes his teeth on his own. This is what I need his doctors to witness, so he can be moved up on the cognitive scale to show progress for the insurance company. In clean clothes, he returns to bed for his evening meal of Bolus. At times, he seems in pain, grimacing and leaning forward in his bed. I ask him if his belly hurts, and he nods. It is confounding that you can injure your heart, lungs, or any other organ and deal with pain and limitations, but when you injure your brain, it affects everything.

Our evening is full of visits from friends and family. At one point, with Scott and several of his friends in the room, Zack decides to stick his finger in his nose. Scott corrects him, telling him not to pick his nose and finally swipes his hand away. Zack just looks at him and smiles cockily. He slowly creeps his left hand up the front of Scott's golf shirt, and then, buttons it up to the collar. Quite impressive, since it was done entirely with his left hand.

The nurse announces that visiting hours are over, so his friends say goodbye, and Zack lays back in bed. He squirms from side to side, grimacing and seeming to be in a lot of pain in his belly. I dim the lights, and Scott stays, trying to comfort Zack. He holds his hand and reaches for mine as he softly begins to pray. He proclaims that things will be better tomorrow, and if not tomorrow, the next day. He reminds us that God has faithfully taken care of all the little things to prepare us for the challenges ahead. He asks out loud for God to help with this belly pain, and I peek at Zack. His eyes are closed, and he lays very still, as if contemplating every word. Scott is getting choked up, so I intervene, continuing to pray for all of Zack's friends, that they will worship God with a deeper appreciation of the many blessings He has given them. I promise that we will continue to shout for joy, because we know that our God can do more than we could ever hope or imagine. Zack's breathing is steady, and I realize he has fallen asleep. Scott continues holding my hand and pulls me towards the door. He whispers that God will take care of Zack tonight and convinces me I need to go home with him to be with the rest of my family.

It's just starting to get dark when we arrive home. Dylan and the girls are excited to see me and cover me with hugs. Morgan says her parents are sitting on their deck and invites us over to update everyone on Zack's progress. We are fortunate to have great neighbors. The Getzes have helped Scott keep up with the laundry, chauffeur the girls, and comfort him when I've not been around. They are eager to hear about Zack, but the more stories we tell, the more emotional Scott becomes. Suddenly, he stands up and announces that he's going back to Frazier to spend the night. He feels like he needs to be there for Zack.

Scott slips into Frazier after midnight, and the halls are dark. He hears moaning and what sounds like throaty cries. When he gets closer to his room, he realizes that it's Zack. He is awake, sitting up in bed, weeping. Scott crawls in bed, cradling him, and gently asks, "What's wrong, buddy?" Zack murmurs something about a dream. Scott hugs him, trying to comfort him, and asks about the dream. Zack looks him straight in the eyes and declares, "I met God."

After our earlier prayers, hearing this come out of Zack's mouth is overwhelming. Tears begin to flow down Scott's face, and he hugs him, finally asking, "You mean you dreamt you met God?" Zack shakes his head slowly back and forth, then confidently replies, "I met God." He becomes quiet, and they lay together in his bed. Tears continue to flow silently from Scott's eyes, but Zack is no longer crying. He is peaceful and resonant. It seems he just needed to tell someone, and God knew Scott needed to hear it.

Zack mumbles something and touches Scott's face, tracing a tear down his cheek. Neither of them speaks. Zack having nothing further to say, and Scott not wanting to break the spell of the moment with words. He dozes off and is awakened by Zack sitting up, putting his feet on the floor and trying to get out of bed. He would coax him to lay down, but before long, he would try again to get out of bed. Finally, Scott moved to the chair next to the bed and called for the nurse. It was 4:30 a.m., and he was afraid that he would fall asleep and Zack would try to get out of bed. She reviews his chart and realizes that Zack had not been given any Trazodone, which had been ordered in case of restlessness to help him sleep. She gives him a dose through his IV, and he finally falls asleep. Content that Zack won't attempt to get up, Scott makes himself as comfortable as possible and dozes in the chair.

# Week Two, Sunday

It's 8 am., and the rest of the floor is busy preparing for morning rounds. Scott is groggy, with a stiff back from dozing in the chair. He recognizes he could use some real sleep, and he drags himself to the elevator, just in time for the doors to open and his mother, Rita, step out. She agreed to relieve Scott and stay with Zack, so I could go to church with the rest of the family. When Zack wakes up, Rita has a difficult time keeping him from scratching his head wound. She holds his hand, but gets distracted and finds him tearing at his bandage. Nurse Jennifer decides a hand mitt might be the best way to get him to leave it alone. Just before lunch, Mary Beth sneaks in to check on Zack, even though it is her day off. She explains to Rita that she's always thinking of ways to bring the best out of Zack. While they talk, she engages him with bedside stretches and demonstrates how a towel should be rolled up and placed under his pillow on the left side, in order to force him to face midline. Rita complains that he looks uncomfortable, but Mary Beth assures her that this is good therapy, that every recommendation has a purpose.

After she leaves, Zack is restless and constantly tries to get out of bed. He is frustrated, mumbling incoherently, with tears in his eyes. Rita paces the room, obviously upset to see her first-born grandson in distress, and frantically calls out for Jennifer. In an attempt to determine what Zack wants, she asks him several questions, but gets no response. Jennifer glances beyond Rita, to the sunshine dancing on the window, and asks if he wants to go outside. Zack follows her eyes, nods his head, and mouths "yes".

Imagine my surprise when I arrive to find Zack dressed and Rita smiling as she guides his wheelchair around the front entrance. It is good for my soul to see him outside, barefoot and waiting for us to arrive after church. Dylan and the girls are delighted to see their brother lounging in the sunshine like a normal teenager, except for the wheelchair and helmet. The girls skip around his chair, and Dylan keeps asking for high-fives, not discouraged at all when Zack seems to ignore him. Our little group makes quite an impact on the other visitors as we gleefully enter the lobby, Kyle stroking Zack's arm and asking if he wants anything.

In the elevator, Logan is reluctant to let go of my hand, but she also wants attention from Grandma and whines that Kyle won't let her assist Zack. I'm preoccupied with trying to circumvent another argument when we lumber into our stuffy room. An aide files in, to report that the air conditioner was out of commission in several rooms, including ours. On a hot, August day in Kentucky, you don't want to be without air conditioning. It was even hotter for Zack in his helmet. Sweat runs down beside his ears, and he squirms uncomfortably in his chair. Sending Dylan, Kyle, and Logan down the hall to wait in the conference room, Rita gets a cold washcloth to wipe off Zack's forehead when I remove his helmet.

Within five minutes, Kyle races back into the room, announcing that Dylan broke something, and water was spewing everywhere. Apparently, the emergency eye wash station piqued his interest, and ignoring the signs, he activated it and caused it to start flooding the hallway. He was hiding in the conference room as an aide called for maintenance to shut off the valve. God bless him. Our decision early on to limit Dylan's visits was justified. A hospital is just no place for a curious 12-year-old boy with lots of energy. Kyle was indignant that she was going to have to leave now because of the mess Dylan had created, but Rita pacifies them with promises of ice cream.

Sunday afternoons always brings lots of visitors, and the staff is sending them to the conference room to wait. Our room is unbearably hot. The maintenance man was occupied with mopping up the hallway and resetting the eyewash station. It could be several hours before the temperature was tolerable, so Jennifer suggests we take Zack to the conference room in his wheelchair. We are greeted by a dozen of his friends, and Zack is content fiddling with their cell phones. We discover a deck of cards, and I demonstrate how to shuffle. Passing the deck to Zack, he flips one card over at a time, arranging them in random, meaningless stacks. His attention is diverted to the door when Cassie, one of the therapy dogs, comes to visit.

Zack has grown up with dogs, and although he is willing to pet Cassie, he definitely did not like her licking his hand. I notice he becomes more agitated as the chatter starts to drift into multiple conversations. I remember Dr. Kraft's instruction and want to avoid over-stimulation. Commenting that he looks tired and needs to rest, I send Andrew to check on the airflow in his room. He agrees that it was cooling off, so we walk our guest to the elevator and say goodbye. Jennifer eases Zack into bed, and I comment that I'm much more perceptive of when he gets frenetic. This leads to a conversation revolving around the importance of family support, but also recognizing the fragile state of Zack's neurological disorder. Just like finding the perfect balance of nutrition, we must consider his disposition during visits.

Revived after an hour nap, he welcomes a group of all female classmates and appreciates their undivided attention. His friend, Allie, is messing around with his bear. Holding it up to his face, she tells him to kiss the bear. He smiles coyly. She presents the bear and giggles, "Kiss me." Abruptly, he laughs out loud! A genuine, belly-hugging laugh. We were stunned and excited. I grabbed the camera to capture the replay as she continues to make him laugh. Memories flash across my mind of my baby and how content I was as a new mother to capture each expression. Now, I create a new album as Zack comes back to life with laughter. These are the blessed moments I cherish in the midst of chaos.

Just before shift change, we get an unexpected visit from Stephanie, one of our favorite ICU nurses at University Hospital. She had a special connection with Zack, tenderly caring for him throughout the night in my absences. I was so humbled that she hadn't forgotten her favorite patient, taking time to stop by on her way to the hospital. She is amazed with the progress he has made in only 12 days since leaving ICU. I describe the laugh he gave us earlier and the words he has spoken. We have come a long way from demanding a thumbs up. I thank her for the role she played during our most desperate times on 5West. She left encouraged, excited to report back to our ICU family that Zack is on the road to recovery.

It was after visiting hours when Rick Thompson, a friend of Zack's and recent Christian Academy graduate, sneaks into our room. Rick is good for Zack, talking with him like he always has, joking around. Zack is engaged, and before long, he has his baseball glove on, transferring the ball back and forth into his right hand. I scribble in my notebook, reminding myself to tell his therapist that we are making headway with his right-side neglect. Rick is very animated, going to great lengths to entertain Zack, and at one point, unbraids his hair into a big afro. Zack studies him, leans back in his chair and says, "Right on," with a big grin. His face beams as Rick and I double over with laughter. The ruckus blows our cover, and a nurse invades our room to announce Zack needs to return to bed to start his tube feeding. Rick bids goodbye and closes the doors, and we begin our nightly ritual.

It is quiet when I look up and see the door slowly creak open and see Linda. This is the angelic lady who worked the patient information desk at University Hospital, with the warm smile and contagious love of the Lord. The day of Zack's accident, Scott had taken a walk and ended up in the lobby. Distraught and emotional as he stood at the elevator, he turned to this woman he had never met and confessed, "My son is in critical condition in ICU." He quickly apologizes for his outburst, admitting he didn't even know why he said it. Linda confidently said she knew why. Zack needed prayer, and she was our direct line to God. She prayed with Scott that night, right there in the lobby of University Hospital, and reminded him that God says if we ask anything in His name, believing it and not doubting, we will receive it. She prayed, Scott believed, and she has been praying for Zack every day since.

He had not seen her since that first night, even after searching in an attempt to make introductions. Apparently, after our ICU nurses reported on Zack's progress, she made the connection and sought us out at Frazier Rehab. She tells me that it is no coincidence that we finally met on the Lord's Day to praise God for answered prayers. Linda holds my hand and extends her arm over Zack's bed, thanking God for His healing. She hugs me, whispers that God is in control, and disappears down the hall.

Gently closing the door, I allow a sliver of light to enter our room and sit next to the bed. Zack's breathing is steady, and I slowly trace my finger along his arm until I reach his hand. I consider all the people committed to praying for Zack and recognize that we experience the healing power of prayer every day, firsthand. Even those days when it seems that Zack makes no progress, we can feel God's reaching out to us. When we fondly reminisce about the plans we had for him, we are reminded of our mission.

For years, we professed it didn't matter if our children made lots of money, were successful, or were powerful; it didn't matter who they became when they grew up. It would be irrelevant if they didn't trust Jesus as their Lord and Savior. If they possessed all the world had to offer, but did not have faith, they would have nothing at all. Sitting here in the dark, I feel this more than ever. I close my eyes as the tears begin to form. I pray that through his recovery, God creates in Zack an unshakable faith.

Wen I arrive this morning, I find Zack in his wheelchair in the hallway near the nurses' station with Dr. Miller. I am surprised to see him up so early, and our aide Shirley explains that she found him standing next to his bed. Concerned for his safety, she puts him in his chair by the nurse's station, where they can keep their eye on him. This will be the next challenge, since it is dangerous for Zack to be without his helmet, nor should he stand unassisted. Shirley said she noticed him rubbing his leg with tears in his eyes and asks him if his leg hurt. At first, he had no reply, so she asked again, "Does your leg hurt, or are you just unhappy?" Despondent, he answers, "Unhappy." As she describes this conversation, my heart breaks. I kneel down and take Zack's hand. Our eyes meet, and I ask, "You okay, buddy?" A blank expression and no response. Frustrated that I can't decipher what he needs, I wheel him back to our room in search for answers.

Zack is soaking up the sun streaming through our window when Dr. Mook, Dr. Miller, and their intern, Heidi, arrive to remove the stitches in his head wound. He is sitting in his wheelchair as they disinfect the area and examine his head. They offer no pain medication, and I hold his hand, reminiscent of our bedside procedures in ICU. He moans as they dig for stitches in his newly grown hair. Before long, both of us are crying, our heads bent together in solidarity. I glance up to see tears slipping out the corners of Heidi's eyes.

When that ordeal is over, they bring in a new bed. This enclosure has a mesh tent, which zips up on all four sides, to restrain him during the night. It is less restrictive than arm restraints, but should prevent him from getting out of bed on his own. While we are preparing to go to the gym, Amy checks in to see our new enclosure. I am explaining that Zack kept trying to get out of bed, when I notice he has become visibly upset, tears spilling from his eyes. I ask him what's wrong, and glancing at Amy he replies, "No story." Surprised that he was paying attention to our conversation, we discuss his state of mind with more sensitivity. Amy explains that this is part of Phase Four...coming into his emotions. He may cry and not know why. Unfortunately, we can also expect him to show signs of frustration and depression.

As she walks with us to the gym, Amy informs me that Mary Beth has the day off, so Debbie will be assisting with occupational therapy. Just as we reach the elevator, the door slides open, and Scott steps out. He notices a difference in Zack's demeanor and decides to accompany us to therapy. Debbie is waiting for us when we reach the gym. After a brief introduction, they take Zack to the mat to stretch the muscles that haven't been used in a while. He tolerates this well, so they sit him up and introduce a small ball. Positioning it at eye level, they instruct him to grab it. He tries, his arm shaking as he attempts to reach up. He knows what to do, but can't make his body do it. Frustration overtakes him, and he starts to cry. Scott hasn't seen him struggle this way, and he cringes. His hands grip the side of his chair, as if to prevent himself from leaping out to grab the ball himself. Recognizing that Zack's emotions are getting the best of him, Amy discards the ball and helps him to a standing position. Seizing the opportunity and unable to stop himself, Scott comes forward and asks for a hug. Zack puts his left arm around him and pats his back, while Scott chokes back tears. It is an impassioned scene and clearly demonstrates how badly Scott wants his son back.

As Scott leaves for work, Debbie tells us that Zack showing empathy for his dad is a positive sign. I walk Scott to the elevator. He punches the button and turns back to watch Zack. When he finally speaks, he mutters, "I can't…" before his voice trails off into nothingness. He doesn't need to finish the sentence. His eyes reflect the pain that his voice can't bear to admit. I hug him, gently nudging him into the elevator, and promise that Zack is improving every day.

When we returned to our room, nurse Jennifer strides in with his new neck brace. She adjusts the Velcro closures to get the right fit. It works well at keeping his head up, but Zack hates it. He already has to deal with the sweaty helmet, and now, they want him to wear this hot thing around his neck. It looks like torture. Jennifer tosses me a knowing look, and as if reading my mind, removes both the neck brace and his helmet. Jennifer smiles and says, "Let's go camping." She transfers him to the bed and zips it up for a short nap before speech therapy. When it's time to go to downstairs, I intentionally leave the neck brace in our room. Once in Kathy's office, Zack eats ice and drinks water from a cup with no problem. She brings out some lemon ice to try, which he eagerly devours. Pleased with his efforts, she announces that he is scheduled for a swallow test this Wednesday. She explains that in a controlled environment, he will be given food and liquid to swallow while they x-ray him, ensuring it's going down the right way. If he passes the swallow test, we will be able to give him certain things to eat by mouth in very small bites. Kathy is anxious to get this eating thing out of the way, so she can start working with him on speaking. Right now, he speaks only when he wants to and not very often. We need him to start consistently answering questions and expressing himself verbally.

In our afternoon PT/OT session, he is taken to a private room, where there are less distractions. I'm asked to wait in the gym, which leaves me feeling a bit dismissed. While I wait, I watch the other patients manage stairs and balance on large balls. I recognize that they are much further along in recovery and wonder how long they have been here. I glance at the clock, mentally reminding myself that our insurance will only allow 60 days of acute rehab therapy, and we are already on day 11. I close my eyes and recall his condition when we arrived. He couldn't stand or even hold his head up. He didn't talk, smile, laugh, or cry. He couldn't throw a ball or hug his dad. I know that Zack has made great strides in a short time; I just hope we see exponential progress moving forward. I'm still lost in my thoughts when Amy wheels Zack back into the gym. He is holding a balloon in his lap, pinching it between his fingers. She explains that they were hitting it back and forth to him, but he was far more interested in the annoying sound it made when he rubbed his hand across it. I smile, flashing back to last Easter. I remember my kids playing with balloons, and Scott threatening to pop them if they didn't stop with the maddening noise. Some things never change.

Rick Thompson from Christian Academy is waiting for us in our room when we return. He is intent on playing ball, and they toss it around for several minutes. When Zack seems to lose interest, Rick asks if he can take him for a walk in his wheelchair, and I welcome the opportunity to return phone calls. I can hear his animated voice as Rick describes who might be in each room that they wheel past. They run into Scott in the hall on his way to our room, and he asks Zack to wink at him. BAM! Without hesitation, he winks. Scott is excited when he bounds into the room to announce this new trick Zack has mastered. He is in a much better frame of mind than when he had left the gym this morning. We are showing Zack pictures of his friends, pointing out and naming each one from the posters they made, when a new therapist, Elizabeth, knocks on our door. She introduces herself and explains that Zack will start art therapy tomorrow. They plan on working it into his evenings twice a week for 30 to 45 minutes. Art enables people with a brain injury to express themselves in different ways. They talk about being angry, frustrated, confused, and sad, and this can be expressed on paper. I am curious to see how Zack will respond. Scott comments that he has to leave to pick up the girls and watch Dylan's football practice. He asks Zack for a kiss goodbye, and he complies. We stand him up and Scott gets another hug and pat on the back. Intuitively, Zack is comforting him. That is just what Scott needs right now.

After several other visitors and a long nap, Zack appears restless when he wakes up. Scott's mom attempts to pacify him with his baseball, but he is not interested. Deciding another walk might be a good idea, Rita quickly volunteers. She strides off down the hall, but returns only a minute later. Zack had started crying, and she couldn't figure out what was wrong, so she brought him back to me. I assure Rita it was nothing that she did and explain the ramifications of this new emotional stage. We are beginning to realize what a long, grueling process lies ahead. As he recovers, we will experience things that won't be pleasant. There will be times when visitors won't be a good idea, and we will have to limit them. The only consolation is that these phases are temporary. As Rita prepares to leave, we notice that Zack is watching the Monday night football game on TV. It's comforting. He seems very much like the teenager we knew, ignoring us while the game was on.

When it is time for him to return to his bed, I stand him up and notice how much taller he is, towering over me. He hugs me and gently rubs my arm as I help him into bed. I am struck by his tenderness and whisper a prayer that God will grant us as many unexpected smiles as tears. I remember the hug he gave his dad in the gym and pray strength for Scott as he contemplates a future that is so uncertain. Zack's breathing is steady, and I realize he has already fallen asleep. I move to my chair, open the laptop, and hope to respond to some messages. I read an anonymous note on the blog that starts,

> I'm Kristy, and I was one of the people who was in the waiting room the day of Zack's surgery. I walked in that waiting room that day, and I happened to be standing nearby and overheard everything (not trying to be nosy), and I started to cry. I had no idea who he was, nor did I know anything about your family, but my heart ached for you all, and I just started to pray. I am so relieved to hear about how much he has progressed. What an awesome God we have. I'm just so amazed at all of God's power and know he has a wonderful future in store for your son. Zack has already blessed so many people, and he doesn't even know it, yet."

Silent tears slide down my face as I slowly close my laptop. I decide to ride home with that message ringing in my ears. I kiss Zack goodnight on his cheek and walk my familiar path to the parking garage. Pulling out into the darkness, I feel God's presence as I drive home in silence, pondering what future He has planned for Zack.

Zack is at his new morning position, parked by the nurses' station in his wheelchair when I arrive. Aide Shirley commands him to hold his head up, and he doesn't dare disobey, or she will put that awful neck brace on him. Shirley has a way with Zack, and he always seems to listen to her. She has a commanding presence, and I wouldn't want to cross her either. I wheel Zack to our room and decide to let him try my laptop. Pushing him up to the table, I show him how to place his fingers on the keys. He is focused on the screen and slowly punches the keyboard. It only takes him a minute to become agitated when he can't make his fingers do what he wants. I divert his attention to my phone and explain that I need to call home and check on the kids. Once he hears me talking, he holds out his hand and whispers my instructions to Dylan, "Stay out of trouble." As we are hanging up, I hear Dylan shouting to the girls that he talked to Zack. His gaze turns to the windowsill, where I have placed his ball. "Want to play baseball?" I put his glove on his left hand and give him the ball, moving back about six feet. He fingers the ball with his right hand and throws it perfectly. Baseball is the key to getting him to use his right arm. I am aware that Zack is sitting up straighter and holding his head up. His frustration over the keyboard seems forgotten, and we toss the ball around until the clock signals it's time to go to therapy.

As we move to the gym for our morning session, I stop at the elevator, and Zack pushes the down button with no prompting. We slide into the elevator, and I bend down to eye level, announcing, "This is going to be a good day, Zack." When we enter the gym, Amy grins and invites me to attend this session with them. She shows Zack how to move his feet while holding onto his wheelchair and walks himself into the private therapy room. With less distractions, she takes a different approach to therapy. Propping her foot on Zack's chair, she waits for his reaction. He unties her shoe, but gets frustrated when he can't tie it back. She quickly diverts him to a puzzle, and he manages the different shapes easily. I watch his face as he doodles with a pen and paper. He shows little emotion, but his eyes are captivated as he slashes colors across the page. When he is satisfied with his artwork, he pushes the paper towards Amy and quizzically raises his eyebrows, looking for affirmation.

I sit quietly in the corner, not wanting my invitation rescinded for interfering, but desperately wanting to praise his efforts. Amy asks him to stand up, and she retrieves the balloon that was hidden out of sight. She throws the balloon, intentionally with an awkward punch towards his right side. He catches the balloon while standing up using his right hand. He runs his thumb across the latex and looks coyly at Amy, as if challenging himself to pluck an irritating tune from this balloon. He hits it back to her, and she instantly directs it to me. Now, the three of us hit it back and forth, forcing Zack to use his right hand when it comes from my direction. With our game complete, Amy leans back in her chair, and Zack imitates her position, casually leaning on his elbows. The tone in his right arm is almost undetectable as he high-fives Amy on our way out. It was a great session.

There is a big grin plastered across my face as we float back to our room. Purposely pointing at the clock, my fingers formed into a gun, I shoot it and announce, "No problem." I feel confident that if Zack continues progressing at this rate, acute rehab hours won't run out, as predicted. Kneeling to remove Zack's sneakers, I glance up to find him gazing out the window to his right. Therapy is making definitive gains on his right-side neglect. After a short nap, we head to speech therapy with Kathy. She moves him up to a table, slides a piece of paper his direction, and hands him a pencil. I watch as he takes it with his left hand. She asks him to draw a circle. He draws a complete circle with his left hand. His brow is furrowed, and he stares at his hands before switching the pencil to his right hand. He tries to write with his right hand, but just scribbles and drops the pencil. Noticing the sweat trickling down his forehead, I comment how stuffy her office feels, and Kathy agrees to remove his helmet. She hands me a small towel, and before I can respond, Zack plucks it from my hands and wipes his forehead. Kathy brings out a single serving cup of applesauce and hands him a spoon. He reaches for the cup, and after initially pulling away, Kathy presents it to him. Politely, she reminds him to eat slowly. Zack eats an entire serving of applesauce pretty much by himself.

I was in a great mood heading down to the gym for our afternoon PT/OT. Mary Beth immediately starts to work with him, putting bolts through holes and screwing the nuts on them. He uses both hands. They decide to try him on an aerobic step to see if he can take a step up. He does it with no problem. Amy asks Mary Beth if she wants to try walking. They tell Zack if he holds his head up, they will let him walk. With one on each side of him, holding his hands, he is off.

My heart is singing as I watch him walk, three times all the way around the basement area, not just the gym. With laser focus, Zack keeps his head up, and for the most part, looks straight ahead. When his concentration drifts left, they let him collide with the furniture, so he understands what happens if he is not watching where he is going. Requiring his attention to avoid collisions also reinforces that his midline is straight. He walks like a man on a mission, and we are all giddy with excitement. This is definitely a Kodak moment, but I don't have my camera, and my vision would be clouded by the tears of joy, which are now inching their way down my face. His gait is decent, except that he slightly drags his right toe at times. They let him walk up three steps and down again, commenting on his stable balance.

They guide him to the model bus used to teach patients how to adjust to different heights of stairs and to use handrails. There is a bench that vibrates to simulate a real bus. Zack explores the bus, easily managing the stairs and properly using the handrail as instructed. He walks to the back of the bus and sits on the bench. Mary Beth activates the seat, and when it starts vibrating, he smiles, then laughs until tears stream down his face. He reminds me of a baby seated on a running washing machine for the first time. His laughter is contagious, and we all join in until Mary Beth flips the switch off. Zack slowly exits the bus, as if not wanting to leave an old friend behind. He strides confidently, holding their hands, as they direct him to his wheelchair. Amy pats him on the back, commending him on his efforts. As I wheel him towards the elevator, Mary Beth and Amy smile fondly and wave. For the first time, Zack waves back.

I was itching to get back to our room and call Scott. Our nurse, Dana, is in the hallway outside of our room, and I enthusiastically relay our progress in therapy. Zack pulls his wheelchair behind the nurses' station. He is very interested in Emily— a young, pretty aide—who is busy inputting data into the computer. He kept pulling his chair up next to her and was practically pushing Dana out of the way. He is obviously flirting with Emily, and we laugh as he tries getting as close as possible.

"Alright, lover boy," I tease, "time to go to your room." Dana reminds me that we have art therapy, and we make our way down the hall to the conference room. There are a few other patients spread out at the long table. Our therapist offers him colored markers to draw on his choice of construction paper. He selects a red marker and red paper. He draws a circle, not quite round, and puts the marker down. Picking up a green marker, he scribbles inside the circle, filling it in. He continues for a few minutes, drawing various random shapes, filling some in with other colors. When he starts nervously bouncing his left leg, I recognize that art therapy is over for today. We take his Picasso and proudly hang it in his room.

It's early evening when Scott arrives with Kyle, Logan, Rita, and our neighbors. Zack is practicing his newly acquired ability and rolling around in his wheelchair. Somehow, shuffling between Scott and I, he rolls over my toe. I am wearing flipflops, so I holler and jump up, holding my foot. Zack looks at me and grins, then he breaks out into a full belly laugh. My toe still throbbing, I can't help but smile, rejoicing in this side of his newfound emotions.

Kyle keeps us amused with her antics as she tries to make him laugh. Logan, however, still appears a bit afraid of Zack and shrinks away from him. She is not used to her brother being in a wheelchair, nor seeing him so emotional. I toss her a nerf ball and tell her to play catch with him, and that seems to put them back on familiar footing. After hearing me describe our afternoon gym session, Scott decides that he has to see Zack walk. He pleads with Dana until she agrees, returning with a canvas gait belt. She secures it around his waist, demonstrates how to support him and allows us to take him once around the corridor. Scott is animated, hardly able to contain his excitement over Zack walking. After we return to the room, we have to fight off protests from Kyle wanting to take her brother for a walk. Scott announces it's time to pick Dylan up from football, so they reluctantly say their goodbyes, and he hugs Zack before walking out the door. Ten minutes later, my phone rings. Scott is choked up and, between sobs, tells me how blessed he feels to be walking beside his son again.

It is late, after visiting hours, when two of Zack's classmates manage to slip into our room. Dale and Addison present a football signed by the entire team and a Christian Academy football jersey. Zack holds the football and looks at all the signatures. He makes sure the laces are turned just right and cradles it like a running back. Holding it over his head like he's going to throw it, he poses for pictures with his friends. Zack inches his way towards the door in an attempt to get out of his room, so Dale and Addison take him for a ride through the hall in his wheelchair. They return, with Dana following close behind, throwing me a chastised look. Addison reveals that Zack threw him the football using his right hand. I comment that all he needs is the right incentive; his friends and balls, he remembers throwing, and of course, pretty girls. I wink at Dana and point towards the nurses' station. She smiles, but rustles the boys towards the door, explaining that visiting hours are over. Zack gives high-fives to them as they leave, and it's apparent that he doesn't quite want to let go of their hands.

He's tired, and Dana prepares him for bed, zipping him up before she leaves. Zack seems to fall asleep immediately, and for the first time, I can hear him snoring. It is like music to my ears. I have a peace that radiates from my soul and feel honored to take part in God's perfect plan. A few days ago, someone posted a message about how quickly our teenagers grow up, and in a weird way, we are lucky to have Zack growing up before our eyes, like a baby, one more time. They remind me to cherish these moments, and that's exactly what I am doing tonight.

With Zack snoring softly in the background, I silently pray for all the parents of teenagers who are agonizing over sending them off to college or driving alone for the first time, or sitting up late at night waiting for them to come home. That was us only 33 days ago, and I know how quickly one phone call can change that forever. I ask God to give them patience, wisdom, a keen ear to hear everything, and unconditional love for those strange beings with under-developed frontal lobes, that think they know everything and are indestructible. I whisper a final prayer for Zack to glorify God with complete recovery and float home on cloud nine.

Zack is captivated by the bustle at the nurses' station when I arrive before 8:00 a.m. He watches the staff as they shuffle past, and I imagine that he's waiting for his cute little aide to arrive. This morning, we have Shirley, who is in her mid-forties and much larger than the petite Emily. She tells me that earlier, Zack assisted with getting dressed, pulling on his own pants. Then, she barks, "Hold your head up," and he immediately snaps to attention, lifting his gaze. A slight grin inches across her face, extinguishing her tough image, as she reminds me that he needs to brush his teeth. I wheel Zack to the room and retrieve his toiletries from the bathroom. Once I get him started, he brushes his teeth using his right hand. My niece, Sherry, stops in on her way to work, and I explain that Zack is walking now. I notice him smiling and beaming, and I declare that we will be walking more in therapy today.

His grin remains as we enter the gym. Amy approaches and asks, "How are you doing today?" Zack responds, "I'm fine." Amy raises her eyebrows in surprise, then announces that she has a job for him. They walk him to the model car in the therapy area and asks him to help them wash it. With a bucket of water and sponges, Mary Beth demonstrates the process. He catches on quickly, meticulously reaching across the hood and chasing after the water as it drips down the side. Periodically, he stops to peer inside the car, and then, diligently continues working.

When his chore is complete, they have him carry the bucket of water in his left hand as they assist him to the bathroom. He bends down to dump the remaining water into the bathtub, attempting to tip it with his right hand. Slightly frustrated that he can't make his right hand work the way he wants, he uses his knee to nudge it until the water empties into the bathtub. This time, Mary Beth arches an eyebrow in amazement, and then, challenges him to a thumb war. After several battles, with Zack winning each one, she asks, *"Do you always win?"* He grins and nods. I am delighted, thrilled with each new accomplishment. Just last week, he was moaning as his right arm quivered, confused by the signals from his brain. Today, he washed a car and finds a way to compensate when his arm won't cooperate.

When we return to the room, Zack recuperates from therapy with a nap, while I make preparations to move to our new room. It is only slightly bigger, but we will benefit from every inch now that he is wheeling himself around. I would like to keep my toes. It is also on the opposite side of the nurses' station, with full view of our door, so they can keep an eye on him—or perhaps discourage late night visitors. As Zack dozes, I transfer his posters and hang up the pictures of his friends. Shirley moves his clothes, hanging them in the wardrobe, and places his toiletries in the bathroom. She delivers a small table to set up my laptop and explains his enclosure bed will be moved while we are in therapy.

After we have all his personal belongings moved to our new room, I wake Zack up for his afternoon sessions. Arriving at Kathy's office for speech therapy, she explains that in group rounds this morning, they discussed changing his medication. Amy and Mary Beth reported that the tone in his right arm had improved enough to decrease his Baclofen. Since this muscle tone inhibitor causes drowsiness, they agree this side effect now outweighs the advantage. Kathy requests that they increase the Bromocriptine, an arousal drug that stimulates the brain, which will help with speech. She reminds me that even with decreased Baclofen, he will still require frequent naps, since his energy is quickly depleted from therapy. Zack grabs Kathy's hand and pulls it towards his mouth. She corrects him, twice repeating not to bite her nails. Zack looks at her tearfully and replies, "I won't." This is the first time that she has heard him speak. She treats him to some Graeter's ice cream cake, which he devours like a starving child. This is followed by a Nutri-grain bar. She wants verification that he can handle thicker food than applesauce, since his swallow test is tomorrow. If he passes this test, he will get a lunch tray. The thought of Zack finally getting to eat a real meal, after a month of no food, warms my soul.

His afternoon session in the gym was tiring. Zack squats, picks up bean bags, then stands to place them in a basket over his head. He works tirelessly, switching from his left to right hand, over 15 times. We move to a makeshift basketball hoop and have him shoot baskets until he is out of balls. This is not an exercise of accuracy, but rather to encourage him to use his right arm, but several balls found their way into the basket. Finally, Amy announces that they are taking a walk, but they do not hold his hands. He wears the canvas gait belt, which Mary Beth grips to ensure he maintains his balance. After several trips around the gym, I can tell Zack is worn out, and he gladly returns to his wheelchair.

Exhausted, Zack falls asleep almost immediately when we return to our room. I am rearranging the pictures I had hung haphazardly when Dr. Mook checks into our new room. Since I had arrived after morning rounds, he wants to catch me up on their decisions. He reports that Zack's head wound is healing, in spite of the fact that Zack keeps picking at it. We discuss the Rancho Scale, and he agrees that Zack is a strong four. He says his schedule will now include speech therapy in the morning, as well as the afternoon, even though he is still listed as a sub-acute patient. We review the changes to his medication, and Dr. Mook explains the drawback to Bromocriptine is the potential to hallucinate. He says we will know immediately, especially if Zack starts swatting at bugs or talks about monkeys. This should be interesting, considering he has only recently begun to talk.

Several friends saunter in just as Zack is waking up from his nap. He still appears tired, but is coaxed into his wheelchair when Nurse Jennifer arrives with a cup of ice. She demonstrates how to use a spoon to dip the ice out of the cup. Initially attempting it with his left hand, he switches the spoon to his right. Not satisfied with the amount of ice the spoon can carry, he tips the cup upside down and shakes the ice into his mouth. He manages to chew the entire cup of ice with no issues, so I feel confident he will pass the swallow test. The last remnants of sun dances through our window, beckoning us outside. I suggest we walk his guests downstairs, and Kaitlyn volunteers to push his wheelchair. We move through the lobby and find a spot outside to watch the sunset before bidding them farewell.

When we return to our room, I find a random baseball game on TV. I ask Zack if this is what he wants to watch, and he nods sleepily. Tuning in the game, I plop down in my seat. When I look over at him, he is leaning back in his chair, asleep. I recall how hard he worked in the gym today and gently wake him. As I am transferring him to his bed, he snaps his fingers. I ask him to do it again, and he smiles and snaps twice. His fine motor skills in his left hand are intact. I find one of our Vine CDs and quietly play "In the Beauty of His Holiness". Sitting here in his room, lit only by the sliver coming through the crack in our door, I prayerfully admire my son.

I see beauty when I look at him now. Those beautiful eyes with their intent gaze. Zack is in there, and we are waiting on God's perfect timing to give him back to us. Immensely thankful for each new skill that he masters, we praise God for His mercy. He could have chosen to take Zack from us completely, but, instead, is using him to glorify Himself through Zack's recovery. During this process, God allows us to see the impact his recovery is making on the lives of others. I pray that one day, Zack will share that he has no regrets. That drawing others to God and recognizing the power of prayer was worth every struggle of his recovery—that he will shout to the world, "Heaven came to rescue me!"

Zack is parked at the nurses' station chewing on a straw when I arrive. He looks like the familiar teen I had known before the accident, slouched down in his chair with his legs sprawled out in front of him. I tell him he looks too big for that chair, and he replies, "I'm not too big for this chair." Nurse Jennifer chuckles and says he's getting feisty. She had been throwing his baseball with him and asked him to put his glove on. He threw the ball and announced, "I had it on earlier." I cover my mouth to hide my snicker, and Jennifer shows me the back of his chair. She explains that he had succeeded in undoing all of the straps on his chair, and when she was occupied, he had taken a walk by himself. They found him a moment later on his bottom in the middle of the corridor. Asked if anything hurt, Zack had shaken his head and said, "No." Dr. Mook was called to examine him and declared him "fit to be tied", so now, he has a new restraint that fastens behind his chair where he can't reach. He is not happy about it.

An aide takes him to be weighed and the results confirm a good balance has been reached. He is getting enough calories to put on some weight, and he's up to 137 pounds. They inform me that his Bromocriptine has been increased to 10 milliliters, which should encourage him to talk. When we get to his room, I find a tennis match on ESPN and take the opportunity to check my messages. On my drive in this morning, I had been a little downcast, which happens sometimes when I'm driving, and my mind wanders to fonder memories. But God is so good. Just when I need it, He sends me reassurance through messages from strangers. Zack receives a huge card from the freshman class at Oldham County High School, a group of teenagers who don't even know him, encouraged by a mother who found our story online. Tears spill over into my conversation with Scott as I read him the gentle words of God sent through compassionate Christians. At times, we are blessed and allowed to see God's plan unfolding in moments like these, recognizing that Zack's choices and resulting situation is impacting many other teens. Again, I hear God whisper, "Wait until tomorrow."

There was a water-main break in the basement, so the gym is flooded. Mary Beth and Amy have us walk up a flight of stairs to the fifth floor. Amy places beanbags throughout the corridor, and Mary Beth demonstrates how to properly squat to pick them up. This was the workout that wore him out yesterday, but he traverses the hallway multiple times to return each one to the basket. They direct us to the Endo lab for his swallow test, where Kathy introduces us to Dr. Schwab, radiologist. They x-ray Zack as he swallows, starting with applesauce. They proceed with a fruit cocktail, a cracker, and finally, water. Kathy explains that his swallow was slow at times, but I point out he is tired from his PT/OT workout. He passes and is put on a soft diet, finally able to eat real food. Nothing chewy, crunchy, or hard—so he can't have pretzels, his favorite snack. No straws are allowed, since liquids will go down too fast, and no mixed consistencies—so cereal and vegetable soup won't be part of his diet. They have to keep track of every calorie, so his food intake will be closely monitored to determine when they can eliminate the tube feedings. Kathy promises a lunch tray, and we head back to our room like royalty preparing for a feast.

After waiting an hour for his lunch to arrive, Zack grows impatient. He stares at the door and announces, "They're late." He had been sitting at his tray table for over an hour when someone from nutrition delivers his lunch. He gobbles up mashed potatoes, green beans, and a grilled cheese sandwich. He eats every bite, and finishes off a glass of iced tea. For the most part, he feeds himself with his right hand with minimal assistance. After lunch, we are back in speech therapy, but Zack's reactions reflect the fact he skipped his nap to eat real food. He becomes exasperated when unable to identify common items like banana, Coke, and newspaper, but he is talking. He whispers and mumbles, so you can't always understand what he is saying. Kathy agrees that when we get on a normal lunch schedule that allows for a nap, he will perform much better.

With the water leak cleaned up in the basement, we are back in the gym for afternoon therapy. Mary Beth and Amy have taped playing cards to the wall above his head, and he's instructed to pull them off. I notice that without the Baclofen, the tone in his right arm and shoulder are presenting problems. He struggles to raise his arm over his head, complaining that "it hurts" and "I can't". His brain is not sending the correct signals to pick up his arm. Amy describes his aching as psychosomatic pain, or sensory pain, from the brain. I thought he might cry, but instead, he shows aggression, pushing them away when they prompt him to reach for the highest cards. He says repeatedly that he wants to sit in his chair. Mary Beth comments that they may have to E-stem—electronically stimulate the muscles to contract.

Zack practically jumps in bed when we return from the gym. He takes a well-deserved nap until his dinner tray arrives. Food is the one incentive that trumps sleep. I'm amused that mashed potatoes and green beans don't elicit a complaint, since we had them for lunch, but he consumes them like he's starving. Impatient with his right hand, he predominately eats using his left and frequently picks up pieces of chicken with his fingers. With this only being his second meal, I will forego the lesson on table manners. Zack is licking his fingers when his friend, Nick, from Christian Academy, ambles in with Scott. They ask to take him on a walk, so Nurse Kendra secures his gait belt, and they stroll down the hall. He pauses to look in each room and flashes a peace sign to the patients who acknowledge him.

We get several visitors, mostly his friends from school, and after an hour, Zack begins to get agitated. Scott decides visiting hours are over when the Packers football game comes on. He runs all the kids out, so he can watch the game with Zack, and then, informs me that I was leaving, too. He suggests I pick the girls up and watch the end of Dylan's football practice, something I haven't had the opportunity to do since the season started. On my drive home, I think about all the good people who have offered to help us.

The Christian Academy cheerleaders bought my kids their school supplies, delivered in brightly decorated bags that included candy. Neighbors are cutting our grass and doing the laundry. Strangers are providing meals. Aunt Penny and Uncle Jay took the kids shopping for new backpacks and Dylan's first middle school tie. Everyone proposes ways to ease our burden, and we are truly amazed at the Christ-like example they unselfishly display. I shake my head and offer a prayer for those who experience traumatic despair and don't have the Christian support system that blesses us daily. I know Gods heart aches for them, and He is using us to show those victims how trust in Christ will ease their suffering. To know that your cries pierce the ears of God is a comfort we long to share.

I am surprised to find Zack still in bed when I arrive, until Nurse Dana tattles on Scott for keeping him up later than usual watching football. Wound up and unable to sleep, they gave him Trazodone at 4:30 a.m., and the effects are still in his system this morning. She persuades Zack to get out of bed when his breakfast tray arrives. We encourage him to dress himself. Dana places his feet inside each leg of his sweats, and he pulls them on. Zack manages to get his arms into his t-shirt, and I pull it over his head.

As he stands up, Dana reminds him that he has to wear his helmet, so he plops back down, staring longingly at his breakfast. She snaps the strap under his chin, helps him into his chair and wheels it up to the tray. Picking up the fork with his right hand, he digs into his scrambled eggs. Arriving during Zack's feeding frenzy, my friend, Teri, is impressed that he eats his entire breakfast on his own. It's almost comical when he finishes the last bite, pushes away from the table, and leans back in his chair like a champion.

"Come on, Zack, let's show Teri what else you can do." I retrieve his gait belt, secure it around his waist, and Zack stands up, towering over me. With Teri assisting, we take a short walk down the corridor and run into Dr. Mook and Heidi, who follow us back to the room. I proudly announce that Zack ate his breakfast completely with his right hand, and Teri gives him a high-five. Removing his helmet, Dr. Mook examines his head wound and comments that it looks better. As he is putting his helmet back on, he shakes his finger and says, "Don't pick your head." Zack looks guilty and replies with one validating word, "Itches."

His morning PT/OT therapy starts by focusing on fine motor skills. Mary Beth correctly places a pencil in his right hand and asks him to write his name. She demonstrates each letter, and he copies the Z and A before getting irritated. His interest no longer in writing, Amy suggests they take a walk in the stairwell. With Mary Beth leading the way, Zack trails her up five flights of stairs, followed by Amy, who watches his feet and reminds him to use the handrail. Occasionally, his right foot doesn't quite clear the step, and he falters slightly. As we are returning to the basement, we run into Sarah Cahill, his case worker who is responsible for progress reports to our insurance company. She asks Zack how he is doing, and he flashes her the "okay" sign, casually strolling into the gym. A random encounter… or perfectly timed by God.

After the stairs, Amy states that we need to work on weight bearing and situates Zack on his hands and knees. This position is really difficult for him, and his entire body seems to tremble. He was struggling and becomes angry, screaming, "I hate this!" It was heartbreaking for me to be silent. Mary Beth challenges him to hold the position while they count to 20. He tolerates each number and finally chimes in at "16, 17, 18, 19, 20. No more horsey!" and collapses on the mat. They pat him on the back, commending his efforts as I remove his helmet to wipe his forehead. He takes the towel from me and rubs it all over his head, letting out a big sigh of relief. With that torture over, we make our way to our next session.

I steer Zack to the speech therapy office, where Kathy hands Zack a deck of cards. She explains that he needs to sort them into stacks of red and black. She watches him, somewhat amazed, as he also places them in numerical order and divides the colored stacks into four suits. I confess that Zack loves to play cards, so she promises to teach him a game. Confident that he will be a quick learner, as long as she uses the cards with diamonds, hearts, spades, and clubs, and not the ones with pictures of random items.

When we return to the room, he is so exhausted that he virtually falls into bed with his sneakers on. His nap is shortened when lunch arrives, and he devours a turkey sandwich. He has barely finished his applesauce when it's time for our second speech lesson. We are punctual, arriving at 1:30, but Kathy is running late. Zack is tugging at his helmet, so I remove it and ask what's wrong. Glancing down at his feet, he replies, "Sometimes I don't understand Kathy's games." I was dumbfounded. I snatch my little notebook out of my back pocket and thumb through the pages until I find what I'm searching for.

In my conversation with Dr. Kraft, he explains that "working memory" doesn't begin until Rancho Level 6. I will have to request a follow-up chat with him on how Zack is able to recall Kathy's games. Zack breaks my concentration, complaining, "Tell Kathy to come on." I assure him that she will be here any minute and distract him by putting his helmet back on. Just as I take my own chair, Kathy rushes in, apologizing for her tardiness. Zack responds to numerous questions, but always in a low whisper. She gives him some lemon ice in a cup to help with his slow swallowing, and he continues to answer her queries. When his cup is empty, he hands it to Kathy and says, "Thanks for the dessert."

In the gym, we are greeted by Amy and Sherri, another occupational therapist. They work his right shoulder. Amy electronically stimulates the muscles to make them contract, which will send the proper signals back to his brain. Zack is sitting on the elevated mat, and Sherri has him bend to pick up bean bags with his right hand. Then, he has to cross his body and drop it in a basket on the left. It is tough for him, and after only a few successful attempts, he starts to get emotional. The further he has to reach to pick up a bag, the more the tears flow—but he doesn't quit. Once he drops the last one into the basket, he leans back, exhausted, but this time, he props himself with his right elbow. Amy points to get Sherri's attention, and I realize the significance of this posture. Slowly, his brain is recognizing his right side, rebuilding neurological connections.

We had just settled in our room, when our pastor, Dave Stone, arrives with his children, Savannah and Sam, who attend school with Zack. He smiles at them, and Dave teasingly asks Zack who is better looking—to which he quickly replies, "Savannah." A tall, pretty brunette with a warm smile, Savannah blushes and her brother chuckles, punching his dad in the arm. Dinner is delivered, and Sam says grace. As soon as he hears *Amen*, Zack grabs the brownie on his tray and takes a big bite. He would have demolished the whole treat in a few seconds if I hadn't rescued it. I am directing him to the more substantial food on his plate, when Scott's parents shuffle in, with Rita offering candy Zack is not allowed to have. I walk Dave and his family to the door, reminding Grandma that Zack can't have anything crunchy or hard. She has always treated her grandchildren to candy, and she agonizes over not being able to indulge him.

Zack had several other visitors before Marissa, an old girlfriend, and her mother come to Frazier for the first time. She had been to the hospital shortly after the accident, but had not seen Zack since he had begun therapy. They were astonished at his progress, marveling that he was walking and communicating. The recreation department had delivered a portable TV with video games, and I show Zack their various choices. Of course, he selects Nintendo Baseball, and I offer the other control to Marissa. She is not adept at computer games, and the first time he strikes her out, Zack laughs uncontrollably. I feel so blessed to have these positive emotions, even if the negative ones are exaggerated at times. Marissa's Mom reminds me that their church continues to pray for Zack. She reveals that one of the ministers left for Scotland and his recent letter announced that the church in Glasgow, Scotland is also praying for Zack. His story continues to travel around the world. When it's time for Marissa to leave, Zack gets upset and doesn't want to release her hand. He says he does not want them to leave, and tears form in her mother's eyes as Marissa promises they will visit again. I imagine how unbearable it will be for me the first time Zack cries and doesn't want me to leave.

The rest of the night, it's just Zack and me. We toss the baseball and see how many shots he can make in the basketball hoop attached to his bed. I'm encouraged that he uses his right arm and doesn't seem to have the tone he fought with earlier. We watch sports on TV until Dana comes to give him a bath. He stands up, and as I move out of the way, he unexpectedly hugs me. I thank him, and he kisses me on the cheek. I am overwhelmed at his tenderness and whisper a prayer, asking that this sensitivity be a permanent blessing. Once he's in bed, I scoot my chair close and hold his hand while we watch TV. I sense him staring at me. He pulls my face towards his, caresses it, and gives me another kiss. I feel as though my heart will burst through my chest. How many mothers wouldn't love to have their teenage son be so affectionate? I am enormously blessed to have this time with him and as tragic as it seems sometimes, I think I will miss it. Leaning back in my chair, content to just sit and hold my son's hand, I remember the premonition I had yesterday. God whispered, wait until tomorrow.

Dana greets me in the hallway when I arrive to inform me that Zack had gone back to bed after getting up at 6:00 a.m. Dozing on top of the sheets, fully dressed except for his sneakers, I tease him awake with a kiss on the cheek. When his breakfast is delivered, he wastes no time cleaning his plate. He has a healthy appetite, and Dana reviews information on nutrition, explaining that his weight has to be closely monitored. During this phase of recovery, large cravings develop, and he should be prevented from overeating. She claims he can't really tell when he's hungry and may not remember the last time he ate. I do the math, my maternal instinct to feed my child prompting me to count on my fingers the number of meals he has eaten. This breakfast was number five, and he hadn't eaten for over a month. When he stands up, I see a scrawny boy in need of a lot more meals before I will be concerned about curbing any cravings.

Scott dropped Dylan off at football practice and made arrangements for Morgen to stay with the girls, so he could join us this morning. Weekend sessions are inconsistent, and Kathy is off today. Beth initiates speech therapy by sliding a paper in front of Zack, handing him a pencil, and instructing him to write his name. He just stares at the paper, placing the tip of his pencil in the center. She prompts him by demonstrating a Z, and he traces a shaky letter on top of hers. She continues and sketches an A, but his fingers won't cooperate. He gets defeated, inhales sharply, and drops the pencil on the table. Getting the point, Beth moves on to the cards. I smile and give a thumbs up to Scott, recalling how well Zack did yesterday in sorting the deck. She explains that she wants him to separate them into red and black, but Zack ignores her and keeps shuffling the deck. He tries to stack the cards on his lap, but several fall to the floor. Bending down to pick them up causes more cards from his lap to tumble to the carpet. Zack becomes emotional, and when Scott hears him whimpering, he buries his face in his hands. He can't bear to witness his son break down. Sensing the changing sentiment engulfing the office, Beth suggests we try simple card games in our room and dismisses us.

Our morning in the gym doesn't go much better. His frustration continues when Mary Beth tries to get Zack to read large words. She tells Scott that this is a common reaction caused by apraxia; he knows what to do, but just can't do it, which initiates the frustration and emotions. Familiar with Zack's disposition, she directs him to a table containing puzzles, and selects one that requires placing various shapes in their corresponding holes. Zack was unable to do this puzzle a few days ago, but, after a few mistakes, successfully completes it. With his confidence rebuilt, she stands him on one side of the gym and places beanbags in a straight line in front of him. He squats, picks them up and places them in a basket. This is an exercise he obviously does not appreciate, and before he has finished, he is weeping. Scott can't stay seated and is pacing behind Mary Beth, fighting back his own tears. He asks if he can hug Zack, and Mary Beth rebukes him, telling him to take a seat. She patiently explains that if we stop every time it gets hard, we will not make any progress. She sympathetically throws him a nerf ball and tells him that he can help Zack shoot some baskets. When we leave the gym, Scott gives Zack a pep talk in the elevator, explaining that he has to work hard to get better. Dropping Scott off in the lobby, I think he may need an inspiring boost of his own.

Before feeding him, they put Zack on the scale again, and he has lost more weight. I really didn't need a scale to point that out, but I am upset that he is down to 127 pounds. He must be burning a lot of calories doing the beanbag squats. When lunch arrives, he wastes no time in attacking it. He is still eating when we start getting visitors. Taylor Barton, whose father is part of Southeast Christian worship team, delivers a song he had written and recorded for Zack in Nashville. It's titled, "I Come Running", and the melody haunts me. Tears travel down my face as he croons about God walking with Zack and holding his hand when hope was lost. When the cassette stops, it is a moment before I can gather my thoughts enough to hug Taylor. I am at a loss for words, touched that this artist would write a song for a boy he hardly knew. I fold the lyrics and place them in the envelope with the CD. I hope one day, Zack can hear Taylor perform this song at Christian Academy Chapel.

He is barely out the door when we are surprised by another visitor. Matt Rivard cautiously knocks on our door and presents Zack with a stack of baseball cards. He has been keeping up with Zack's progress, but this is the first time he has seen him since his brief visit at the hospital right after the accident. There is no indication that Zack recognizes him. The last time Zack saw Matt's face, it would have been filled with terror, as they careened with a guardrail the night of his accident. Matt was the driver. It was an awkward visit. Matt mentioned he was leaving for college, then stammered and changed the subject, realizing that Zack would not be returning to school this fall. I know he was grateful when I ended the conversation by pointing at the clock and announcing we were expected in the conference room.

Art therapy did little to pique Zack's interest. Not a fan of paint on his hands, he used his construction paper more like a napkin than a canvas. Glue didn't prove to be a better catalyst for his artwork, since he was more interested in eating it, than becoming the next Picasso. My emotions came bubbling up again while hearing the stories of the other patients participating in art therapy. A young football player, injured at practice and unable to walk. A girl not more than 12, missing both legs, amputated above the knees. A father with a brain injury, transferred to Frazier from another state, virtually alone, with no family support. As I wheel Zack back to our room, I consider how devastating it must be to suffer a debilitating injury and have no one to dry your tears or share in your victories.

Zack recuperates from art torture with a quick nap until friends arrive. At first, he is content to sit in his wheelchair, but when we turn the music up, he attempts to slow dance with Tiffany. It looks more like a walking hug, but it's still a welcomed departure from the frustration of therapy today. After all of his guests depart, I find a movie on TV, but Zack seems upset. He keeps mumbling something, but I can't understand his jumbled words. He speaks in a low whisper and becomes increasingly frustrated when I ask him to repeat himself. I am kneeling in front of him, reasoning that I might understand him if we are eye to eye. He takes my chin in his hand and brings my face to his for a kiss. "You're so sweet," I purr, leaning over to offer a hug. "Do you want to take a walk outside?" He nods, and we make our way to the elevator. It is still unbearably humid at 7 p.m., so our walk is brief. Zack is perspiring when we return to the room, and he plops in his chair in time to catch the end of the movie. I seize the opportunity to update the website and check messages. Zack rolls his chair next to me and watches me type, hypnotized by my fingers flying across the keys. I ask him if he wants to try to type "Zack", and I nudge the keyboard in front of him. He gently places his hands on the console, but can't manage to press more than the "s" over and over again. He tries so hard to make his fingers work and ends up in tears. He clutches my hands and with soulful eyes pleads, "Promise to help me type."

He doesn't want to let go and kisses my hands repeatedly. Now I start with the waterworks. I close my laptop and focus on Zack. He is restless, muttering again in a low whisper, and I strain to make out his request. After several tries, he manages to say, "I want Rita." I am puzzled, since he never calls her that; it's always Grandma. I get her on the phone and explain that Zack wants to talk to her. He is crying. He listens and says, "I love you," in response to her affections. He says goodbye, hands me my phone, and stares off into the corner. My phone still in my hand, my eyes travel to the corner that captures his attention. Rita has been here nearly every day, often sitting in that very corner. She reads her newspaper, pays her bills, drinks her coffee, takes Zack for rides outside, and just watches. He must recognize that she has occupied that spot but wasn't here tonight. We sit in silence, with me trying to imagine what is going through his mind. He has cried and said he was sorry. He seems tortured by some phantom pain, and it drains me emotionally. It has been a difficult day for Zack, and now, when it's time to sleep, he seems afraid. I request Trazodone to help him sleep and comfort him until he finally closes his eyes. Reluctant to leave, I hold his hand and watch him sleep. If he were smaller, I would pick him up and rock him, like I did every night when he was a baby. I close my eyes and picture Zack as an infant. Wrapping my arms around my body, I rock as tears fall on my lap. I whisper to God, "*This is your child, made in your image, perfect in every way. He is injured, but you are the great physician and I know you can heal him.*" I reach for my Bible, open to the Old Testament, flip a few pages to Isaiah 40, and meditate on these promises;: "He gives strength to the weary and increases the power of the weak. Even youths grow tired and weary, and young men stumble and fall; but those who hope in the Lord will renew their strength. They will soar on wings like eagles; they will run and not grow weary; they will walk and not be faint." Softly, I close my Bible and wipe my tears on my sleeve. "Make him an eagle, Lord," I murmur. I pray that he sleeps peacefully, and that tomorrow will bring us laughter. I request some extra tenderness to give to the rest of my family—especially Scott, who seems lost in all of this.

Zack slept peacefully last night after the Trazadone kicked in. Another Sunday finds me fortunate that Rita has volunteered to keep him company, allowing me to attend church with the entire family. She describes taking him for a wheelchair ride outside and talking about Hilton Head, our favorite family vacation destination. Zack has been enjoying the sandy beaches in South Carolina since he was born, and she was hoping to spur some memories. Failing to get a response, Grandma tells him about his family, reminding him that he is the oldest and her first grandchild. "Do you know you look just like your Dad?" He nods as she continues to question him about his siblings. With prompting, he says each of their names and then responds, "I love them." Uplifted by their conversation, Rita wheels him back to the room just as a minister from Southeast Christian Church arrives. He prays with Zack and offers him communion, which he readily accepts. It is impossible to know if he grasps the sanctity of communion or just wanted to eat the bread and drink out of a tiny cup.

Nick and Trey, two close friends from school, were already keeping Zack company as he finished his lunch, and I stroll in after church. When every speck of food is consumed, he pushes the tray aside, stands up, and gives me a welcoming hug. He lumbers towards his buddies, and I fully expect him to embrace them, but he playfully leans over and smacks Trey. It wasn't hard, and his quick laugh indicated that he was just goofing around, but I was taken aback. Initially, Trey pauses with his hand touching his cheek, but then the three of them cackle and continue teasing one another. Teenage boys. I am nearly forgotten, and they toss nerf balls at each other, finally saying goodbye with a masculine side hug.

With it being Sunday, I was surprised when Amanda, one of the weekend occupational therapists, ambles in carrying a stack of puzzles. She introduces herself and explains that her goal is to encourage Zack to use his right hand. There are physical benefits to using puzzles in therapy, since they require fine motor coordination. For someone recovering from traumatic brain injury, the cognitive benefits are even greater. Puzzles are games of problem-solving, strengthening visual processing, perception, organization, sequencing, and concentration. Amanda selects a pattern puzzle, and although it doesn't seem difficult, Zack must focus to complete it correctly. Each one gets more complicated, and when he gets tired, he instinctively switches to his left hand. When he places a piece using his left hand, Amanda removes it, reiterating that he must use his right hand. Instead of crying, his eyes narrow, and he concentrates until his right hand cooperates. After an hour, he successfully completes all the puzzles.

There was a parade of visitors solidifying our Sunday routine. It seems that all his friends made it a priority to spend time with Zack today. In addition, Mrs. Funderberg, Christian Academy Middle School principal, stops in with her family. She asks Zack if he remembers her, and he nods yes, but I honestly think he was just being polite. We discuss his progress, and she graciously volunteers to assist in preparations for his return to school. I am bolstered by her positive outlook. When she leaves, it is with a promise to continue praying for complete recovery.

Admissions delivers news that we are being moved to a new, model room. It is right next door, much bigger and painted a bright yellow. I'm excited that it comes with a mini fridge, where I can store the food that friends insist on bringing me. The timing of her announcement was ideal, since I had plenty of kids to help with the move. I ask a few to entertain Zack, while the rest help me clean out the closet and transfer all the posters and pictures adorning his wall. Rick Thompson, a born entertainer, takes the task to heart. Spinning a CD to show off his dance moves, it doesn't take long before the music wafts down the hall, alerting the staff to our party. Nurse Dana marches in, presumably to curb our revelry, but stops in the doorway to observe. I approach her to apologize, and she stops me with a hand up. She points to Zack, who has a big grin on his face, and tearfully comments, "That's the most I've seen him interact with people." Dana returns to the nurses' station, assuring them I have it under control.

As Rick spins around on the floor and others join in the break dancing, I have to keep reminding them we are in a hospital. Periodically, I turn the music down, only to have someone go behind me to crank it up. I can't chastise them, because I am delighted to see Zack enjoying this time with his friends. I am also amused as his female friends, jockeying for the best position as they place their pictures on his wall. Finally settled in our new room, I notice that Zack has grown quiet and suspect he is tired. I suggest they take their party somewhere else, so Zack can rest. He high-fives them as they leave.

Zack seems eager to take a nap, but only sleeps 10 minutes before he is ready to get up. His inner alarm clock must be intact, because dinner arrives as soon as his feet hit the floor. He devours his meal, with me frequently having to tell him to slow down: it won't run away before he can eat it. Once his tray is removed, we flip through baseball cards, and my friend Donna talks with him. He got emotional for seemingly no reason, and Donna patiently asks him what is wrong. No reply, so she inquires if he's just in a bad mood. I suppose she asks one too many times, or Zack just had enough, because he glares at her and says, "Quit asking about my *!@#&* mood!" Fill in whatever word would thoroughly embarrass a mom to hear thrown flippantly at her dear friend. Fortunately, Donna understands that we have been firmly entrenched in this new phase I have been warned about.

Survivors of brain injury do not have the filter that we learn as a child. They will make inappropriate comments and often resort to cussing. The staff explains that it happens to all of their patients—even the sweet old ladies who never use foul language, end up sounding like sailors. Needless to say, I was shocked, having become accustomed to my tender, affectionate son. I correct him, agreeing that it's hard, but ask that he set an example for other people and not use bad words. He nods, but I know he won't be able to stop himself. This is another phase that will have me chasing apologies, but it signals that he is progressing.

Checking the website, I am delighted to receive a message from Auckland, New Zealand. Prayers are being lifted up on his behalf around the world. No doubt these petitions contributed to the wonderful day full of laughter. God granted us more smiles than tears. I sit here and think about the songs from church this morning, and the words come to me, "So blessed I can't contain it, so much I have to give it away." It is true, we are blessed, and I want to share the source of our sanctification with everyone. I recall sitting between my girls during the service and a soloist performing an inspirational song. She sang about our trials not being easy, but God sees us through the storm. Logan looked up at me, and sensing that I may cry, patted my hand, and rubbed my arm to comfort me. I am amazed at how compassionate my six-year-old has become, and then, I glance at Kyle. She has a tough exterior, but now, she wipes away tears as she listens to the words that tell us to "Hold on to the hand that comforts me. He will carry me." Like most siblings, they fight and aggravate their big brother, but they love Zack wholeheartedly. They are acutely aware of how this has impacted our family. We are all changed as a result of his accident, and I see positive transformation, in spite of the turmoil. Peering at my son through the mesh of his enclosure, I see an average teenager being steered through an extraordinary mine field.

I close my eyes and picture his friends; full of life and finally realizing that they are making decisions that will affect them for the rest of their lives. Immediate gratification without thinking of the consequences, produces painful lessons. I am grateful that we have a loving Father who offers forgiveness when we make foolish choices. I pray that Zack will understand why he has to suffer through this now. I plead with God to give him wisdom to teach others, through his testimony of God's forgiveness and grace, how seemingly innocent choices can change so many lives. I want Zack to be the thunder that heralds the impending storm, and then, points them to the one that calms the seas.

Tired from tossing and turning all night, I'm emotional as I approach this dreaded day. All weekend, it loomed in the back of my mind, as I prepared to wean myself back to work. Zack must sense an impending change, because he is upset, sitting in his chair at the nurses' station, when I arrive. When his tray is delivered, he calms down and turns his attention to breakfast, eating the entire meal with his right hand. Today, he starts a new form of therapy, called Activities for Daily Living (ADL), which Mary Beth conducts in our room. He completely dresses himself, including putting on high top tennis shoes and tying them. I am impressed, since I have difficulty with this particular pair of sneakers. He uses both hands, ties them properly, and only shows mild frustration with his right foot.

Dr. Mook and Dr. Miller make rounds and ask him questions. They want to know who I am, does he know me, or am I a stranger? Zack roars with laughter and says I am a stranger. He thinks it's very funny, and Dr. Miller appreciates his humor. Dr. Mook inspects his head and comments that he will schedule an appointment with neurosurgery to examine him as well. The swelling has decreased, but there is still some protrusion. It will be at least a month before his bone flap can be put back, so the irritating helmet remains.

Firmly believing in the theory of family support, I have made arrangements with Donna to fill in for me during therapy while I'm at work. I give her instructions and hand over my precious notebook, so she can record his progress in my absence. We decide to distract Zack and walk him to the conference room when I slip into the elevator. When the doors close, the lump in my throat comes flying out of my eyes in tears. It's like the first time I left my baby in daycare all over again. It will be impossible to concentrate at work, and I will be riveted on the clock until I can return at lunch. Zack watches the door, so Donna asks him questions to engage his attention. He confidently explains that his patient arm band says, "ball player", and repeatedly glances at the door during their conversation. When he notices her jotting things down in my notebook, it upsets him, and he wants to go back to his room.

Once in the gym, Mary Beth instructs him on how to put various size screws in different holes and bolt them using both hands. With relative ease, he determines the proper hole for each screw, but gets angry and throws them down. Based on his reaction and the vision problems that accompany brain injuries, Mary Beth believes he might be seeing double. She notes it in his chart, so Dr. Mook will schedule an eye exam. Amy gives him a large box and requires him to carry it to the model grocery store. They scatter boxes and cans on the floor throughout the mini store, where he is required to pick them up and put them in his basket. He gets very frustrated and doesn't want to participate. After some coaxing, he gets better at scanning the floor to find the merchandise. He picks them up easily, reinforcing their opinion that his vision is the problem. Amy asks him what he wants to do next, and he replies, "I wish I could tell you." Giving Mary Beth a knowing look, she asks him if he knows where he is. He doesn't respond. "You are in the hospital. You were in a bad car accident." Zack's lip puckers up, and the tears flow. They comfort him as he continues to cry. Amy's arm is flung across his shoulder while Mary Beth holds his hand, explaining that we need to tell him where he is, but leave out the details of the accident.

Kathy begins speech therapy by encouraging a slow swallow with lemon ice. Once he finishes his small cup of ice, she describes the orientation questions that we need to review every day. We are to tell him who we are, what day and time it is, how the weather looks, where he is and why. She reiterates that details of the accident aren't appropriate right now and would, inevitably, upset him. Donna is wheeling him down the hall when I step out of the elevator. He flashes me a big grin and takes my hand as we stroll to our room. Scott decides to break for lunch and joins us as they are delivering his tray. When Zack checks out his meal, we all approve with a resounding, "Yum!" He thinks it's funny, and in an instant, he is laughing out loud. He finds the simplest things very humorous. Unfortunately, it also doesn't take much to bring on the tears.

After lunch, I make the slow, torturous walk with them back to speech therapy. This time, Zack realizes I am leaving and starts to sob. Heartbroken myself, I calmly explain that Donna is just filling in for therapy, and I will be back before dinner. He won't let go of my hand and pulls me towards him for a hug. Donna stands behind his chair, caressing his arms, and points to the clock, noting what time I will return. Finally, he settles down, and I leave. At least my body leaves, but my heart lay broken on the floor in that room. My pace is swift as I walk towards the elevator, not allowing me to look back, or I may not have the courage to leave. I am grateful that my coworkers are supportive, and I need not explain the smeared mascara on my cheeks.

The second session of speech therapy brings out the dreaded picture cards. Zack has difficulty identifying the objects on the flash cards, and when Kathy introduces word cards, he checks out completely. He is unhappy, tired, and says he "doesn't want to play Kathy's games." They review the orientation questions, and he silently stares at the floor. Separation anxiety will hamper therapy, so we will brainstorm with his therapist to find a solution.

In the gym for afternoon PT/OT, Mary Beth and Amy agree that the private therapy room might produce better results. They believe the open gym provides too many disruptions, especially with Zack watching the door as he pines for me. Mary Beth presents colored pegs and demonstrates how to put them in the coordinating colored holes on the pegboard. He is intently focused and places all the pegs with few mistakes. He announces that he's finished and stands up to leave, glancing around the room, as if looking for something he missed. When they open the door, he walks straight to his chair, signaling that he is ready to go. Walking back to the room, Donna chats him up, but Zack responds only with nods.

When I return at 4:30, Donna informs me that Scott has wheeled Zack down to the cafeteria to look at food. I'm anxious to see my boy, so we head downstairs just as my sister, Rosemarie, steps off the elevator. The three of us are talking in the hallway outside of the cafeteria. Zack can see me, and his smile of recognition lights up my heart. As our group meanders through the corridors, taking the long way back upstairs, Scott asks Zack if he knew he had been in a car accident. He looks at us with soulful eyes, his smile withers, and he nods. His acknowledgement is another positive sign of recovery, but it's tear-jerking at the same time. Back in the room, we bid farewell to Donna, thanking her profusely for her support. Zack is obviously tired and nearly jumps in bed. He naps until dinner arrives, and I have to drag him out of bed to eat. Normally, food is an incentive for him, but tonight, he hardly enjoys it. He is emotional and fatigued, constantly trying to get up and walk to his bed. As soon as the last bite is done, he falls in bed and is asleep within minutes.

Several of his friends make an appearance, and he seems to get a second wind after an hour nap. They take him for a ride around the corridor, and I can hear them laughing. Creeping back into the room, they snicker under their breath as they explain that Zack stuck his foot out and tried to trip a nurse. Zack looks at me and roars with laughter, outwardly amused by his own antics. He is quite entertaining as he delights in his friends' company, even demonstrating how he can tie his own shoes. I sit in the corner and observe, wondering what his friends must think of a teenager who boasts about tying laces. Then, I notice how patient they are, attentive to his changing behavior, always laughing with him, not at him. I'm so grateful they show concern and affection for him, praying for his recovery, not here to witness some side show.

Zack high fives his friends as they leave, and I convince Nurse Holly to give him a shower, instead of the usual sponge bath. It is not an easy task, since the helmet must stay on, and they have to keep water from entering his stoma. He seems to appreciate it, and for the first time in 39 days, I feel like he is really clean. In fresh clothes, he relaxes in his recliner as we watch TV. At times, he gets emotional and tries to tell me what is wrong, but it is a mumbled whisper and hard to decipher. It frustrates him even more when I keep asking him to repeat himself. I will be relieved when we can communicate better, so I can understand his needs. I am struck by the irony that it's the same for every parent of teenagers: lack of communication and trying to figure out what they need.

It is comforting to know that our Heavenly Father always understands us and knows exactly what we need, even when we don't. He answers prayers not even uttered and provides comfort, even as we push away.

Zack's eyelids become heavy, and I gently walk him to bed. He peers at me through his lashes as I trace my fingers lightly across his face. I ask God to give him restoring sleep and to help him have a voice. I pray that both of us can adjust to my absence, since I need to return to work, and that our family can manage the routine of school again. Tears begin to well up in my eyes as I remember his grip on my hand when I tried to leave today. I scold myself internally, recognizing that Zack can sense my insecurity, and I need to set a strong example. Softly tiptoeing out the door, I listen for God's voice, and He reminds me of his promise in Isaiah 30:15... "in quietness and in trust shall be your strength."

When I arrive this morning, Zack is asleep. He had been up early, cruising the hallways, and talking to everyone in low, muffled whispers. His breakfast tray lays untouched, and as I glance at the clock, I know he will have little time to eat before speech therapy. I'm able to coerce him out of bed by reminding him that he has an appointment with Kathy. He devours his eggs and sausage entirely too fast, so he is ready when Kathy walks in for speech therapy in our room. She asks if he knows his name, and he replies with first, middle, and last name. Unaware of his middle name, she looks to Donna for confirmation and checks it off on her list. She asks him how old he is, and he responds that he is 16. Checking her notes, she explains that he's is not 16 yet, but will be on his birthday. Moving to more difficult questions, she states that this is August and wants to know what month comes after August. He confidently replies September, a smile creeping across his face. He tells Donna, "She help me talk," and waits for the next question. Kathy reviews all of the orientation queries: date, weather, where he was, and why. He correctly answers several questions and says he wants to take her for a walk.

With Kathy guiding him down the hallway, they unexpectedly run into Amy, and he offers a hug. Amy continues to walk him to the gym for PT/OT, and they review the alphabet. Using oversized blocks, she asks him to find various letters. Zack perfectly recites the alphabet, but has trouble selecting the letters she calls out. He becomes frustrated and pushes Amy away when she prods him to find a letter not in his name. A seasoned therapist, Amy knows when it's time to move on, so they play baseball until his mood improves. She comments how much better he is throwing with his right hand, although abnormal tone still makes it hard for him. While Mary Beth goes to find a larger ball, Zack glances at the door and says, "My Dad is not picking me up." The Bromocriptine is stimulating him to talk a lot more. With a bigger ball, Mary Beth demonstrates how to kick it and maintain balance. Zack masters this task in minutes, so they proceed to the stairwell and walk several flights. He is worn out by the time he leaves the gym.

Down for a quick nap to recuperate, Zack is not thrilled about getting up to eat lunch. I had to help him eat—at times, almost spoon feeding him, since he kept trying to return to bed. Nurse Dana delivered promising news that he had graduated from tube feeding since his calorie intake by mouth is sufficient to gain weight. They cannot remove the gastric tube from his stomach until six weeks after placement, which was on July 22nd, but at least he won't have to deal with tube feedings in bed during the night. With lunch complete, Zack stands and walks to the bathroom. He stares at himself in the mirror and wants to take his helmet off. Standing close behind him in case he stumbles, I watch as he rakes his hands through his hair, as if trying to style it. He becomes upset after he sees his surgery stitches and laceration. I explain that he is getting better, and we should just keep the helmet on until his hair grows out and covers the scars. He checks his teeth for bits of food and turns his head from side-to-side. He is starting to be interested in his appearance again, another sign of recovery. He yanks his pants below his waist, a habit of most teenage boys, and walks out of the bathroom, satisfied.

Back in Kathy's office for afternoon speech therapy, she has him identify basic shapes— like a square, circle, and heart. He struggles with the more difficult ones like parallelogram and trapezoid, but is able to recognize five out of twelve. Honestly, I'm not sure I would have fared much better. If he is never able to point out a rhombus, I don't believe it will hamper his quality of life. We return to the gym, and Amy gathers the metal pipes, demonstrating how they fit together. They show him a picture, and he must duplicate the design using the pipes. Zack excels in this activity, completing every diagram they offer, smiling as he presents each finished design. Quite proud of himself, he leans back in his chair and nods his head in approval. Mary Beth has him sit on the floor to see if he can get to a standing position on his own. No problem. He stands up easily, without being shown how, and they commend him. It is amazing how many simple movements we take for granted. How intricately God has woven our bodies together. How the brain and body work together. Spend one day watching these therapists work with patients and tell me we are the product of random selection or chance.

As we wheel back to the room, I pat Zack on the back, telling him how impressed I was that he knew how to put the pipes together, and he carries a grin through the hallway. He glances in rooms as we pass, and I smile, thinking he would like to announce to everyone his success in therapy. Rita is reading the paper when we roll in the room and greets Zack with "Hello, darlin'." She fondly referred to him that way as a toddler, and he would always reply, "Me not the darlin'!" I guess it was wishful thinking that he would respond that way now. Rita entertains Zack with jokes, and when she starts with the knock, knock routine, he immediately responds with who's there. As Rita is leaving, Scott comes in with his friend Chris, who has worked for him for years. Scott tells Zack that Chris had been worried about him since he saw him in the

ICU at University Hospital. Zack stands and extends his hand to Chris. They shake hands, with Zack nodding, as if to say, "I'm okay now." Chris bites his lip to keep from crying.

To witness him standing and talking is quite the shock, when only a month ago he was comatose. Scott is amazed at how clear-minded his son seems. He asks Zack if he knew what a "wet willy" was and licks his finger. Zack laughs and covers his ears. He responded to several questions, and I notice Scott's bottom lip begins to tremble. When it's time for him to pick up the girls, he pulls me out in the hallway.

We are hardly out of earshot when he collapses in my arms, weeping uncontrollably. Through his tears, I decipher that he is overwhelmed with how well Zack is doing. Dana sees us from the nurses' station and starts heading in our direction. I wave her off and explain later that he was just overcome with emotion, ecstatic to have his son back. We step back in the room, and Scott says goodbye. Without skipping a beat, Zack replies, "See ya, brother." I didn't need to see him to know that Scott was bawling as he staggered to the elevator. We feel enormously blessed as Zack progresses each day. We hardly know what to pray for as God answers it before we ask. He knows the desires of our heart and our innermost thoughts.

Several classmates stop by, expounding on how much they miss Zack, especially on this first day of school. He smiles for pictures with them in their uniforms, and then, cries when they leave. I comfort him, but his bed is a bigger draw, and he flops down for a nap. When dinner is delivered, he does not want to leave his comfortable refuge. I have to drag him out of bed to eat, since missing a meal is not an option now that his tube feeds are over. Once at the table, he is so hungry he decides it is faster to eat with his fingers. I have to keep correcting him and putting the fork in his hand. He couldn't get his right hand working fast enough, so I would put the fork in his left hand, and he would transfer it back to his right. Getting frustrated, he attempts to go back to his bed several times, and I would redirect him back to the table, reminding him not to eat with his fingers.

His anger bubbles to the surface, and he gets up from the table, aggressively puffing his chest out. When I tell him to sit down and eat without using his fingers, he gets furious and pushes me, shouting, "I don't want anything!" Fortunately, Nurse Holly enters the room and steps in to settle him down. I was shaken, taken aback by this belligerent side I had not experienced. She ushers him back to his bed and explains that this aggressive stage could potentially get a lot worse. Frequently, therapists are sent to the emergency room after confronting a violent patient. But she reminds me that this is just a phase, hopefully short-lived, and an indication of progress. As his brain rediscovers emotions, everything is exaggerated, including anger. She eases my fears by clarifying that the aggressive phase typically last through Rancho Level Six, and then, a light bulb will just go off inside him that will control the anger. Then, he will be the one asking us questions.

There are a few more visits from friends, but many are busy with adjusting to school routines. When the last of his friends are leaving, he gets emotional. He walks up to me and says, "Don't leave me. Hold my hand." It was heartbreaking to see him afraid to be alone, but I am grateful the anger towards me has disappeared. There is an innate fear, because he doesn't understand what is happening to him. We take a walk to the nurses' station, and he tells the staff that Carolyn and Kristen came to see him. He gets upset when I foolishly correct their names to Avery and Taylor. I shrug my shoulders in defeat as his lip pouts and tears fill his eyes. Holly puts an arm around his shoulder and whispers in my ear,

"You'll learn." She walks with us back to our room, and I find a ballgame on TV. She suggests that we go ahead with the Trazadone to ensure he sleeps tonight, commenting that more frustration will surface when he's tired. As she leaves to retrieve his medication, I think I would like a dose myself. Many nights, although my body is weary, my brain just won't shut off.

Turning the TV off and dimming the lights, I hold Zack's hand until he falls asleep. I'm exhausted, but continue to sit in my chair until I find myself whimpering. The tears just won't stop, and I cry out to God, *"Don't walk with me, Lord. I need you to carry me now."* My strength is spent, and I consider sleeping right here in my chair, but wisely remember the nightly interruptions. I lean in and softly kiss Zack's cheek. "Goodnight, darlin'," and make my way home.

Breakfast has already been delivered by the time I slip into his room. Zack glances up, flashing me a smile of recognition and continues eating. Scooting my chair across the floor, I settle down next to him, gesture to his near-empty plate and comment that he must have liked his meal. He nods and slowly slides his chair back as he stands. I ask him to sit down, but he points across the room and replies, "I want to shut the door." I fumble getting out of my chair, stating that l will take care of it. "Should I?" he asks as he inches towards the door and collides into Dr. Mook. "That's a sensible question, Zack." Dr. Mook exclaims. He moves to check out the breakfast tray and leans against the windowsill. He studies Zack for a brief moment and confirms that Zack is a strong four and will be moving into Rancho Level Five. He requests that we limit visitors to two or three at a time, and none during meals. We can expect to see increased aggression as he becomes more frustrated with mastering utensils. He explains that his emotions are "labile"—meaning Zack will be easily angry, easily frustrated, easily happy, with every sentiment exaggerated. I'm nodding my head in agreement, but thinking to myself that we will have to create a visiting schedule, or the hall will be littered with teens waiting to see their friend.

Assisted daily living coaching begins with Mary Beth instructing Zack on how to dress himself. He has no trouble pulling on his pants and slips his shirt over his head, finding the holes for his arms. Bending down to put his shoes on, he becomes discouraged when he can't tie his right sneaker. He tries over and over again, getting increasingly exasperated. Mary Beth patiently explains that when he gets so frustrated that he can't function, he needs to ask for help. Zack sits back in his chair, a concerned look on his face and lifts his foot towards her. "Please help me." As she is tying his shoe, we discuss what happened at dinner last night when he got aggressive with me as I corrected him. There is a pained expression on Zack's face as she advises me not to get into battles with him over eating, but instead, use diversion. Getting off her knees, her eyes meeting his, she says "Tell him he's 15 and shouldn't eat with his fingers." We are both silent, waiting for his reaction, when Donna strolls into the room and lightens the mood. Zack seems relieved and stands to give a hug to his rescuer. I check the clock and remind him I have to leave for work, but will return for lunch.

Kathy arrives for speech therapy and has Zack sit across from her. She asks him to count to 10, and with confidence, he rapidly fires off the numbers. Explaining that she wanted to play the opposite game, she lifts one hand and says, "Right," and then the other and says, "Left". Placing his elbow on the table, he leans in, ready to respond. She starts with "up", he responds, "Down," and they continue with night/day, off/on, girl/guy. All seem to come readily to his mind. When she asks him to identify items in his room and gets to the CD player, he turns it on. The song that Taylor Barton wrote for him begins quietly. He turns up the sound and watches Kathy's face as the music fills the room. He seems hypnotized by the melody, and when the song ends, he reaches over to take her hand. The mood in the room seems almost spiritual. He responds to a few more questions, but it's clear the song's message has hijacked their session. When their hour is over and Kathy praises his effort, Zack gives her a hug and politely responds, "Thank you."

At morning PT/OT in the gym, Mary Beth produces fencing swords and stands to face him. She playful jabs in his direction, and he steps back, throwing up the sword in defense. He looks confused and shakes his head, not wanting to fight back, as if afraid to hurt her. Zack lets the sword drop to his side and slowly hands it back. Mary Beth raises an eyebrow and smiles, commenting that most patients go after her with a vengeance. There is a long balance beam set on the floor, and he carefully maneuvers across it several times. Amy takes his hands and helps him walk it sideways, one step at a time. Reaching the end, he pushes Amy away and attempts it on his own, but now, he has to start with his right foot, which poses a problem. He struggles to reach midway, and then, turns around and proceeds with his left foot leading. Now, it's Amy's turn to raise an eyebrow at his ingenuity.

Lunch has just been delivered when I rush into his room. Zack asks, "Where have you been?" When I explained that I was at work, he scolds, "What took you so long?" Obviously hungry, he puts down his fork and picks up a green bean, popping it into his mouth. Frustrated that I won't let him continue to eat with his fingers, he starts to cry, but finally agrees to use his utensils. When he is finished, he stands up and hugs me, melting my heart with, "Thank you for making me eat." I am struck by his appreciation, and it makes it harder to go back to work. I walk with him, and we part at the elevator, grateful that he doesn't cry when I leave, and Donna escorts him to speech.

Kathy works through more opposites and tells him to count to 10 out loud. He raises his voice and counts, continuing until he reaches 20. "That's really good, Zack. I need you to keep using your voice." He responds to multiple questions, his voice audible and no longer a whisper. As they head to the basement, he tells Donna, "I talk loud." She laughs and replies, "So does your mom." When they get to the gym, Zack heads straight to the balance beam, but Amy redirects him to a table covered with bottles of various sizes. She tells him to take all the tops off, and as he complies, she scatters them around. Now, he must find the correct size and put all the tops back on. He attempts to force one that is too small for the bottle, but before being corrected, finds the right size, and screws it on.

His fine motor skills are excellent—at least, with his left hand. Mary Beth clears one side of the table and brings out flashcards. She shows him the days of the week and asks him what they say. He purses his lips, gets very upset, and slams his fist on the table, shouting, "I don't know!" This is where his frustration reaches a peak. He was an honors English student, and now, he struggles to read.

I expected visits from his friends to slow down now that school has started, but several guys arrive before dinner. Reviewing the new rule that Dr. Mook introduced, allowing only three visitors at a time, I start a sign-up sheet. Many of his friends come every day, or at least several times a week, and I want to ensure they all get to spend time with him. Zack can learn things from his friends that the therapists can't teach him— namely, how to be a teenager. When dinner is delivered, they make their way down the hall just as Scott arrives with Dylan, Kyle, and Logan. The kids rush to greet their brother, and Scott reminds me that it's Wednesday. I had agreed that today, he would stay with Zack, allowing me time at home with our younger ones. Ignoring the disruption, Zack continues eating, while I give his dad instructions. Scott waves me off and takes the baseball from Dylan, placing it on the windowsill. Zack studies him and remarks, "I love you because of your personal quest." We don't know where that came from, but Scott is delighted.

My ride home with the kids seems very noisy after my weeks with Zack. They are all talking at once, reminding me they need my help with homework. We stop at Walgreens to pick up a prescription and run into our neighbor. Chuck lives across the street and tells me there has been a parade of teens passing by our house, their cars decorated with "I love ZH". He has noticed them on several occasions, praying outside of his bedroom window. I think it's apparent that many teenagers have been impacted by what has happened to Zack. They realize that the decisions they make today can impact them for the rest of their lives. They have a friend who is living proof of that. I don't know why God chose Zack to teach this valuable lesson, but to spare his life and use his recovery in such a powerful way is humbling.

Walking into my house before the sun has set seems strangely odd for me. Logan drags me to her room to show off her new backpack. Before long, things seem back to normal as I referee an argument between Kyle and Dylan over the TV. We settle at the kitchen table to review homework, and I find my mind drifting back to Frazier, wondering what Zack was doing. Snapped back to reality by the shrill ring of my phone, I glance down and recognize Scott's number. Zack announces, "I'm okay," and I hear Scott coaching him in the background. A lump forms in my throat as I fight back tears. My girls stare at me, a hint of fear in their innocent eyes. "It's Zack. He's fine." The noise increases as they fight over who gets to talk to him.

When each has had their turn, we pack away homework and settle into a familiar nightly routine. I read a bedtime story to Logan and find Kyle in her room, laying out her clothes for school. After answering a hundred questions on when Zack will come home, I finally kiss her goodnight and check on Dylan. He has the dog in bed with him, and I decide not to argue about it tonight. With the house quiet, I walk around, aimlessly turning off lights. I don't quite know what to do with myself and consider calling Scott again. Instead, I fill up the tub and soak in a hot bath— something I haven't had the pleasure of doing for over a month. Steam rises up and mingles with the tears that stream down my face as my heart longs to be at Frazier.

On my way to the room this morning, I run into Dr. Miller in the hall, and we discuss Zack's progress. He is pleased that Zack is talking more freely, and reports that he is much calmer today than yesterday when he had to chase him around the room for an evaluation. Dr. Miller reveals that as he makes rounds at a pediatric office, patients often ask him if he knows Zack when they discover he works at Frazier Rehab. Everyone seems to know about the amazing recovery of this teenage boy. We want them to know the great physician who is restoring him through the power of prayer.

I discover Zack fully dressed, lying in bed, laughing at some comment from Nurse Dana. Leaning down to hug him, he smiles at me and says, "I've been waiting to hug you, sweetie." He takes my hand and pulls it to his mouth for a kiss, and my chest feels as if it may explode with emotion. The breakfast tray is placed on his table, and Zack licks his lips in anticipation, hopping out of bed to take his seat. Pausing as he runs a finger across a piece of sausage, he shoots me a knowing look, stabs it with a fork, and pops it in his mouth. While he continues to eat, I show him pictures of his siblings and ask him who they are. He identifies Dylan and Kyle, but when I get to the picture of Logan, he says she is his mom. I snort and tell him to stop teasing me because he knows Logan is not his mom.

"I wouldn't tease you if you weren't sitting here. These questions are silly."
I lean back in my chair and consider his response.

"Do you think all the questions are silly? Even the questions Kathy asks?"

He places his fork, balancing it carefully lengthwise on the side of his plate, as though it's one of his therapy drills, and licks some ketchup off his finger. He slowly nods his head. Before he has a chance to respond verbally, Dr. Mook strides in and confirms that our family meeting is arranged for next Wednesday at 1:00 p.m. This is a mandatory meeting for all those who will be involved in Zack's care and his team of doctors. They will discuss what we can expect over the next month, and their plan for addressing the physiological, psychological, and neurobehavioral issues that arise.

Morning speech therapy takes place in our room, and Zack is very talkative. When Kathy arrives, he politely says good morning and helps clean up his tray as she takes a seat at the table. She runs through the orientation questions, telling him what month and day it is and why he is here. When she asks, "What is the name of this place?" he replies, "One ugly bed." Even Kathy has to chuckle at that description. Zack keeps looking at the clock, wanting to know when he would leave for PT/OT. Kathy notes in his chart that he is acutely aware of his therapy schedule, and then explains that she wants to play a memory game. She selects the pictures of Kyle and Logan and wanders around the room, placing them in different spots out of sight. She continues to ask him questions, diverting his attention from where the pictures were hidden.

After 20 minutes, she asks Zack to bring her the pictures of his sisters. He stands up rubbing his chin but looks directly at the drawer where she hid Kyle's photo. He retrieves it, and then, moves the newspaper aside on the desktop and locates Logan's photo. He presents both pictures to Kathy, extending his hands, as if presenting a gift, a big grin spread across his face. She is delighted, checks the clock, and notes the time in his chart. "Very good, Zack. Can you count for me?" Without faltering, he begins counting…in Spanish! Uno, dos, tres, all the way to 10! When he is finished, he says, "Wow!", amazed at his own ability. She responds, "My name is Kathy," in Spanish. Zack replies, "Mi nombre es Zack."

She shakes her head, incredulous, and scribbles in her chart. She asks him what comes after January, and he recites each month and announces the year is 2005. He cocks his head to one side, as if remembering something, and says he had a dream last night. We wait anxiously for the details, but he claims he can't remember it. When it is time to leave, Zack stands up, hugs her, and thanks her. Kathy seems surprised by his affection. She pauses in the doorway and opens her mouth to speak, but flashes a smile instead, her hand placed over her heart. Zack lumbers over to his bed, plops down, and grins, "That was fun."

In the gym, he is given tiny pegs and instructed to place them in tiny holes using only his right hand. He is not happy and protests, periodically rubbing his eyes. He acknowledges that his vision is blurry, but he completes the tedious chore and pushes the pegboard across the table as far away as possible. Deciding to focus on more physical tasks, Amy shows him how to stand and pass a ball between his legs. No problem. When directed to pass it behind his back, he turns around in a circle, not understanding her directions. Amy laughs apologetically and demonstrates how to hold the ball behind his back, passing it from one hand to the other. He attempts it, but complains, "It hurts."

The abnormal tone in his right arm still presents problems, so Amy fashions together a weightlifting bar and requires him to lift it above his head. He cries out loudly, but is determined to complete 10 arm lifts. Once he is finished, he collapses on the mat, breathing heavily. "That was hard." Curious, he saunters over to the bar and wants to know how much weight he was lifting. Amy answers it was seven pounds. My strong athlete, who had regularly lifted weights for football, now struggles to lift seven pounds.

Zack kicks his shoes off and dives in bed after his strenuous workout. He is coaxed out of bed when lunch is delivered, but he doesn't finish his meal. He complains that he is full and staggers back to his bed. Recalling what Dana had said about monitoring his appetite, I conclude that he had eaten enough. My opinion made no difference, since he was asleep within minutes. I pick at his remaining food and notice that his lanky body is almost too long for his bed. It seems the food he eats isn't putting on bulk, but is certainly adding inches to his height. His hair grows fast, and soon, the surgery scar will be hidden, even when he takes his helmet off. He looks so relaxed that I regret having to get him up for speech therapy. Staring down at him, I try a soft approach, "Come on buddy, it's time to go to the gym." He stretches and rolls over, his back to me. I rub his arm, trying to persuade him to get up, but he only grunts. Not wanting to elicit an aggressive confrontation, I step to the nurses' station and ask Dana to help me. She strides in with a more authoritarian approach. "Zack, you're going to be late. Let's go." Arching his back, he throws one leg over the side of his bed and sits up. His eyelids are half-closed, but he remains upright while Dana puts his sneakers on. She helps him stand up, and he shuffles to his chair. He's ready to go, but not happy about it.

Wheeling into the gym, Zack still appears tired. Mary Beth leads him over to the cabinets, where they have removed everything, and explains that he needs to organize where the items should be placed on the shelves. Zack meticulously stacks all the games on one shelf and separates the balls according to size. He loads small boxes on the top shelf and larger ones on the bottom. After rearranging a few items, he stands back with his arms folded across his puffed-out chest, pleased with himself. Amy places an arm around his waist, congratulating him as they walk to the makeshift basketball goal. She tosses him a ball and says, "Show me what you can do." He makes several baskets, some leading with his right hand. His confidence built up, Mary Beth guides him to the puzzle table. He sits down and is reminded that he can only use his right hand. Pausing at times before selecting the right piece, he slowly completes the puzzle. He stands up, yanking his pants down well below his waist and struts back to his wheelchair. "I'm tired. I work hard." Both therapists walk us to the elevator. Zack leans lazily to one side and thrusts his arm out for a handshake, "Good job."

Praising Zack as we wheel back to the room, I comment, "I bet you're ready for a nap."

He replies, "I want my bed."

Since he didn't finish his lunch, when dinner arrives, he is hungry and doesn't need to be told to get up. He pads to the table, pulling on his pants again, and drops in his seat. I'm amused that he almost seems to be on autopilot when it comes time to eat. He finishes every morsel, never once using his fingers, and tips his Boost drink up to consume the last drop. Dana comes in to collect his tray when I'm helping him with his sneakers.

No sooner than when she is out the door, several friends peek in. They followed the rule about not coming during mealtime, but now, four guys crowd into the room. Deciding it would be best to take our group on a walk, we proceed down the corridor. We wander through the halls until we reach Jewish Hospital and run into Nicole and her dad, on their way to visit us. Nicole was one of the girls in the accident with Zack. As backseat passengers, none of the girls were seriously injured.

After a few minutes of awkward conversation, we are rescued by Averi and her mom. I had learned from his friends that Averi and Zack were an item in the weeks leading up to the accident. Averi had visited at University Hospital and nearly passed out in the hallway after seeing Zack's condition. She is almost giddy that he is talking with her, and its comical watching Zack ignore his male friends, while relishing the attention of the girls. At one point, he gets out of his chair and yanks his pants down, embarrassing the girls. I comment that we need to get back to the room and usher Zack back to his chair.

As we traipse through the hall, I admonish Zack, whispering that he can't pull his pants down in public. We wheel onto our floor and stop by the nurses' station. Zack stares at the wall, pretending not to hear me, as I explain to Dana his odd behavior with his pants. She is not surprised and reminds me that he is working his way through several stages, and each of them have their specific challenges. She agrees that we should correct him when it happens and keep a close eye on him until we get over this hurdle. Hoping this stage isn't replaced by one that is more obnoxious, I take Zack to the room, and he scrambles into bed. He acts tired, but isn't content in bed, going back and forth to his chair all evening. Reasoning that a shower might help him to relax, I call for Dana one last time. While they are in the bathroom, I straighten up his linens and pull my chair next to the bed. When he is clean and settled under the covers, I ask him if we can pray. He closes his eyes, and I begin to recite the 23rd Psalm. I finish and request that he say it with me. I start, "The Lord is my shepherd," and he follows with, "I shall not be in want." We continue through the entire psalm, alternating verses until I finish, "I will dwell in the house of the Lord forever."

He starts weeping and asks, "What if Jesus leaves me?" My heart shatters. "Don't be afraid, Zack. Jesus will never leave you."

He searches for my hand and clutches it, his fingers intertwining with mine. His eyes remain closed, and I squeeze mine shut to hold in the tears. I can hear my heart thumping in my ears as I imagine Zack waking and being in fear. His hand relaxes, and I open my eyes to see his steady breathing. He is calm, sleeping peacefully, and I can't help wondering what his dream was about last night. I bow my head and pray that tonight he dreams of green pastures and quiet waters. I beg Jesus to wrap his arms around him, so he will not be afraid. Sniffling, not wanting to wake him, I search my heart for a verse that I can pray over him. I am given Joshua 1:9, "Have I not commanded you? Be strong and courageous. Do not be afraid; do not be discouraged, for the Lord, your God, will be with you wherever you go."

The lights are off in his room when I arrive this morning, but Zack is not asleep. Dr. Miller makes rounds, turns on the lights, and examines him in bed. He reports that the team has discussed starting him on Zoloft, an anti-depressant, since he is moving into a phase during which depression is a common side effect. As Zack progresses, he will likely battle increased depression, because he will be aware of what happened to him, what he can no longer do, and what he is missing out on. Already, he is concerned about his appearance, taking off his helmet to examine his head. Dr. Miller states that he would be on the smallest dose of the anti-depressant, and they don't expect it to be an ongoing medication for him.

Breakfast arrives, and Zack is all smiles as he digs into scrambled eggs. I am extremely grateful to spend mornings with him, since he seems to be the most talkative and can usually find something to laugh about. I propose taking a walk before therapy, and he replies "Not right now, probably later. I have eggshells on me." He is a messy eater, and little bits of scrambled eggs are scattered on his lap. Recently, I have noticed that he picks tiny pieces of lint from his clothes and doesn't want to wear a shirt that shows remnants of a meal. Becoming meticulous about his appearance could be a positive side effect of his brain injury. The dietician stops by with information about the feeding group scheduled for next week. Zack will eat one meal in the conference room with Mary Beth and several other patients. They will work on eating with his right hand, how to enjoy a meal in a social setting, and new foods will be introduced.

Kathy comes for speech therapy and reviews 20 yes/no questions. These are relatively simple; Do fish swim? Is ice cold? Can dogs fly? He misses eight questions, and she explains that he has signs of aphasia, a language disorder caused by damage to specific parts of his brain, making it difficult to recall the names of common objects. Kathy offers this simple description of aphasia. All of us have filing cabinets in our heads. Animals in one, food in another, apparel in another, etc. For Zack, it is like all the files have been dumped, requiring him to find each one and store it in the correct cabinet. Aphasia is why Zack told her he had bricks for breakfast, instead of bacon. This disorder also causes his frustration with her picture flash cards. He knows what the items are but can't recall their names. He may also make up words and get upset that we don't understand what he's saying. Working through identifying objects will be a major focus in speech therapy.

An exercise bike is introduced in the gym for physical therapy. Zack accepts the challenge and rides for seven minutes, working up a sweat, but is not impressed. He complains to Amy that he could show her how to ride a real bike, if she would take him to the park. How glorious to think of going bike riding in the park when a few weeks ago, I was praying he could learn to walk again. Mary Beth moves him to another area of the gym, points to a plastic disk with a hole, and hands him a golf club. Dropping the ball in front of him, she explains that he has to hit it into the hole. Without a demonstration, Zack studies the hole, and then, kicks the ball in that direction. Mary Beth points to the club and says, "What's this for?" It takes a moment for him to regain his composure after laughing at his own mistake. She drops another ball and shows him the correct grip. Focused like a laser, he takes several shots, and finally makes a hole-in-one from 10 feet away. He cheers, giving both therapists high-fives, and holding the club over his head. He grins ear-to-ear for the rest of the session. Before the accident, Scott had taught Zack how to play, so he will be ecstatic to learn that golf was on the agenda today.

An hour siesta before lunch helps Zack maintain his positive mood, and I don't have to drag him out of bed. He eats everything except dessert, stands up, and brushes crumbs off his pants. I know he's going to head back to bed, so I ask him to sit with me while I finish my lunch. I question him about his favorite thing to do in therapy. He pauses, and I can see him trying to come up with the right answer, his brain spinning. Finally, he stands up and holds an imaginary golf club, taking a perfect swing. Teasing, I inquire, "Is that baseball?" He furrows his brow and glares at me. "It must be golf." He grins, nodding his head.
"Golf!" he shouts and takes another swing.

Afternoon speech therapy presents an obvious challenge. Kathy brings out the flashcards and lays several on the table. Some contain words, and others are the objects that match those words. This requires him to know what the object is called and be able to read the word. Even though the words aren't difficult, he can't seem to match them up, and becomes increasingly frustrated. He shakes his head, looks away, and tears well up in his eyes. Kathy slides the cards into a desk drawer and changes her strategy. He follows instructions as she requests that he touch his nose, tap his foot, point to the wheel of his chair. When it's time to go to the gym, he gives Kathy a kiss on the cheek. I think he was rewarding her for putting those darn flashcards away.

Mary Beth starts occupational therapy by writing a number and having Zack copy it. They get up to six before he loses interest and tells her he is bored. He requests they do something else and scans the gym, looking for his golf game. Mary Beth has other ideas and produces a piece of paper covered with black dots. She hands him a red marker and explains that he has to draw a circle around every dot. A very tedious task that he completes without complaining. She comments that he seemed to circle all the ones on the left page fairly quickly, but slowed down substantially with the dots on the right. Drawing a line down the center of the page, she asks him about the ones on the right, and he says they are hard to see. Another notation about vision difficulties is marked down in his chart.

When we get back to the room, Zack says he is very tired and wants to take a nap. I try persuading him to stay up, since it is nearly time for dinner, but he is asleep before I finish praising his efforts in therapy. I slide over to my makeshift desk and review the scribblings in my notebook. I'm trying to find the date when Mary Beth first started commenting about his vision issues and run across several notations about how the brain recovers while you sleep. I glance over at sleeping beauty and vow I will not discourage his naps in the future. Seizing the opportunity while he sleeps, I google information on aphasia, which probably wasn't a good idea. Before long, I'm wiping tears away as I learn there is no cure for this disorder. I pour over articles on the various types of aphasia and realize this could greatly impact his life. The more I read about it, the more distressed I become.

When dinner is over, Zack's friends start to stream in. Lauren and Trey bring him a mix tape and pop it in the CD player. As they listen to music, Zack is bobbing his head and tapping his fingers on the arm of his chair. By the second song, he is up dancing, and the party begins. His friends are such good therapy, and our room is filled with laughter. Several other kids arrive, and it was hard to follow the rules of only two or three at a time. Word spread quickly, and on a Friday night, everyone wants to see Zack dance. I finally had to close the club down, so my mom and sister, Colleen, could have some time as well.

Mom is in her 80s and doesn't get to visit unless someone drives her downtown, so I want to make her time worthwhile. It pains her to see Zack struggle, and this is her first opportunity to witness him walking and talking. As soon as she lays eyes on him, the waterworks start. I find a Kleenex, sit her in my chair, and give her the baseball. Zack wheels his chair in front of her, and they toss the ball as Colleen's chatter fills the silence. Mom could care less what they talk about, for she is delighted to see him out of bed, no longer attached to a monitor. She must have kissed him a half a dozen times before shuffling out the door, sniffling as she went down the hall.

With visiting hours over, I go to the nurses' station to inquire about my missing camera, and I'm introduced to a few mothers of new patients. One despondent mom invites us to meet her son, John, who is paralyzed from the waist down, so I sprint back to the room. At first, Zack is reluctant to leave his recliner, but hearing there is a boy his age down the hall, he eagerly follows me. John is a big, 14-year-old athlete, and his mother fusses over him as we enter the room. Zack approaches the bed and shakes his hand. After some awkward teenage introductions, he tosses John his baseball. There is not a lot of conversation between them, but his mother plies me with questions. Her son has a serious spinal cord injury, and she fears he may never walk again. My heart skips a beat as I am taken back to University Hospital, where I had feared my son might be bound to a bed forever. My lip trembles, and I stare at the floor, fighting back tears.

When I have the courage to speak, I tell her how far Zack has come in the weeks we have been here. I describe his condition when we arrived at Frazier as devastating; not able to hold his head up, feed himself, talk, or walk. Gesturing at Zack as he stands throwing the baseball, I say, "Look at him now." She watches as her son returns the ball to Zack and wipes tears off her face with bare hands. I put my arm around her shoulder. "I understand exactly how you feel. You can't give up hope. God has performed miracles here for Zack." A pained smile graces her face when I ask if I can pray for them. I take her hand and ask God to give her peace and bless her with patience to wait on his timing. I plead courage for John to fight hard through difficult therapy. When I look up, Zack is standing still, his head bowed and eyes closed, listening to our prayer. I release her hand, and she moves over to John, caressing his arm while she plumps up his pillows. Zack starts wandering out the door, so I hug her and promise to pray for them.

I slip out the door and follow him down the hallway. He strolls three doors down and turns right into our room. Scampering after him, I tell him I am proud of how he talked with John. He offers a small grin and climbs in bed. Approaching the bed, I help Zack take his helmet off and affectionately rub his head. He closes his eyes, and I whisper a prayer, asking God to give me more opportunities to offer hope to other hurting families. I pray that depression doesn't overwhelm Zack or hinder his progress. I think of his friends who are leaving for college, and I plead that they will feel God's presence and not be tempted to lose faith. By the time I say amen, Zack is asleep. I feel deeply grateful to be where I am, no longer terrified like John's mom. Our future is uncertain. Zack faces huge deficits he must overcome. But, we have a history of how God answers prayer in amazing and unexpected ways.

The girls had been begging to spend the day with Zack and were writhing with excitement when we bound into his room. He is lying in bed with the enclosure zipped up. With eager faces staring at him through the netting, I try to move the zipper. It doesn't budge—definitely stuck. I point at Kyle to tell her not to touch it and rush to the nurses' station to solicit Holly's help. Naturally, as soon as I'm out the door, Kyle tries her hand at the zipper. Zack glares at her, glances at the door, and scolds her, "Don't touch it!" She backs up and folds her arms behind her, trying to look innocent when I scramble in with Holly. Tugging on the zipper, Holly complains that this always happens at least once on her shift with these beds.

She finally frees him, just as breakfast is delivered. Always curious, the girls hover around the tray, commenting on what looks good. Zack couldn't have a bigger incentive to get out of bed than his little sisters ogling his food. He eyes them suspiciously and puts his forearms protectively around his plate. I'm beginning to wonder if it was such a good idea to bring both girls here at the same time. While I'm distracted, getting the weekend schedule from Holly, Zack gets in a hurry and tries picking his scrambled eggs up with his fingers.

Kyle was having none of that and commands, "Don't eat with your fingers!"

To which Zack retorted, "Shut up!" I snort, shaking my head. Some things never change.

Now that he was busted, Zack continues to eat breakfast using his fork, paying close attention to me sorting his laundry. When I get to his socks, he points at the cabinet and advises, "That's where we keep them." He turns his attention to Logan, who has found his bear. Several of his female friends had brought him this bear with a recording of their voices saying, "We love you, Zack!" Now, his little sister was repeatedly squeezing the hand that activated their sweet sentiment. Wrestling the bear from Logan, I offer another distraction and tell the girls we are taking Zack for a walk. He looks relieved as I lead them into the hallway, away from what little precious belongings he claims in his room.

As we make our way in the direction of the nurses' station, Holly approaches us with a blood pressure cuff and a small paper cup of pharmaceuticals. Zack has started to take all his medication by mouth, swallowing one pill at a time. Considering he is on multiple prescriptions, we watch as he gulps water with six different pills. The girls crowd around as Holly wraps the latex cuff around his bicep and compresses the bulb until it tightens around his arm. As the needle settles on the gauge, Zack is very concerned with the numbers. She releases the pressure on the cuff and slips it off his arm, registering the reading on his chart, while he gawks over her shoulder. She smiles and announces that he got an A+ on his blood pressure. Zack takes a deep breath, nods his head in agreement, and replies, "That's what I was going for." Deciding he had passed the first test of the day; he trails the girls as they skip off down the hall. We make it around the corridor to the elevator when he decides he is tired of chasing after his sisters and makes his way back to the room.

Lounging in bed, Zack pays close attention as I remind the girls we are in a hospital, and they must not run around disturbing the other patients. I rustle up paper and some colored markers, settling Logan at my little desk. Kyle is hanging around his bed, waiting for Zack to require something that she can assist him with. He leans over and remarks, "I'm going to give you a message," and then, he talks gibberish. She giggles, "What?" He repeats himself several times, always with the same garbled message at the end that I can't translate. Sensing that she might be missing out on some profound statement, Logan hops over to the bed and discovers the bear hidden beneath his sheet. She can't resist playing the recording. Exasperated Zack pleads, "You can take my bear, but go away. You all are annoying."

He keeps glancing at the clock. I read his mind and tell him we go to speech at 11:00, and the girls would be staying here. Abruptly, he decides it's time to go and jumps out of bed, striding towards his wheelchair. As I was unlocking the brake on his chair, he begins to fall. Kyle is screaming, and I lunge towards him, but he tumbles to the floor. Fortunately, his helmet prevents his head from hitting the floor, and I am immediately at his side. My heart is racing, adrenaline rushing through my body as Zack begins to cry. I screech at Kyle to run get Holly and lay Zack flat on his back. Logan huddles in the corner, whimpering as she hugs his bear to her chest. Kyle returns panting, with Holly hustling in behind her, and now, she is also in tears. We fuss over Zack, asking him if anything aches, and he moans that his back hurts.

A resident, who I had never seen before, is here within minutes to check him out. He rotates his arm and shoulder, quizzing Zack for signs of injury. He removes his shirt and discovers that his shoulder blade is slightly red, but nothing appears to be broken. Zack has calmed down, moving his arm without pain, his range of motion unaffected, so we determine an x-ray isn't necessary. Terrified, Logan is still slumped behind the recliner, tears streaming down her little face. Holly and the resident help Zack into his chair, since I'm too shaky to even stand. Kyle moves close by my side, clinging to my arm as we kneel at his feet. Once my nerves are under control, I move to my chair, and both girls are immediately on my lap.

I assure them that Zack is fine, reminding them that is why I stay here to take care of him. Zack regains his composure and focuses on the clock, ready to leave his sisters behind and head to therapy. I peel the girls from my chair and direct them to the art supplies, instructing them to make a poster for his wall. Scott is supposed to have picked them up by now, and I'm afraid if we wait any longer, we will be late for our session. I caution them not to leave the room or touch anything until their dad gets here. Before we reach the elevator, he rounds the corner and meets us in the hallway. I give him the short version of the fall while Zack gazes up with puppy dog eyes, seeking sympathy from his dad. Scott wants to walk with us to speech therapy, but I remind him we have two little girls alone in his room that need his attention. Convinced that Zack is not injured, he reluctantly parts as we step into the elevator.


Erin is covering in speech therapy this weekend, and although we have seen her before, it's only been on a weekend. She starts with "opposite" questions that are way too easy for Zack. He breezes through these with no problem. Erin moves on to "fill-in-the-blank" questions. Almost spontaneously, Zack has an answer for every question, and some were quite creative. He is cooperative, calm, and extremely polite.

However, there are clear signs of aphasia when she asks him to identify the objects in the dreaded flashcards. Not wanting to dampen the mood after such a strong start, she switches to a deck of playing cards and instructs him to sort them according to suit. I lean back in my chair, a knowing smile creeping across my face. My boy knows cards! Zack separates the deck in half and shuffles, as if preparing for a card game. He taps the cards together on her desk and very quickly separates the deck into hearts, clubs, diamonds, and spades. Then, he leans back in his chair and looks at Erin, a satisfied expression on his face. She was impressed and dismisses us five minutes early, commending Zack for his cooperation and effort.

He is quiet on our way back to the room, appearing to be deep in thought. When we wheel into the room, Zack gets upset before he ever gets out of his chair. He glances around the room and sputters, "Why are we in this place?" I kneel next to the chair, rub his arm tenderly, and explain that we are here so he can get better. His solemn eyes meet mine as he replies, "I want to get better". He breaks our gaze and walks to the window. The sun is bright, throwing shadows on the pictures of his friends that grace the adjoining wall. He surveys the posters briefly, and then, stares out the window. After a minute, he says, "I'm feeling bad." I embrace him, recalling what Dr. Miller said about depression, and redirect him to the recliner.

Before I am settled in my own chair, he complains that there is nothing to do and moves to his bed. He lays there silently, staring at the ceiling, before becoming emotional. When I approach the bed to ask him what's wrong, he shakes his head, his eyes brimming with tears, unable to give me an answer. I glance at the clock and ask him if he's hungry. "I'm very hungry!" Noticing his tray is not on the table where it should be, he hops out of bed and walks towards the door, looking for the food cart. As soon as he enters the hallway, I notice him falter, become dizzy, and grab onto the doorframe. I am at his side in a flash, supporting him as I yell for Holly. Slowly assisting him back to his chair, I describe to her exactly what happened. She says that he may just need to eat, explaining that he no longer gets insulin shots, and his blood sugar could be low. Holly follows me into the hallway to look for the food cart and dashes off to get him some chocolate pudding from the nurses' station. Zack is pleased to eat desert before lunch. When his tray arrives, he gobbles down his lunch and takes a well-deserved nap.

When we head to the gym for occupational therapy, I remind Zack that Mary Beth is off today. I tease him, saying I think Brook was going to take it easy on him, since it is Saturday. "I don't think so." Zack was right. She produces a worksheet with letters jumbled all over the page and tells him to locate the "N", and circle it with a red marker. He shifts the paper in several directions and studies it, his chin resting on his hands, elbows on the table. He finds the scattered letters very confusing and pushes the paper back to Brook, unable to complete the exercise. He sits back in his chair, bouncing his knee nervously as she manually writes multiple letters on another sheet. She slides it across the table, and this time, asks him to circle the "Z". He stares at the paper and starts to cry, "What happened to the eyes?" I comment that Mary Beth believes he has vision issues, and Brook agrees he needs to be tested.

Deciding to try him on the vision board, we move to a smaller office, and she dims the lights. He sits at a table in front of a large board, covered with tiny lights. Once activated, a single light illuminates, requiring him to turn it off with his finger before the next light comes on. Brook records his time, starting with his left hand. He triggered 27 different lights with his left hand in 60 seconds, but only 10 with his right. All of his deficits seem to be associated with the right side, including his vision issues.

Several friends spend their Saturday afternoon hanging out in our room. Andrew is complaining about the extensive amount of homework he must tackle, when suddenly, Zack stands up, instantly losing equilibrium, swaying to his left. Robbie and I sprint to his side, to prevent him from falling. Lowering him back into his chair, I shout at Trey to alert Holly, and the rest of us fuss over Zack. As Holly enters the room, she immediately comments how humid it is. Shining a light in his eyes and checking his pulse, she carefully examines Zack. She asks if he had anything to drink recently and hurries off to retrieve apple juice from the nurses' station. They must stock a mini store in that office. Once Zack is finished with his juice, he engages his friends in a card game.

A contented smile graces my faces as I consider that my boy resembles his friends, only with a helmet instead of a baseball cap. Even though he has lost a tremendous amount of weight, he is not much scrawnier than Andrew. I'm so grateful that their camaraderie distracts him from the depressing mood he expressed earlier. When it's time for them to leave, Zack walks them to the lobby, but takes the long way around the other side of the nurses' station. He is reluctant to part with his buddies, and when we arrive at the elevator, he gestures and solemnly implores, "Are you getting in there?" The boys shuffle their feet and stare at the floor before nodding their heads. "That sucks." We watch the door slide shut and traipse sluggishly back to the room.

Fortunate to tune into a golf match on ESPN, Zack is preoccupied when Taylor and her dad swing by. I welcome the distraction, since I find televised golf extremely boring. I'm drawn into their conversation when

Zack hushes us as Tiger Woods approaches the green. He mentions that he's a big fan of Tiger, and later comments on his admirable bunker shot. Though not a golf enthusiast, I recognize how much more coherent he is, and his desire to communicate is enhanced when things interest him. I much prefer the sports-engrossed teenager over the despondent son I comforted earlier. While Zack is absorbed in the match, I call Scott to confirm our plans. His Aunt Penny and Uncle Jay coerced us into a night off by offering to stay with Zack, so we could enjoy dinner with the Jahas. Rita was taking our other kids to a movie, so we couldn't deny the opportunity.

Although I enjoyed a delicious meal, my mind kept drifting back to Frazier. I felt unnaturally guilty to be out in the world, while Zack was confined to the hospital. Reading my mind, Donna whispers that the guys can take care of the check, and we sneak off to see our favorite patient. When we slip into the room, Penny has the lights dimmed, but Zack is awake. He is surprised to see us, and after walking his sitters to the door, we describe our night out. We answer questions about our meal, and he is comical, wanting to know all the details. I reveal that tomorrow is Sunday, and Daddy would be filling in for Grandma while I attend church.

His sneaky grin makes me wonder what Scott does with him when I'm away. He was in an exceptionally good mood, pulling my arm to draw me close, until I was lying in bed next to him. Commenting on his strength, he teases, "You know how easily it would be to break you?" We laugh, and I tenderly kiss his face. He seems embarrassed by the affection, taking my hand, and wiping the kiss from his cheek. We are very blessed. To think that God could have easily decided to take him home, but instead, chose him to be a witness to so many young people. It seems like we have been doing rehab forever, and yet, only yesterday, we were arguing over curfews. Donna kisses us both goodbye, and I relish the last few minutes of the night with Zack. He closes his eyes as I pray for his friends, imploring that they seek God's guidance now that they have seen first-hand what has happened to one of their own. I peek at Zack, asking for courage that he will see this through to the end, and that his testimony will be to the Glory of God.

Sleeping later than usual, Zack is roused from bed when breakfast is delivered. When Nurse Jennifer comes to retrieve his tray, he has newspapers wrapped around his shoulders. Amused, she asks if he is cold, and with teeth chattering, he requests a blanket. He is quite resourceful in his own unique way. Grandma Rita, filling in so I can attend church, asks if he would like to take a ride. Always anxious to get out of his room, Zack says he wants to go outside. Mr. Sweetness wants to pick a flower for his mom. On their walk, she asks him if he was going to get married. He smiles, "Yes, on October 5th, and I'm going to have five kids." He entertains Grandma all morning with his creative answers. At times, he is clear and communicates easily, but then the aphasia kicks in, jumbling up his words.

Dr. Boran and Dr. Shaw make a rare Sunday visit and inquire about his EEG. Familiar with his injury, but only seeing him briefly in the past, they are impressed with his progress. Unfortunately, they leave just before Zack has another attack. He had fallen asleep in the recliner, watching TV and upon standing, it hits him, more violently this time. Rita is unable to catch him, and he falls to his knees. Scared, he starts to cry and becomes very upset. Rushing to the nurses' station, Rita returns with Jennifer, and they get him back into his chair. A quick examination reveals no injuries, but that does nothing to calm his fear. Seizing Grandma's phone, he calls me as I'm leaving the church parking lot and demands to know when I will be there to take care of it.

I arrive as he is finishing lunch, and he is still upset, complaining that I need to fix him. He is accustomed to me taking control and talking to the doctors to resolve his problems. I told him not to worry about it anymore, that it was my job, and I would take care of it. He looks at me with concern written all over his face and tells me that we have to get out of here. Trying to relieve his fear, I ask him where he wants to go, and his answer pierces my heart. "Home." I feel so inept, knowing I can't grant that wish, nor is it the answer. I wrap my arms around him and attempt to divert his attention by suggesting he brush his teeth. His anger melts, and we are a team again. "When are we both getting out of here?" I promise that we can go home as soon as he graduates from therapy, and I will be here to encourage him every day.

Steve Smith from Southeast Christian Church comes to give Zack communion, and we discuss his attacks. Steve is an E.R. doctor at Baptist East Hospital, and upon hearing me describe when these spells occur, he believes it is blood pressure-related and not seizures. My gut tells me his reasoning is correct, and before he leaves, we pray that God will give us the answer today. He is barely out the door when Dr. Puri arrives with the results of his EEG. The pediatric neurologist on call, Dr. Puri, explains that there was some irregular activity on the right side of his brain, but nothing significant. It only indicates that if Zack were to have a seizure, it would most likely originate on the right side.

He confirms the problem stems from orthostatic hypotension, a sudden drop in blood pressure due to position changes. The dazed look in Zack's eyes is due to not enough blood circulating to the brain. He describes that when you recline for long periods of time, blood pools in your calves. When you stand up, the blood rushes to your head to feed the brain, but it isn't happening fast enough in Zack's case. I'm relieved to learn that the condition is common in tall, thin teens, especially ones experiencing a growth spurt. There is also a genetic factor if a parent has low blood pressure. Zack fits this profile perfectly, since he has recently shot up in height, lost a lot of weight, and I have always had low blood pressure. Dr. Puri will prescribe Florinef, a drug that regulates blood pressure by helping the body retain fluid. He suggests that we instruct Zack to first wiggle his feet before standing, then pump his legs up and down to drive the blood to his brain. Recommending 10 to 12 glasses of fluids a day to aid circulation, he thinks Gatorade would be a good choice. Zack has been listening intently, and when Dr. Puri concludes, he immediately looks to me for confirmation. I smile and nod my head, confirming we have our answer. I'm so grateful that Dr. Puri took the time to stop in and explain everything, instead of just prescribing medication. These attacks won't scare us any more, now that we know their cause and how to combat them. As Dr. Puri heads to his next patient, Dave Stone and his family arrive. Zack stands to greet his pastor, and I march with him, so he understands the procedure. I explain our behavior and how God answered our prayer today with simple instructions on how to stand up. Dave, tall and lanky, jokes that maybe he should try marching, too.

After dinner, Zack is putting in the room with the golf club and mini green his dad had surprised him with earlier. He makes a hole in one from 20 feet away and wants to call Scott to celebrate. Passing him my phone, I ask if he remembers his dad's number, and he dials it with no hesitation. He brags on his golf skills and asks if they can go fishing. No doubt, Scott will be delivering a fishing pole next. When they hang up, I ask Zack if he remembers my cell phone number, and he recites it instantly. He then repeats our home phone number, but can't remember his own, saying he doesn't call himself.

His friends begin to drift in, two at a time, in keeping with the visitation guidelines. They are curious if Zack can recall their cell phone numbers and ply him with hints to help him remember. I can't help but laugh when we all march in place every time Zack stands up. A melody has haunted me today, and the song finally comes to mind. "Onward Christian Soldiers" will be our mantra while we battle orthostatic hypotension. Sunday is always full of visitors, and those who haven't seen him in a week are shocked at his progress. As each one leaves, they vow to keep praying for his recovery understanding the difference it has made.

As night falls, Zack is lying in bed watching TV as I update the website. When I glance up, he motions for me, saying that he wants to see the computer. I slide next to his bed, hand him the laptop, and type his name, moving the cursor to the middle of the page. He places his fingers on the keys and slowly types, "zackistheonlywaytoshowyou". The hairs on the back of my neck stand up as he nudges the computer in my direction. He indicates he's finished, and I ask him what it means. He just shrugs his shoulders, leaving me to decipher the meaning on my own. I stare at the sentiment, the cursor blinking in tune with my racing heartbeat. My eyes filling with tears, bounce from the screen to Zack's face.

It dawns on me that perhaps God has revealed to him that His discipline may seem harsh, but Zack is the only way to show His healing power. He has come so far in such a short period of time, defying the experts who concluded his future was dim, that we know the hand of God has been at work though out his recovery. Prayers have lifted him up since day one. I am reminded of the song we sang in church this morning; "You said ask, and I'll give you the nations to you. Oh Lord, that's the cry of my heart." People from many nations are praying for Zack. I know that is not what the lyricist meant with this ballad, but we can no longer sit in church and not apply every scripture and song to our situation. We feel so blessed that God has drawn us into His word so intimately. We know the meaning of Him as our shelter and believe we will have life more abundantly. We weep for those who go through similar tragedies and don't know Jesus. They have no shelter in the storm. We are wrapped in His loving arms, and each day, he sends us new hope. I hear him whisper to me still, "Just wait until tomorrow."

Massive rain and a six-car pileup on the freeway make me late this morning. Zack has finished breakfast and is hanging out at the nurses' station, joking around with the staff. We head to his room to get dressed, and he announces that he wants to go swimming. I usher him to the window and explain that although it is summer, the pools would be closed in this downpour. We watch the drops beat against the window, and he replies, "We can't swim in that." I'm glad that it's the weather that denies him and not me. When Kathy arrives for speech, he is still fidgety and keeps gazing out the window. He grins when he completes sentences with complex endings, but becomes hypnotized by the rain and starts throwing out random answers that make no sense.

When we move to PT/OT in the gym, he still seems preoccupied. Amy changes his stance as she hands him the baseball, telling him to step forward and throw it like a pitcher. This position requires rotating his right shoulder with more control before he releases the ball. They trade the baseball for a football, and he has to alter his grip, as well as move his arm higher over his head. Watching him master these throws, I daydream, wondering if he will ever play either sport again. He loved baseball, and I know his goal would be to pitch again.

When Mary Beth takes over, she asks him about his weekend. He answers, "I fell down. My accident is getting better." He remembers more about yesterday's events than they expect, and she notes his comment in the chart. Still preoccupied, he can't write his name, but is very interested in beating her in hangman. Every therapy is turned into a competition. She brings out some coins and explains he can keep all the ones he correctly identifies. He turns each piece of silver face up and sorts them into groups, using only his right hand. Pinching the coins with his index finger and thumb, he works his fine motor skills as he picks them up to drop in a jar.

Mary Beth joins us for lunch in his room, and Zack immediately digs into a pile of mashed potatoes, burning his mouth. His tongue hangs out of his mouth, and he reaches for a drink. He is upset and emotional, but soon forgets and takes another big bite, burning his mouth again. This time, he is mad at both of us, claiming we aren't paying attention. He scolds us for not stopping him, but Mary Beth reminds him that a 15-year-old should know when the food is too hot to eat. Zack looks to me for his defense, and when I offer nothing more than a stifled smile, he ignores his potatoes for the remainder of the meal.

After Mary Beth leaves, I get the sense that he's ignoring me as he slips into bed for a nap. He is in a foul mood when he wakes up, complaining of a scorched tongue. We return to the gym, and his emotions bubble over. Anger gets the best of him when he can't complete the instructions on making a paper airplane. He removes his helmet and throws it across the room, demonstrating the mood swings that accompany this phase of recovery. But unlike other patients, Zack apologizes quickly and retrieves the helmet himself. It is hard not to sympathize with his frustration, and I find myself wanting to hold him. He sits on the edge of the platform and puts his helmet back on, expressing regret at losing his temper. Mary Beth pats his knee, her heart melting at his sentiment, and suggests they try the computer game. I'm amazed how quickly his mood changes, and he conquers the game with his best score yet.

Amy brings out the elongated skateboards and challenges Zack to beat her in a race across the gym. As she is clearing the course for their duel, Sarah Cahill motions for me in the hallway. She explains that the order for Florinef to regulate his blood pressure has been approved, and there are additional insurance papers for me to sign. Taking the clipboard, I express my relief to finally have an answer for his spells and scribble my signature on multiple forms. Opening the door to the gym, I expect to cheer encouragement to Zack as he battles with Amy, but find them both sitting quietly in chairs against the wall. As I approach, I can sense that something isn't right and see his tear-stained face. I move to my knees in front of Zack and look at Amy for an explanation. Her hand is on Zack's shoulder as she describes them racing the skateboards, lying on their bellies, around the gym.

One moment, he was laughing, propelling himself forward, and then, he suddenly stopped, hung his head, and started sobbing. At first, she thought he might have run over his fingers, but he was not injured. I take both his hands in mine, examine his fingers, and look him in the eyes. "What's wrong, Zack?"

His brow furrows and tears spill slowly unto his cheek. He leans forward and whispers, "God showed me the world." My heart skips a beat, and I survey his face.

He is solemn and soulful as I press him further. "What did you see?" His lip quivers, and he slowly shakes his head back and forth. He seems reluctant to answer and murmurs something I can't understand. "Was it bad?" I prod earnestly. He only nods. Amy goes to retrieve his chair, and I slide into the seat she vacates. "Are you okay?" He watches as his therapist walks away, and his eyes drift off towards the ceiling. "Zack, are you okay?"

As if coming out of a dream, his gaze drops, he turns, and smiles his response without uttering a word. Amy helps him into his wheelchair, and his demeanor changes; he seems himself again. I wheel him into the elevator, and when the doors slide shut, leaving us alone, I ask him again. "Zack, you said God showed you the world." Fearing I may lose the opportunity to recover this vision, I nearly shout, "What did you see!" He looks at me quizzically, like he can't understand why I would ask him such a question and offers no explanation. My brain flooding with questions, my heart aching for an answer, I scrutinize his face and realize he cannot articulate whatever was revealed to him. His encounter with God is a mystery.

Back in our room after therapy, Grandma Rita entertains him with knock-knock jokes. He endures her corny attempts to make him laugh and refers to her as "Grandma Goofy". That produces rounds of nicknames, where I become "Momma Hot Stuff". I'm not sure if he meant it as a compliment or a backhanded reminder of his hot mashed potatoes. Big John, the 14-year-old patient from Mayfield, KY, wheels himself in and presents Zack with an over-sized, bean-filled baseball. As they toss it around, I realize that John's friends rarely visit, since their hometown is over three hours away. Knowing how critical friends are to his recovery, I'm torn between two emotions. I feel such gratitude for the many teens who visit us every day, but it is tarnished by the sorrow I feel for John, knowing he sits in his room alone.

Their game of catch ends when the dinner tray arrives. This time, Zack is careful, testing each bite with his finger to ensure it's not too hot. I demonstrate how to blow on his food, and he fills up his cheeks in an exaggerated attempt to imitate me. Before long, we are laughing between each bite. With his meal complete, he's restless and requests that we take a walk. As we wheel down the hall, he is astutely aware of the patients who occupy this floor. He glances into rooms as we pass, nodding politely if they acknowledge him. When we get to the elevator, he seems reflective and states, "They never take walks."

We are quiet on our ride down in the cab, and I feel it is disheartening to consider how much more enhanced their recovery would be if each patient had our level of support. I contemplate asking him again about what God might have revealed in the vision, but inwardly conclude that it will remain a conundrum. Moving through the lobby towards the front door, I'm thankful the rain has stopped, and we can go outside. August in Kentucky is humid and sticky after a summer downpour. After lapping the block, Zack announces he is desperate to return to his room for a shower. I understand that his helmet makes it feel hotter than normal, but I'm the one needing a bath after pushing him up the ramp to the entrance.

Refreshed from his shower, Zack carefully selects clean clothes and waits for his friends to arrive. After 10 minutes of staring at the clock, a smile flashes across his face when Tiffany appears in the doorway. He dutifully marches in place upon standing, but is impatient and sounds more like he's stomping on bugs. We decide to try something new that Mary Beth had suggested would be good therapy. I demonstrate how to tip my chair backwards, so it's balanced on two legs. He takes over, holding the chair with his right hand while we consider what he could do with his left. Mary Beth had felt like catching a ball would be too difficult, but Zack wanted to try it. After several tosses, he shows off by increasing the difficulty and stands on one foot. It's a maneuver that both Tiffany and I can't do as well as Zack. When his buddies arrive, I walk Tiffany to the elevator, and when I return, the boys are engaged in a raucous game of catch. They laugh and tease each other, claiming that Trey throws like a girl. Zack has been melancholy, but now, his spirit is uplifted as he chills with the boys. I'm content to fade into the corner, observing teenage testosterone. This is the kind of behavior he can't learn in therapy, and we are blessed by faithful friends who teach him every day.

Scott calls and wants to switch places, so he can spend an hour or two with Zack before he goes to bed. He's anticipating his own discussion about the world God showed him. He puts Dylan on the phone to convince me I need to take them out for ice cream, and I hear the girls begging in the background. My ears fill with their pleas, and I'm convinced they deserve more of my time. Andrew and Trey agree to stay until I can get home to relieve Scott, and I swing by the nurses' station to let Kendra know of our plans.

On the drive home, I ponder the many moods Zack exhibited today and wonder if the Zoloft will make a difference. I let my thoughts dance around the encounter in the gym. Will these images be exposed to him again? Will he ever be able to describe what he saw? Whatever was revealed, it left him sobbing. I shiver as I imagine the turmoil that would have elicited such a reaction. The sun is setting as I head east, and I glance in my rearview mirror in time to glimpse a rainbow. God's promise after a storm encourages me, and I accept it as a sign that the world is still under His control. I have faith that the God of the mountain is with us in the valley.

The rain is back again this morning, but I avoid traffic by leaving a little earlier. Zack is awake and ready to get up and eat breakfast. As I release the safety ring that locks the zipper on his bed, my foot hits the garbage can. When I move it out of the way, I notice an odor, and upon closer examination, I realize it contains urine. What! I question Zack, and he confesses that he had to go to the bathroom. When he couldn't get the zipper open, he improvised and somehow peed in the garbage can. I explain how to use the call button again, but he just grins and says that his way is faster. Fearing that this might become a nightly habit, I move the garbage can across the room. "Use the call button."

I'm not sure if this is expected behavior for his stage of recovery, or if he is just being a teenage boy, but I need to put a quick end to it. He gobbles down his food entirely too fast and is getting dressed when Dr. Mook makes rounds. He reports the gastric tube will be removed Friday morning, so our worries about Zack fiddling with it and spilling the contents of his stomach will end. We have time before speech therapy, so Zack wants to take a walk and reveals that his nurse let Scott walk him to the cafeteria last night. He wants to go look at the rain and is not satisfied with viewing from the window.

After getting permission from the nurses' station, we take off down the hall, and he impatiently punches the elevator button. Glancing back down the corridor, he whispers, "Let's leave, let's just get out of here." This is his mantra every day now. He talks about going home or anywhere, just as long as he can get out of here. Trying to sound as positive as possible, I remind him he has therapy today, and he scowls. It's so hard when he feels trapped. I start to explain how important therapy is for his recovery when the elevator door slides open, and we see Kathy. She's surprised to see us in the lobby without his wheelchair, and Zack explains we are going to look at the rain.

We part ways, and his pace picks up as we head towards the front of the building. I have a strange sensation that if I didn't stop him, he would walk right out the door and go anywhere but here. There is a covered walkway outside that leads to the ramp, and we lean against the wall and silently watch the rain beat against the pavement. The smell of wet cement and the spray of rain that splashes up the curb as cars drive by reminds me of the days we holed up in the snack bar at the ballpark, waiting for a baseball game to resume. I wonder what memories this brings to Zack's mind, or if the weather will hamper his mood today. When he finally breaks the silence, mumbling "Let's go," I fear I will have to chase him down the sidewalk, but he slowly drags himself to the door.

The dreaded flashcards threaten to defeat him when Kathy instructs him to divide words into categories. He struggles to recognize the myriad of words identifying fruit, animals, colors, and clothing. He gets frustrated, repeatedly glancing at the clock, but he doesn't give up. When she switches out the word cards for picture cards, he does much better, but his frustration returns when he is unable to identify all the letters of the alphabet. Zack was an honor roll student, an astounding whiz at math, and excelled in English and literature. Now, he finds it difficult to identify simple words, and the expression on his face breaks my heart. When speech is over, he lays down in bed with a grin and says he's glad she's gone.

He would prefer physical challenges and is ready to move to the gym for PT/OT. The exercise that Amy has planned is not one he expected. Pushing a cart around the gym, he must fill it with heavy weights, picking them up with his right hand. When he has recovered all the objects, he must push the heavy cart up a ramp. The wheels get stuck, tipping the cart over and spilling weights everywhere. He groans loudly and begins picking everything up, almost near tears. Amy asks what happened, and he angrily growls, "I don't know." She shows him how to tilt the cart to push it over the hump. Physical tasks now involve a degree of problem solving that would emulate life circumstances. Zack looks at the clock and tries hard to tell time, ready to move on to whatever Mary Beth has arranged for him. He stares at the hands of the clock, knowing where they need to be when PT is over, but he can't verbally express the time. Aphasia robs him of even this simple skill he mastered in kindergarten.

Before they begin any activity, Mary Beth asks him what happened with the cart, why it fell over, and how it made him feel. He says, "It scared the crap out of me!" He continues to explain that he didn't tip it over on purpose, and he won't do it again. His willingness to cooperate and apologize for events out of his control is endearing. She instructs him on how to complete a more complicated puzzle than he has attempted in the past, and it gets the best of him. He cries and shakes his fist, but then expresses regret at the outburst. He doesn't want to get upset, but he can't control it, and that makes him angry.

Mental gymnastics wear him out, and he is ready for a nap when we return to the room. He lays in bed and contemplates his situation. I can sense his apprehension as he calls me over to reveal his plan. He explains that he wants to leave, that I was driving, and Donna would sit in the back seat and help take him home. I was both amused and saddened that he felt it necessary to come up with an escape plan, but then, I pointed to the rain still pouring down outside. I tell him that people are driving like maniacs out there and it really isn't safe. He considers my statement, his brow furrowed with worry, and he announces, "We have to get you away from those maniacs." In spite of his desperate desire to leave here, he is still concerned about me. His tenderness covers over all the eruptions of anger at his inability to read, tell time, or complete a puzzle.

After lunch, he is relaxing in his recliner, and Grandma Rita asks if she can sit next to him and hold his hand. He says it would be better if she didn't touch him, but she is persistent and asks if she can rest her hand on his knee. No, that doesn't suit him either, and he also turns down her request to place her hand on his chest. As he begins to lose patience, she asks, "Can I tell you that you're handsome?" That produces only our second smile of the day, but clearly lifts his mood. Mrs. Funderburg stops in to show me some vocabulary lessons she thought would be helpful and tells Zack she will return on Saturday to work with him. She asks him if there is anything he wants, and his only request is "a convertible to get out of here". I will have to warn visitors that he will now be singularly focused on going home, and I envision a battle each time his guests leave without him. Mrs. Funderburg asks him if he knows who she is, and he replies, "Judy", laughing boldly, which raises eyebrows for both of us. Her first name is Judy, but he has never referred to the assistant principal in such an informal way. I wasn't sure how he even knew her first name, since he has only heard me refer to her as Mrs. Funderburg.

I wasn't sure how she would react, but she leans down and says, "I love you."

He smiles, "I love you, too," and his eyes drive the sentiment into her soul. As she turns to leave, a tear escapes her eye, and she whispers to me how sweet he is. I think of how she and others would have described him before the accident, and I doubt that "sweet" would have made the top 10. He has always been kind, but that characteristic was often overshadowed but his competitive nature.

Returning to the gym, he continues to work on strength, endurance, and balance with Amy. He battles lifting 10-pound weights with his right hand, complaining that it's hard, but pushes through as many repetitions as she demands. Mary Beth informs him that he will possibly go home in three weeks and asks what the first thing he wants to do is. His answer is surprising—"Sleep." It makes me laugh when I think of all the naps he takes, but I guess he is tired of them being interrupted. Sleep is when the brain heals, and I've been cautioned that fatigue can be a lifelong battle for those who survive traumatic brain injury.

As we make our way to his room, we meet Nick Snoddy in the hallway. Nick has been a classmate of Zack's since elementary school, and they played football together. He has been out of town and hasn't seen Zack in several weeks, so his reaction reminds me of just how much progress has been made. He looks as if he has just witnessed Lazarus rising from the grave when Zack greets him with a handshake. Zack leans in and mutters something, and then, announces that he and Nick need to leave. I inquire where they might be going, and he swiftly answers, "Out of here!" His friend isn't sure how to respond and is relieved when our dinner tray arrives. Fortunately, hunger will distract him from his desire to escape—at least, until the food is gone.

After dinner, other friends begin their evening ritual of hanging out in our room. They pass his bean-filled baseball around, and Zack keeps asking if they want to go bowling. It was a favorite pastime before the accident, and he challenges Andrew as he walks to the door. He tells me goodbye and promises to come back if I let them take him bowling. They stand dumbfounded, not sure how to respond, but I interject that there are other friends already waiting in the hall. As the line of visitors forms outside our door, I decide to take the entire group to the conference room.

I'm likely to be chastised by Dr. Miller when he learns that our party has grown beyond the allotted two or three, but I plan to play dumb, claiming we weren't in his room. Anything to help Zack not feel trapped here. The kids find a deck of cards and gather around the table, while I try to hide on the couch. They play Go Fish, and Zack deals, counting in Spanish. He is in his element, just hanging out with friends, but he keeps looking at me and saying, "Bye, Mom," or "Goodnight." There is no way I can leave and still explain to Dr. Miller that I had control of the situation. Before long, it becomes obvious that he needs to rest, and we bid farewell to his friends. He doesn't want them to leave, but he confesses he is tired and wants to take a nap. On cue, they remember their homework assignment, swearing to be back tomorrow.

A short siesta is all he requires before the restlessness begins again. Mr. Greener from Christian Academy shows up just in time and teases that he brought Zack his homework. He's not bothered by this imaginary threat, and says he wants to go back to school. No doubt, he would agree to attend school even on the weekends if it meant getting out of here. Zack walks Mr. Greener to the elevator, and when the doors slide open, he tries to leave with him. All the way back to the room, he wants me to explain why he can't leave. We walk to the nurses' station, and I enlist Jennifer in our discussion, hoping she can offer a better explanation, since he is becoming increasingly impatient with mine. She has the cure, as she checks his chart and informs me that he will start on Lexapro tonight. She hands him a small white pill and a glass of water, explaining this mild anti-depressant will help with his anxiety. Not wanting to inhibit the depression that is a natural part of recovery, Dr. Miller decided this milder pharmaceutical may help take the edge off. He has read the reports of his restlessness, particularly at night. I walk him around the halls as we wait for an aide to give him a shower. If I stop or take him back to the room, his constant reaction is, "Let's go."

This behavior is plaguing me with mixed feelings about him coming home. We will no longer have the staff to intervene, and I fear he may get frustrated with Dylan and the girls. There won't be the structured environment he has become accustomed to, and I don't know how easily he will adjust. It scares me to think he may get up in the middle of the night, and the responsibility is nerve-wracking. I remember when we brought Zack home from the hospital as an infant. We were first-time parents, living out of state, with no family to offer advice. I was nervous, constantly second guessing every decision, and calling my pediatrician— sometimes, three times a day— with tearful questions. I feel that same kind of apprehension now.

Knowing that every moment we need to be certain that he is not doing something that could result in a fall and reinjury to his head. He is so precious to us, and as I imagine all the things that could go wrong, I am reminded that God is in control. I feel certain that he would not spare Zack's life and send him home without preparing us. My confidence is bolstered when I recall how fearful I was to leave University Hospital ICU. Gods plan transitioned us perfectly to Frazier Rehab, and he will see us safely home when the time is right. God has gone before us, and

He is never caught off guard. I breathe a sigh of relief and place it all in God's hands.

Rising earlier than usual, I pack my car and check the list to be sure nothing is forgotten. Today is Zack's 16th birthday, and even though he can't leave Frazier, we still have a party planned. This is the day that every high school student looks forward to, and I can't help but feel somewhat downhearted. I should be driving Zack to the licensing bureau to get his driver's license, not watching him struggle through therapy. I try to push the melancholy feelings aside, but an inner voice keeps questioning if he will ever be able to drive. Pulling into the parking garage, I chastise myself for focusing on the ability to drive, instead of being grateful that he didn't die in the car accident.

Juggling packages, I ramble down the hallway and slip into his empty room. His breakfast tray has been delivered, but obviously not touched, so I peek out the door towards the nurses' station. He is holding court with several attentive nurses, who laugh at whatever comments he throws their way. I stow his presents in the closet and join his fan club in the hallway. As I approach, he announces that we are leaving to go buy him a car, because today is his birthday. Reminding him that he doesn't even have a permit, I divulge that I have presents for him, but he would have to open them after therapy. As we walk to his room, I explain that he has to take a difficult test in order to drive, and he hasn't even practiced for it yet. This seems to curb his desire to drive for the time being, since he doesn't want to get a "bad grade". By the time he sits down, his breakfast is cold, and all he wants to eat is toast with plenty of jelly. No problem. I have a feeling there will be plenty to eat as the day progresses. When Kathy arrives for speech, his preoccupation with driving returns. He manages to include a car in every sentence completion, and most answers make little sense, but he finds them very funny.

In the gym, Amy capitalizes on his obsession with driving and has him wash the windows on the Frazier car, inside and out. He sits in the driver's seat while she questions him about what kind of car he wants. Considering a Mercedes convertible is way out of our budget, I need to start offering up suggestions more in line with a Honda Civic. Mary Beth brings out a deck of cards and challenges Zack to a game of Blackjack. He deals like a Vegas pro and beats her in several hands, but soon becomes fixated on the clock. Confessing that he didn't eat breakfast, he keeps checking the time, so he won't miss lunch. She decides to cut him a break and release him early, but only after he writes his name. Sliding a piece of paper in front of him, she hands him a pencil, and he carefully spells out his name in cursive. Then, he adds a huge "16" that fills up the rest of the paper and slides it back, grinning like a Cheshire cat. As we head back to the room, we are stopped by several therapists who wish him happy birthday. It seems the entire Frazier staff knows that he is turning 16 today, and they want to make him feel honored. Right now, the only person he's interested in seeing is the one bringing his food.

As he relaxes in his recliner after lunch, we hear a commotion in the hallway. Jennifer parades in with a birthday cake, trailed by Emily, who is carrying a handful of balloons with streamers, and half the Frazier staff. All the nurses on 4South, his therapists, Dr. Miller, several aides, and even the cafeteria lady who delivers his tray sing him a happy birthday.

They cheer as he blows out a single candle, and I serve him a big piece of chocolate chip cheesecake. They file out the door, and when he's finished eating, I hand him a package. Gleefully tearing into the paper, he pulls out a U of L Cardinal hoodie and slides it over his head.

As he prepares to open another present, several friends from Assumption High School timidly knock on the door frame. My gift is forgotten as he welcomes the girls with a flirtatious smile, and they present him with a giant birthday card signed by their entire class. They also bring a cake, this time lighting 16 candles while they serenade him. Flocking around his chair, they point out signatures on the card and declare that their class has been praying for him since his surgery at University Hospital. It is apparent that Zack doesn't know who two of these young ladies are, but appreciates their attention.

He leans back in his recliner with a cocky grin on his face as they autograph his helmet, already covered with names. I watch as they fawn over him, their exaggerated compliments overshadowing any thoughts of driving. As he walks them to the elevator, I place their cake in our mini fridge and search for a bare spot on the wall to hang his oversized card. He returns, plops in bed, confessing, "Those females wear me out."

"Well, Romeo," I reply, "if you weren't so popular, you might get a nap before your party." His eyes widen, but before he has a chance to ask questions, Kaitlyn and her mom stride in with more balloons and his favorite dessert—Key Lime pie. This sends him to the table, where he can't resist having a small piece. He reads their silly card and hands it to me, pointing to where he wants it placed on his wall. I'm still trying to make room for the last one.

Grandma Rita stumbles into the room, carrying two large bags full of giant character hats, with comical faces and brims that say, "party animal". Exhausted from her long trek from the parking garage, she collapses in a chair and hands me a third bag containing three dozen squashed glazed donuts and multiple bags of candy. There is now enough sugar in this room to put an entire kindergarten class in a coma. She tosses Zack a bag of Twizzlers and promises there is more to come. Checking the clock, I start the feel the pressure of an onslaught of teens soon to arrive and want Zack to open a package that arrived from California. His cousin Amanda sent it to our house for his birthday, and I am excited to see what it contains. Slicing the packing tape with scissors, he pulls out a personalized autographed picture of Tiger Woods winning the Masters, a golf glove, a cap, and the newly released Tiger Woods PGA Tour video golf game. Amanda knew that Zack loved golf, so she reached out to her high school friend and sent him this fabulous package. She hasn't seen Zack since he was two years old, but she certainly made an impression today.

As his friends start to arrive, I call Scott and tell him to order additional pizzas, and we head to the conference room. He is presented with a pair of white, Nike tennis shoes, signed by all his friends and several homemade CD's containing a mix of his favorite songs. Another cake arrives—a large sheet cake with his picture on it and "We Love You" spelled out in blue icing. As I jog back to the room for more paper plates, their singing drifts down the hallway and melts my heart. I know I won't be missed, so I take a brief moment and gaze at all the cards, posters, and drawings that grace nearly every inch of his walls. It dawns on me that I could not have planned a party that would be more appreciated, even if we were at home.

Memories flash across my mind's eye of birthdays at Chuck E. Cheese and the skating rink, but none of them compare to this momentous celebration at Frazier... that almost never was. When I return to the conference room, Scott has Dylan and the girls carrying in boxes of pizza and two liters of soda. Our famished guests devour four large pepperoni pies in no time, and we cut the cake. His friends trade silly hats, each taking pictures with Zack and jockeying over the pink, fuzzy pig head. They parade through the corridor and out to the courtyard, hanging out until dark. As the party dwindles, and Scott heads home with the kids, I clean up the conference room, carrying his presents back to the room. Zack never got a nap today and fatigue is getting the best of him. He sits in his recliner and examines his new sneakers. "Why did they mess up my shoes?" I point out the names of his friends, little hearts, and short sentiments. "They love you, Zack. They want everyone to see that when you wear them." He has always been meticulous about his clothes, and although he appreciates their gift, he still isn't thrilled that they scribbled on his shoes. I divert his attention to the box full of Tiger Woods paraphernalia and ask if he wants to try on his cap. Removing his helmet, he puts on the hat and checks himself out in the mirror, tugging on the brim until it's situated just right. Spinning around to face me without his helmet, he looks like any one of the teenage boys here earlier. Then, he takes off his cap and peers in the mirror, a grimace revealing his thoughts. His hand slowly moves across the right side of his head, where his missing skull shouts its deformity, even though it is covered with hair. He is never without his helmet, except when showering or sleeping, so he hasn't really examined his head. "I don't like this," he says as he points to the indention. I explain that the skull forms the shape of his head, and once his bone flap is put back on, he will look just fine. Satisfied, he says he is ready to go to bed and doesn't even bother with a shower.

Making room in the mini fridge for his Key Lime pie, I realize there is no way we will eat all this cake. I shuffle to the nurses' station with one that was never cut and leave it for the staff. When I slip back into the room, Zack is already asleep. I stand next to his bed, contemplating the last 16 years of his life, not knowing what the future will look like. My precious son may not be able to drive a car, but he certainly is driving a message. Every teenager who celebrated with us today has witnessed the power of prayer, and their faith has been renewed through this experience. They understand that when you let go, God does his best work. His strength is made perfect when we are weak. It's a message that never fails.

As soon as breakfast is over, Zack is pestering me to take him on a walk. Moving like a man on a mission, he heads straight to the elevator and punches the down button. Stepping out into the lobby, we make our way through the connecting corridors that leads to Kosair Children's Hospital, with Zack leading the way. He smiles and nods a greeting at the medical staff that crosses our path. When it's time to circle back to Frazier Rehab, I challenge him to find his way back to the room. He does well to maneuver through the myriad of hallways until we come to a set of elevators he doesn't recognize, and he asks me to save him. Guiding him back to the lobby elevators, he punches the correct button for our floor and is able to find his way to the room. He checks the clock and insists we have somewhere to go, arguing that we are going to be late for his appointment.

Our debate ends when Kristi enters the room, announcing that she is filling in for Kathy's morning speech session. She reviews yes/no questions, and he misses most of them. He doesn't do any better on sentence completion. He is not taking it seriously and laughs at his own silly answers. He won't pay attention and seems preoccupied. When she switches to object/word matching, which is much more difficult, since it involves reading, he answers them correctly. Kristi had hidden two items before she started the questions, and she asks Zack to find them. He retrieves them immediately, but identifies a penny as a concubine. Kristi had to laugh, which only encourages him to be silly in order to entertain us. This is the confusing nature of speech therapy for someone who has aphasia and a sharp sense of humor. It's hard to tell when he's trying to be funny and when he really can't recall a word.

Once in the gym, Amy works on path finding, walking him around the basement corridors. When it's time for him to show the way back to the gym, it goes well, until he gets to the elevators, which confuses him again. I think about the many times I have visited various hospitals and become lost taking the wrong set of elevators. We don't think about way finding as a skill, but I know several people without brain injuries who can't navigate their way out of a paper bag. When Amy asks him his last name, Zack replies, "Thong," roars with laughter, and waits for her reaction. She rolls her eyes and turns away from him, so he doesn't see her snicker.

Given the opportunity, he could change this session into a comedy hour, a gift he learned from his dad. Mary Beth takes over, and she has him write his first and last name in cursive. After he correctly writes his first name, I cringe, waiting to see what he writes as his last. Focusing to make the cursive letters, he forgets the humor, and thankfully, the thong. Solitaire on the computer proves a bit more challenging than other games. It requires problem solving and attention to colors, as well as numbers. He concentrates and does very well, with frequent exaggerated sighs to indicate the difficulty. When the game is over, he smiles and turns on the charm, asking if he can help them do anything else. I shake my head, commenting that he's just like his dad, which pleases Zack immensely.

The challenge at lunchtime is slowing Zack down, since he is always anxious to get back in bed. His meal usually interrupts a nap, which makes him gobble up his food entirely too fast, always with one eye on his pillow. Sleeping too much during the day means the night nurse will be wearing a path down the corridor taking him for walks. Fortunately, he is conscientious about not being late for appointments, so I can point to the clock to get him out of bed for afternoon sessions. Expecting to see Kristi again for speech, I am relieved to find Kathy in her office. Zack is less likely to fool around, and she will keep him focused. Beginning with object identification, she asks him what you do with a book. He responds, "Read novel."

When she points to the clock and asks what it's for, his response is chilling. One word— "curfew". Arguing over curfews is what led to him sneaking out of the house and getting into an accident that resulted in his brain injury. I will never hear the word curfew and not think of the tragic consequences that brought us here. The clock may forever be a reminder for Zack of the rash decision he made that changed his life. Kathy moves on to sentence completion, and he surprises me again. "When you want to see yourself, you look into the _____."

He answers, "Bible." She doesn't count that as a correct answer, but my heart thinks it's perfect. I hope he always sees himself in the Bible as the one God rescued. I'm still smiling at his last response when she inquires if he has a pet. He sees the glow on my face and develops an answer to please me, "a Christian pet". We have a sweet wirehaired Fox Terrier, but I wouldn't describe him as Christian. I also wouldn't attribute his answer to aphasia, but a response to gain my favor. When we leave her office, he tries to convince me there is enough time for a nap before he is due in the gym. This will be our battle now: keeping him occupied and away from his bed.

Amy wears him out with weight resistance on the pulley rope to strengthen his arms and shoulders. He tosses the medicine ball and lifts it over his head for 20 repetitions. Then, his endurance is tested on the treadmill. Zack is cooperative and doesn't complain, but his moans signal that this is not an easy workout. Mary Beth gives him a break and produces a deck of cards. She says that they are going to play Blackjack, so he takes the cards and begins to shuffle. Amazed at how well he handles the deck, she starts to explain the rules, but he is already dealing the cards. He knows how to play and is enthusiastic about the game. Rejoicing with each hand he wins, he is equally disappointed when he loses. Mary Beth informs me that the team will be discussing a discharge date on Thursday, since our acute rehab hours are slipping away. She feels that he needs another two or three weeks of intense therapy, despite the insurance requirements.

Zack's bed beckons, and he takes a short snooze before three friends interrupt his nap. It doesn't take these ladies much prodding to coax him from his bed. He announces that he is going home tonight, points to Lauren, and says she can drive him. I think at this point, he would leave with a stranger if they agreed to take him home. Escorting the girls to the courtyard, they toss around a ball until the intense sun drives them back inside. They are in the middle of a game of Nintendo when his dinner tray is delivered. We bid farewell to this group, and he digs into his food, hoping to finish his nap before other visitors show up. As I watch him stab as many green beans as his fork will hold, I think about his priorities. He often eats like he's starving, and he falls into bed like he's just completed a marathon. But nothing trumps his friends and the visits he looks forward to every evening.

Proving my point, he says he's finished when the next round of friends slips in, ignoring the chocolate cake that was his desert. This group of girls are interested in playing hot potato and gather in a circle. Standing several feet apart, they pass balls around as fast as possible, trying not to drop one. It is excellent therapy, requiring Zack to transfer the balls from his right to his left hand and quickly receiving the next ball. Laughter bounces off the ceiling, and shrieks can be heard down the hall every time a ball is dropped. The girls have a hard time keeping up with Zack, so when they take a break, he decides to take a walk, and we head back out to the courtyard. I'm tickled when I notice each girl has brought a ball along, and they want to continue the game outside. Four high school students set up in the courtyard, giddy about playing a kindergarten game, with Zack as team captain. This time, they reverse direction and count each time the balls make it back around. The longer they play, the more excited they get, squealing with delight. When a loose ball ends the game, they announce they are champions, completing 51 rounds without anyone dropping a ball. If you would have told me I could entertain teenagers with a hot potato ball challenge, I would have thought you were crazy, but when Tiffany walks up, they are ready to start again.

Without another ball and desperate to join the group, Tiffany produces a roll of tape. I'm quite amused as I watch the six of them shout encouragement to keep the objects moving. After multiple rounds, with the roll of tape always slipping through the fingers of someone, Zack tires of the game and suggests a walk. As we stroll down the hall, he asks me, "What's the schedule for this period?" I tell him we have no schedule right now. "Do we have any more classes?" I remind him that there is no more therapy tonight, and Brooke chimes in that this is recess. It dawns on me that these classmates remind him of school, and therefore, his terminology is fitting.

After a long walk outside, we part ways with the girls and head back to our room. Tasked with keeping him awake until his shower, I make a feeble attempt to beat him at Nintendo. He enjoys winning, but I am not much of an opponent, so it doesn't take long for him to lose interest. Pushing the controllers aside, he asks me again when we are going home. Nothing I can offer will be a satisfactory answer. I'm sure he feels he is capable of functioning outside of this building. He doesn't understand that beating Mary Beth at Blackjack, the girls at hot potato, and me at Nintendo still doesn't qualify him to graduate from therapy. I rack my brain searching for an answer that will placate him. He stares at me, expecting some profound revelation that he is ready to leave. Holding his hand, I remind him that God has a plan, and being here right now is part of it. He sets his jaw in defiance, so I divert his attention to his answer to Kathy's question today.

"Remember that you said when you want to see yourself you look in the Bible. I think God has a reason to keep you hear a little longer. He is with you every step of the way, and we have to trust His plan." His face softens, and he squeezes my hand. I whisper a prayer that God will give him patience and his doctors' wisdom. I confess that I'm a little scared to take care of him without the nurses. When I draw on a scripture verse, I'm not sure who needs it more, but we can both claim it as God's promise in Isaiah 41:10— "Do not fear, for I am with you."

As Zack is finishing breakfast, Dr. Mook comes by to check on him, and we discuss when his bone flap will be reattached. Without intracranial pressure, his head is no longer swollen, but rather grotesquely sunken on the right side. Thankfully, his friends never see him without his helmet, because even with his hair grown in, his appearance is disturbing. This surgery will be performed at University Hospital after we are discharged from Frazier Rehab, and I ask Dr. Mook to request a plastic surgeon close the final incision. If his hair doesn't cover it, we want the scar to be as clean and small as possible.

After his shower, Zack is ready for a walk, so we head to the nurses' station to let Dana know where to find us. We see Jerry, a 27-year-old patient with a brain injury, being assisted with his breakfast. He is unable to walk or talk, and since he was transferred here from out of town, he rarely has visitors. While I speak with Dana, I notice Zack watching Jerry being fed by another nurse. His expression is one of concern and compassion, so when we walk away, I tell him the Jerry is very sick. He pauses, looks back over his shoulder and replies, "I can tell." He is quiet as we stroll down the hall, and at the intersection, turns to look back one more time. I sense that he's about to ask a question when we run into one of the occupational therapists, who has heard of his amazing recovery. She recently returned from a mission trip and is excited to tell us that the church in Romania is praying for Zack. Her enthusiasm is contagious, and when we part, he has forgotten about Jerry.

Kathy reviews sentence completion and is impressed with Zack's answers. Even being plagued with aphasia, his intelligence and vocabulary are apparent. When shown a picture of an object, he is able to identify it and write part of the word, but adds extra letters. When we move to the gym for PT/OT, we are greeted by Rita, who is filling in for Amy. She wants to try a different exercise and tosses him a volleyball, instructing him to hit it back before it touches the floor. Enjoying a new challenge, he laughs if she misses his returns, and never once allows the ball to drop. Mary Beth introduces various sized clothespins to strengthen his wrist and right hand. He has to squeeze each one open for five seconds before placing them on the clothesline. Each one was progressively harder, and I find myself making a fist as I watch his hand tremble.

Zack is ready for a nap after his workout, but eagerly jumps out of bed when Scott joins us for lunch. Assuming he would have an advocate to lobby for his release, he plies him with questions on when he can go home. He complains, "I don't need the stuff they have here. I'm ready to go. When will you leave with me?" Once he realizes his dad is not taking him home, he switches to another request. "I've been waiting to play golf since I got up. You said you were going to get me another golfing surface." Scott talks to Zack a lot about golf and reminds him that Dave and Sam Stone have challenged them to a match when he is able to get out on a course again. I sit back and breathe a sigh of relief that the conversation is centered on golf and not his desire to go home.

With lunch complete, Scott leaves to go back to work, and Zack heads to speech therapy. Kathy tests him with a memory card game, and I'm astonished when he wins. Short-term memory is a common deficit for those with traumatic brain injury, and I'm encouraged that this game doesn't point to serious memory loss. Throughout the game, he keeps referring to "W" and can't seem to get it out of his mind. Kathy identifies it as perseveration: the brains inability to switch ideas appropriately or inhibit response repetition. Fortunately, we haven't seen this occur often with Zack, so additional cognitive behavioral therapy shouldn't be necessary.

Amy has returned for our afternoon session in the gym and puts Zack back on the stationary bike. The resistance is set fairly high, and before his 15 minutes are up, he is ready to quit. He requests, "Can you take me off here? This is poop!" It's hard not to giggle at his descriptions, especially when he's so polite about it. When he stands up, he has a terrible headache. Gripping his head in both hands, he starts to cry, says his head hurts really bad, and his eyes hurt, too. He finds his wheelchair, rests his elbows on his knees, cradles his head, and sobs. Amy sends him back to his room to be examined by the nurse. They check his blood pressure and shine a flashlight in his eyes while he complains the pain is on the right side of his head. I'm always concerned with any head issues, but she finds nothing abnormal. She gives him Tylenol and suggests he take a nap. Zack's countenance perks up at the thought of a lengthy snooze, and he climbs in bed with a smile on his face. The headache is gone when he wakes up an hour later.

After dinner, I return with Logan, and we entice Zack out of bed with a trip to McDonald's. As we stroll through the connecting corridors, he holds her hand while my niece, Sherry, and I walk behind them. Logan barrages him with questions, and he glances back at me to rescue him. He looks relieved when we make it to the restaurant and holds the door open for everyone, including other patrons. I have to intervene, or he would graciously be their doorman for the rest of the evening. He is so polite and sweet as can be. Once we are seated, he offers Logan a drink of his Gatorade and smiles as she takes a big gulp.

He tolerates his little sister much better when she's by herself, without Kyle and Dylan. He listens to her talk and talk and talk, but doesn't get irritated. I'm delighted as he nods his head and throws smiles in my direction. I feel this is a good indication that he can adjust to our hectic life at home. We decide to take the long way back to Frazier and walk outside along the sidewalk. Taking advantage of the extra time, we play a game where I say a letter and Zack has to give me a word that begins with that letter. His answers impress me, and Logan claps after each one. Emphatic for E, quaint for Q, and unanimous for U—every word correctly corresponds to the letter. There may not be a cure for aphasia, and I know he is aptly diagnosed, but this evening, he proves he will not let it define him.

Back in the room, I have to find things to keep him busy and out of bed. When Andrew, Brittany, and Tiffany arrive, he is content to chill out with them and play checkers. They offer to give Logan a ride home, and Zack walks with them to the elevator. I fear that he may beg to go with them, but apparently, the fact that his little sister is tagging along makes leaving less attractive. As we stroll down the hallway, he stops to visit other patients. He plays Nintendo with Mathew, who is five years old, and we meet Chris and his parents.

Chris arrived last Friday, transferred from University Hospital after a traumatic brain injury. He had a flat tire on Interstate 64 and was waiting in his car when he was struck from behind. Having heard of Zack's remarkable progress, they were excited to meet him. They had seen his picture from the article written in the *Southeast Outlook* hanging on the wall at University Neuro ICU and were shocked at how good he looked. We talk at length, and I offer advice, encouragement, and hope. Our mission to reach out to other hurting families remains a priority while we are here. Desperate people long to hear the hope that comes from knowing that God is in control.

Having been denied another nap after dinner, Zack is ready to rest and crawls in bed. It doesn't take long before he is asleep. He must be dreaming, and I scoot my chair close to the bed when I hear him talking in his sleep. He mumbles, and I can make out some of his words: "Well, thank you," he repeats several times. I doubt he will remember this tomorrow, so I imagine what he might be dreaming about. I close my eyes and wonder if God is talking to him, telling him what a good job he is doing. If he mumbles, "Stay the course," I'm likely to fall out of my chair.

We may never know of his conversations with God, but I know God is healing him. He has come so far in two months that it's hard to imagine where he may be two months from now. I think back to Psalm 23 that I prayed over Zack so many times at University Hospital. During that horrific time, I dwelt upon the verse, "You anoint my head with oil," but now I claim, "My cup overflows." His promises are revealed in the many blessings that we have witnessed through Zack's recovery. There is no doubt that all of this was part of His plan. A tragic car accident, a devastating injury, and a miraculous recovery, so that God may be glorified.

Arriving at my usual time, I was surprised that Zack was still asleep. I check with the nurses' station and learn he slept through the night, so I don't hesitate to wake him up. As I'm getting him out of bed, he has an attack that really disturbs me. It has been nearly a week since his last spell, so I feel like we had resolved the problem with medication. Zack isn't bothered by it. He just smiles and moves to the table to eat breakfast. Kristi comes to the room for speech therapy and reviews the alphabet, making him write each letter. He unscrambles letters to make four-letter words and matches pictures to words. Although his aphasia is still very present, he has little difficulty with these drills. As I sit quietly observing, I wonder when he will be ready to move out of first-grade material. At this rate, it will be years before he is caught up to where he was before the accident.

The gym is more crowded than usual, with newer patients starting physical therapy. Amy takes Zack to a mat and has to close the curtain to keep his attention. He's wearing his new tennis shoes, and she tightens the laces before starting him on the treadmill. As soon as his time is up, he climbs down and announces, "I need to sit down and fix my feet." It takes him a long time to loosen his laces to his satisfaction, and Amy was not pleased when he was finished. He can slip them off without untying them, and she doesn't feel it is safe. With time to spare before his next therapy, Donna takes him to the cafeteria for a snack, and they talk along the way. She asks him what sport he is going to play when he is strong again, and he grins. "Jugs!" So, there you have it. My sweet, precious, hormonal teenager is still interested in women's breasts. Obviously, his testosterone level has not been impacted by his brain injury.

Returning to the gym, Mary Beth slides him a piece of paper and asks him to write the date and his name. He has no problem, even writing his signature in cursive. When she asks him where he lives, he is able to identify Kentucky, but has trouble with the city. It's his answer to where he goes to school that I find most amusing. He has been talking about how much he wants to go back to CAL (Christian Academy of Louisville), but instead, tells Mary Beth he attends Kentucky Kingdom. No doubt he would like to go to this amusement park, but he wouldn't learn very much.

Moving to a cabinet, she hands him a file folder with his name on it and asks him to file it alphabetically. Without hesitation, he inserts the file into the drawer in the correct location. Mary Beth can't believe how quickly he responds and comments that it doesn't make sense with the difficulty he has reading. She starts to hand him other files, one at a time. Zack leans back with his arms crossed to assess the situation, and then, as if listening to music, he starts bopping his head as he files them away. She finally hands him the whole stack. He snaps his fingers, says, "No problem," and continues bopping to whatever music is playing in his head. Towards the end, as he becomes tired, he struggles and slows down, but completes the task without error. Mary Beth just shakes her head in amazement and notes it in his chart.

When we return for speech in the afternoon, we are back in Kathy's office. Zack gives a gallant effort on relearning how to tell time, but he struggles. He gets the concept, but his aphasia prevents him from expressing it properly. This deficit is manageable in a rehab facility, but could present real problems integrating back into society. Life beyond these walls won't have compassionate therapists correcting him. She asks him to identify objects within a picture, and he has a difficult time. Sometimes, it appears that to Zack the object is just a foreign something. He just cannot retrieve that word from his brain.

The new tennis shoes are a problem for Amy. She hates that they are never tied properly and doesn't want him wearing them to therapy or on long walks anymore. Zack is not happy that his new shoes are banned, and they discuss it while he's on the stationary bike. She explains that it is dangerous for his shoes to be loose, because he could trip and fall, reinjuring his head. He looks at her and down at his shoes, purses his lip and shakes his head. I can read his mind: all of his friends wear their sneakers loosely tied. To prove her point, Amy moves Zack to the rocker board. It's a wooden board, smaller than a skateboard, where he must stand heel to toe and balance it on the rocker. With his shoes not tied tight enough, his foot slides around inside, making it difficult to balance. It is a perfect lesson that I'm not sure Zack appreciates.

As we are leaving the gym, we are approached by the recreational therapist. Carey explains that Zack will go on some kind of outing next week. Hoping for a trip to the bowling alley, I tell him it is a favorite activity, and one that would be good therapy. When we get on the elevator, it's hard for me to contain my excitement at the thought of Zack getting to go anywhere outside of these walls.

After lunch, Zack is in the gym with Mary Beth, and I head to the conference room for a family meeting. Rita and Donna attend, and I'm not really disappointed that Scott needs to work. He doesn't do well in these serious meetings, and I can relay all the information to him myself. This is a smaller group, and a neurophysiologist discusses how the brain recovers. He explains that Zack is tired because all of his energy is expelled trying to heal his brain, rebuilding neuro pathways. He is likely to be easily fatigued for the next 10 years. He confesses that they used to believe that people with brain injuries weren't capable of learning new things more than two years past their injury. Suddenly, it's as if my ears are stopped up; his voice is muffled as I flashback to this morning in speech therapy. Aphasia makes everything harder, and Zack has a lot to relearn. If he plateaus in two years… my mind snaps to attention when I hear his follow up.

Experts now know that healing and learning continues for life. The neurons continue to develop new pathways around the injured part of the brain. I stop gripping the arms of my chair and relax. The human brain is a masterpiece, and I know the Creator. Slowly, the door opens, and there stands God's current project. Mary Beth escorts Zack to a chair and motions for him to stay quiet while we finish the meeting. He patiently stares down at his shoes, periodically glancing at the clock. When he can't take it any longer, he glares at me and gestures with his head towards the door. He may not be able to express the time, but he knows when it's time to go finish his nap.

Still groggy after I wheedle him out of bed to eat dinner, he is confused about the time of day. As he devours his food, we argue over whether it is 6:30 in the morning or 6:30 in the evening. He wants it to be morning, so he can go to therapy. Insisting I'm wrong, he goes to the nurses' station to ask the time, and they concur that it is 6:30 in the evening. He says they are all lying and demands I take him outside to see if it's dark. Pointing to the light coming through the window, I explain that it doesn't get dark until later, but it is still evening.

Several friends meet us in the hallway as we return to the room. I introduce them to my alphabet game, but instruct them to be creative in the words they chose. Zack lounges on his bed and they gather around, laughing as they entertain each other with ridiculous words. I'm amazed that he has aphasia, a language disorder, yet he masters this game with quick, witty answers. As Zack gets tired, his aphasia really kicks in, and he starts making up complex words, convincing his friends they are real. I don't know what Zack's future holds, but God certainly didn't waste the charm and sense of humor.

The remnants left on the breakfast tray let me know that Zack has already been up, but now I find him back in bed. I rouse him from his slumber with the help of an aide who has come to offer him a morning shower. While he is occupied in the bathroom, Dr. Mook comes in to inform me that we have an appointment on Monday with Dr. Haan at University Hospital to discuss replacing his bone flap. He also reports that the evaluation concludes that Zack should remain here another three weeks before being transferred to Frazier East Outpatient Program. Our case worker, Sarah, will have to work this out with the insurance company, since we only have a week of acute rehab therapy left on the clock that started ticking when we left University Hospital. I fully expect a battle, but this time, Sarah will be arguing on our behalf.

Then, I remember the business card that Jude Thompson gave me on his first visit with his son. As Zack gets dressed, I dig in my purse and find the Anthem insurance card. Calling the office number, I reach Mr. Thompson's secretary—who, oddly enough, knows who Zack is. I leave a message that I need assistance with an insurance issue and hang up, hoping he will call me back. Zack was listening to my conversation and wants to know why we had to go back to the hospital. I explain that we have a meeting next week to schedule his surgery, and he insists we take a walk, so he can "find his bone flap". Not convinced that it is stored safely at University bone bank, he wants to go find a better one.

Once in the gym, Amy has him running on the treadmill, followed by several repetitions of squats and stretches. He seems preoccupied, and she asks him if he's tired. "I'm just confused." She drapes her arm across his shoulder and walks him to Mary Beth, announcing that he would like their next activity. He follows them to the kitchen, and Mary Beth explains that he is going to make cookies. His eyes light up and a big grin spreads across his face as he listens carefully to her instructions. Gathering butter and eggs from the refrigerator, with a little assistance to know what to look for, she shows him how to read the temperature settings for the oven. He delights in cracking eggs into the bowl, and is careful not to include any shells. After all ingredients are mixed together, Mary Beth shows him how to make the dough into little round balls and place them on the cookie sheet. Normally, getting his fingers dirty would be upsetting, but not with cookie dough. While his treats are baking, he has to wash the dishes and put them back into the cabinet. This is the kind of life skill that will come in handy, and I hope he can teach his siblings how to clean up after themselves. When the timer goes off, she shows him how to take the hot tray out of the oven and remove the cookies from the tray. His mouth waters as he reaps the reward of his efforts and quickly devours several cookies.

My schedule is complicated, as I attempt to stay involved in Zack's therapy while returning to work. Fortunately, my office is only 10 minutes away from Frazier, but racing back and forth often leaves me frazzled. Finding a convenient parking spot feels like I hit the lottery, and every red light that halts my progress means I will be running down the hall. As Zack gains weight, I lose it, preferring to skip meals, so I can catch as much therapy as possible. Stepping in for me while I'm at work, Donna and Rita are perfect surrogates. They take notes, filling me in on each therapy I miss. Without them, I wouldn't be able to leave Zack. Since my conversation with Dr. Kraft on the documented value of family support, I have been blessed to have them share in Zack's recovery. It is a prayer I never uttered, but one God knew to answer.

Balance is still a concern, because falling would be disastrous if Zack reinjured his head. Amy is tasked with assuring me that when Zack leaves here, he could walk a tightrope and not fall. She has him stand on one leg with his eyes closed and balance himself for five minutes. This is repeated on both legs until they move to the counter to work on a puzzle, where he must also balance on one leg. Amy watches to see if his balance is thrown off when he has to concentrate on a mental activity. His ability to work both physically and mentally requires a lot of stamina, another trait they measure. Finishing the puzzle, he braces both feet on the ground, announcing, "This is killing me." He doesn't always understand the purpose of these exercises, even though they explain it, but he cooperates with genuine effort.

Thrilled to be back in bed, he's relaxing when Rita sneaks in, her hand behind her back. Zack strains to see what secret might be hidden in her hand while she asks if he knows her name. He replies, "Yes, my appendix." She laughs and his eyes follow her hands as she dramatically produces his favorite red licorice. Only Grandma can get away with giving him this forbidden candy, but she has always indulged her darling Zack. He leans his head back on the pillow and chews the stringy treat. She pulls a piece out for herself, takes a bite, and questions if he likes it.

"It killed me."

Puzzled she inquires, "What do you mean it killed you?"

"I'm dead."

Grinning, she teases, "You don't look dead."

He closes his eyes, throws his head to one side with his tongue hanging out. "I am."

Gazing at him with affection, she asks if he's trying to play dead. With a lopsided grin, he confesses that he planned to play this joke on Grandma, which earned him another stick of licorice. Rita agrees that the mischievous side of his personality is intact, and it pleases her immensely. She promises that she has a joke to play on him later.

They stroll down to the gym, and she teases that he won't know when it's coming, so when they take their seats at the table, Zack eyes her suspiciously. Mary Beth brings out a math worksheet and instructs him to add three-digit numbers together. Once he has mastered a few simple problems, she moves on to multiple numbers, where he has trouble understanding how to carry a number to the next column. Working through several problems, he finally grasps the concept and completes the worksheet. Rita starts hollering, "Woof, woof, woof!"

Other patients in the gym take notice, and Zack gets embarrassed, covering his face. Rita cackles, and seeing the confused look on Mary Beth's face, explains that she owed him a joke. He nods his head and laughs, recognizing that he was just spoofed by Grandma. His sense of humor is definitely inherited. Before they leave, Mary Beth writes a "A" on his paper, and says she is very impressed with his progress. Zack is in a good mood as they walk back to the room, and he reads the signs on each door they pass. Surprised, Rita comments that she didn't know he could read so well. Somewhat indignant, he replies, "Well I'm not that dumb yet." This produces another round of giggles.

Tiffany swings by for her daily visit and Rita, still impressed from the reading lesson in the hall, keeps giving Zack words to read. He is no longer interested in entertaining his Grandma and whispers to Tiffany, "We need to get away from this girl." How quickly he forgets who sneaks the candy in his room. I get the same treatment when Averi and Lauren join Tiffany, laughing and sharing secrets with Zack. They decide to go on a walk, and Zack makes it clear that I'm not invited. They stroll down the hall, around the corner and sit on the therapy mat, where they can talk away from me. They pop back in every ten minutes and shuffle off again.

Zack wants to be away from me, but at the same time feels safer when I'm around. He's a typical, confused teenager. When they finally land back in the room, he wants to know when he can get out of here for good. I tell him he has three more weeks. Disgusted, he huffs, "That's no good. It's cutting into my pal time." I know he would like nothing more than to hop in the car and leave with these girls. He walks with his friends to the elevator, and I lag behind, to insure he doesn't get into the cab with them. Dragging himself back to the room, he announces how tired he is. He explains that he worked really hard in the gym, and his legs are sleepy.

Looks like tonight, I will go home early and get eight hours of sleep for the first time in weeks. We have been here so long that Frazier seems like home sometimes. We are well taken care of by the staff, and it is obvious that they love Zack. God put us exactly where we need to be at this time. We are blessed beyond measure, and best of all, we know it. Others may have more possessions, vacations, or free time, but we have a tragedy that awakened us spiritually. We understand the meaning of "all things work together for those who love the Lord." I kiss Zack goodnight and make my way to the parking garage.

Arriving home earlier than usual, I find Scott on the couch, reading the note from school that had come home in each of our child's backpacks. There are tears in his eyes as he hands it to me, and I read out loud of the fundraiser planned by the high school students. They are selling t-shirts with the inscription "CAL loves ZH", and all the students will wear them to school in lieu of their uniform shirts on October 13th. Christian Academy has never allowed the entire student body to be out of uniform. I've been asked to speak at the middle school chapel that day and will be blessed with hundreds of students unified in support for Zack. It's hard to imagine the emotion I will feel when I look out among a sea of young people all sporting t-shirts with his initials. God has been moving so visibly—and at times, audibly—through our lives these last two months. I believe the whole community will hear his thunder on that day. His mercy and grace will be magnified though the lives of teenagers who have witnessed the power of prayer.

Zack had eaten breakfast, showered, and dressed by the time I reached his room this morning. He was waiting for me to take a walk to the hospital gift shop, because there was something he wanted to buy. Leading the way to the elevator, his pace indicated this wasn't a leisurely stroll, but a mission to purchase a trophy. I don't know where he got the idea, so I ask what the trophy was for, expecting some profound answer. He said it was to look at. Puzzled, I decided to tease him and inquire if it will say, "World's Greatest Mom". Standing in front of the locked door to the shop, he pulls on the handle and replies, "You're not that hot."

I grin, "Well, I'm hot enough to know this place is closed."

As we walk back towards the main elevator lobby, he has a slight swagger and bobs his head, as if listening to music. There is a satisfied grin on his face as the elevator doors slide open, and we share the cab with the lady who delivers his meals. When the doors close, Zack smiles and asks her, "Do you want to hear me sing?" She recognizes him immediately, and without waiting for her response, he enthusiastically starts rapping the 23rd Psalm! Bobbing his head, he belts, "The Lord is my shepherd... I shall not be in want. Psh sssh sssh psh...He makes me lie down...in green pastures...Psh sssh sssh psh...He leads me...beside quiet waters... Psh sssh sssh psh...HE RESTORES MY SOUL! Psh sssh sssh psh." His voice carries out into the hall as the elevator doors open. "When I walk through the valley.... Psh sssh sssh psh...of the shadow of death.... Psh sssh sssh psh...I fear no evil...Psh sssh sssh psh...for GOD IS WITH ME!" He shouts the last verse. I am dumbfounded, she is delighted, and Zack is quite pleased with his performance. He leads the way to our room, still bobbing his head, and I trail him, wondering when the gift shop will be open, so I can get him his trophy.

Kathy is being shadowed today by Katie, a cute U of L student who quickly got Zack's attention. He is smiling ear to ear and keeps glazing in her direction as Kathy tries to focus him on reading. Even though he acts silly and aphasia mixes up his words, she reports that they are making strides in reading and feels a breakthrough is right around the corner. He is stuck on the word "contract" today, and uses it frequently as he searches for the two objects she hid. He finds one easily and hovers around the general area where the other item is located, until he holds it up announcing, "Contract."

When their session is over, Katie follows her mentor out the door, and Zack watches as they walk down the hall. Disappointed and obviously smitten, he pouts, "I wish she could have followed us." We make our way to the gym, and he is still stuck on the word "contract", stating it as he pushes the elevator button. I never know where these words come from, but this morning, I'm tickled thinking he may be needing a "contract" to rap Bible verses.

Mary Beth pulls out Zack's folder and reviews the math he completed yesterday, stating how pleased she was, while tapping her pencil on the "A" she had circled. She slides a blank piece of paper in his direction and instructs him to write the date and his name in cursive. Without further prompting, he remembers how to write a cursive Z, and the rest just flows off his pencil. She tells him to write any sentence, and he prints, "Pat Day is a Lola jockey."

Everyone knows the Kentucky Derby-winning jockey. He is a devout Christian, but I don't think he ever rode a horse named Lola. Mary Beth produces a large cardboard clock, and they work on telling time. Today, as she moves the hands to various numbers, he easily identifies the time. It's as if a lightbulb suddenly went off, or the neurons finally reconnected, and he is notably proud of himself. When they move onto seek-and-find puzzles, he scans each row, looking for the words she requires, but can't find them. It is very hard, but he doesn't get frustrated, and when she points to the general area, he locates the word.

After lunch, Zack wants to take a walk to the courtyard to look for "his people". I explain that his friends are in school, but he insists they are waiting for him outside. Following him to the elevator, we tramp through the lobby to the empty courtyard. Agitated when he fails to find his friends, he takes a seat on a small concrete bench, and I slide in next to him. He's quiet, no rap song exploding to fill the vacant square. He breaks the silence and asks if I like it in this place. I explain that I didn't mind being here, because this place is helping him. He considers my response, purses his lips, and shakes his head. I think he understands that therapy is important to his recovery, but he desperately wants to go home.

His mood is still dampened when we arrive in the gym for PT. Amy takes him to the Frazier grocery store and instructs him to find four potatoes, five oranges, three onions, one corn, one pepper, and some miscellaneous items. He walks aimlessly around the small store, unable to identify the vegetables. He comes back to the table, emptyhanded and confused. She shows him each one and then hides them throughout the market. This is an exercise in short-term memory and concentration, but it is complicated by aphasia. He has difficulty trying to express his thoughts, especially when it comes to food. They sit at the table and she distracts him with some generic questions before allowing him to return to the search. Having had the items identified, he finds them all, with only a little trouble locating the pepper amidst a sea of other green vegetables. These are life skills that will help him maneuver in the real world, but it's depressing to watch him struggle to identify objects that most six-year-olds would know.

After a short nap, he requests another walk, and seems to meander with no particular destination in mind. His mood is somber, and when I ask him what's wrong, he just shrugs his shoulders in reply. The lobby begins to fill with office staff heading to the parking garage, and Zack takes note of the time. Guiding me to the elevator, he decides it's time to go back to the room, announcing he wants to take a shower. His dinner arrives as he exits the bathroom and selects clean clothes. He rummages through the top drawer in search of his cologne, which is amply applied in anticipation of female visitors this evening. As I watch him primping, I am reminded of what Dr. Kraft told me: that intelligence does not change because you have a brain injury. Well, apparently, the instinct to make yourself appealing to the opposite sex doesn't either, at least not for my boy. During dinner, Scott calls, and Zack says to tell his dad that he wants to "return to his residence", instead of go home. Words are swirling around in his head, and he frequently recalls higher level vocabulary that proves Dr. Kraft's hypothesis.

As I flip through the channels on TV, trying to find something that will interest him, he calls me over with something to say. "I want to leave here and not come back. That's how it sucks for me." His revelation steals my voice, and I find myself at a loss for words. The pain on his face is mirrored in my eyes that are getting misty. Promising that his continued efforts in therapy will help him recover and get him out of here, I convince him to take another walk. We put a note on the door, in case any friends stop by and begin our trek outside. We walk around the entire Jewish Hospital campus, playing the alphabet game. His gaze follows a car he thinks he recognizes as belonging to a friend, but they turn the corner and drive away. Feeling certain that someone is probably waiting for him, we return to an empty room. I challenge him to checkers, which interest him only briefly, his attention divided between the clock and the door as he waits for guests to appear.

Reasoning a card game might be more his style, I deal out several hands of Blackjack before he gets antsy and wants to roam. I suggest McDonald's, but when we get in the elevator, he punches the button for the basement. We head to the cafeteria, and while eating ice cream, he prods me on what we are going to do. All of my suggestions are met with a bored stare. My cell phone rings, and I let Zack answer the incoming call from his Dad. He listens a moment, and then, requests that Scott come rescue him because, "This woman doesn't know what to do with me." He hands me my phone, and I confess that I could use his help, since we have had no visitors today to keep him entertained.

His gait is a more intentional on our walk back, since he anticipates his dad's more exciting agenda. I try not to be offended that my company is too boring for him tonight, but in the back of my mind, I look forward to the break. Visiting hours are nearly over, and without his friends, I know he will sink further into depression with Mom as his only companion. He plops in his recliner and agrees to watch TV until his dad comes with something interesting to do. I slip down to the nurses' station to tell Kelly that Scott and I are trading places, before popping my head back into the room to say goodbye. Zack salutes me, and without a word, returns his gaze to the TV.

On the drive home, I analyze how our day went from him rapping Psalm 23, to wandering vainly around in search of happiness. I wish I could walk with him on the familiar streets of our neighborhood or go to BW3 to eat and play the trivia game like we did on Friday nights after football games. Anything besides walking the halls of the hospital looking for a way out of what he has come to believe is his prison. The tears begin to fill my eyes, slipping down my cheeks as I realize we have no scheduled therapy tomorrow. If I don't come up with a stimulating weekend plan, I will be facing his despondent attitude for the next two days. I flip on the radio, and as music fills the car, an idea comes to mind. Maybe we can work on finishing his rap song and I will record it, so he can hear himself sing. I wipe my eyes as I pull into our subdivision and murmur a prayer. I plead with God to send his friends, because the 23 Psalm, as beautiful a prayer that it may be, will not fill up an entire day. Shutting off my car, I close my eyes and whisper, "Restore my soul." God nudges me a reminder to just breathe.

The Brain Injury Alliance of KY had notified me of the "Riverwalk", a walk-a-thon to prevent and raise awareness of brain injury, was happening today and the girls want to participate. Riding with me to Frazier Rehab, they are excited to tell Zack that they are walking in his honor. When we waltz into his room, he is eating breakfast and listens as Kyle explains how far they will walk today. Logan chimes in and shows off the t-shirts they are wearing, and they buzz around him, full of energy. I had made arrangements with Donna to pick the girls up out front, so after a quick shower, Zack leads the way to the elevator. He strolls through the lobby, holding his sisters' hands as they vie for his attention. We step onto the sidewalk just as Donna pulls up to the curb and gets out of the car to greet us. It's a beautiful day, and I wish we could all climb in Donna's car and head to the river. Fortunately, Zack is not disappointed when they pull away without him, since he hopes to entertain girls his own age today.

Knowing I have the daunting task of filling Zack's time, we walk towards the gym as I plan in my head what activities would interest him. Zack immediately walks to the stationary bike and sets the timer for 15 minutes, which allows me to search the cabinets until I find the hand weights. Before we have a chance to work on strengthening his right hand, Tom approaches us with his schedule in hand and reports that

Zack has an hour of OT. He demonstrates an old-fashioned method for strengthening the hands and fingers, brings out two buckets, and begins filling one with water. Taking a small hand towel, he soaks it, and then wrings the water into the empty bucket. He has Zack transfer the water from one bucket to the other, solely by wringing out the liquid-soaked towel. Whipping out a piece of paper, he challenges Zack to see who can make the smallest ball of paper, and the contests are on.

As we leave the gym and make our way to the elevator, Zack asks what we are going to do next and raises an eyebrow when I tell him we have speech therapy in his room. Taking his place at the table, he stares at the clock, expecting Kathy to walk through the door. Trying to be as professional as possible, I pull out the folder with lessons she has prepared for me. Zack's lopsided grin tells me he will cooperate with Mom as his therapist, and I pull out the multiple pictures for him to match to their corresponding word. He lines each of them up perfectly, and I mark a big "A" on the top sheet as his grade. When I introduce a word-finding exercise, his aphasia kicks in, and he struggles, but completes the entire page before announcing that he's tired.

Before he has a chance to rest, Kaitlyn and Tiffany pounce on his bed, giggling that it's time for a milkshake from McDonald's. There are so many trips to McDonald's these days that I could undoubtedly find my way blindfolded, but I don't complain. Whatever makes Zack happy, I'm content to oblige. The staff is familiar with our frequent quests for ice cream. I have long ago given up the fight against straws, and Zack laughs as he makes annoying noises, slurping up the last drops of his shake. Once we return to the room, he makes another attempt to nap when Dylan pops his head into our room. It is consuming, trying to work around his football schedule and tennis practice, but today, Avery and her mom pick him up on their way to the hospital.

The brothers fist bump, but Zack is more interested in flirting with Avery. When Dan and his family arrive, I know the nurse will be concerned about the crowd in our room, so we all make another trip to McDonald's. Zack has picked up 15 pounds in recent weeks, which is not surprising, considering the number of fries and shakes he consumes. As I watch him devour a Big Mac, I notice Dylan staring at his brother, a look of adoration on his face as he stuffs his mouth with fries. Four years his senior, Dylan has always looked up to his brother.

Though forced to wear an unattractive helmet and searching for the right words to express himself, Dylan watches as his brother commands the conversation. He teases Avery and jokes around with Dan, occasionally throwing a fry at his little brother. He asks me if Dan can spend the night, but without waiting for a response, he glares at me and tells his friend that he's not allowed to leave this place, so he can't spend the night. I think back to all the weekends that these boys begged for slumber parties and then it dawns on me to ask Zack a question. "On those nights when we refused your request for a sleepover, did you sneak out your window to meet up?" He looks confused, but Dylan, Dan, and the rest of our group know exactly what I mean. I told Zack that he climbed out his window the night of his car accident and that was why he had to stay here: to recovery from a brain injury.

All eyes are on him, and his reply is classic as he addresses his friend. "You can't spend the night. They don't have windows here." The table explodes with laughter, and the mood shifts away from his tragic mistake.

We part ways in the lobby, and Zack tells me he is taking a nap as soon as we get to the room. He grins as his head hits the pillow, and he is snoozing in no time. I take the opportunity to check my messages, hoping to have a reply from Jude Thompson on our request for more acute therapy hours. Before I have a chance to pull up my email, Sarah Cahill knocks on our door. She strides in and looks at me quizzically. She explains that our request was granted. "I don't know who you called, but the case worker's response was three weeks or 60 days, give them whatever he needs."

My astonishment mirrors hers. I dig for the business card under my laptop and hand it to her. Explaining that Zack played basketball with his son, and he had offered to help with any insurance issues. She looks at me, rocking her head back and forth in disbelief. "Jude Thompson, President BlueCross BlueShield. Amazing." I agree that it's a divine connection. Sarah murmurs something about informing Dr. Mook and heads out the door, seeming bewildered. Staring at the card in my hand, I trace my finger across the title. "President" I whisper to myself and smile. He never returned my call. He just approved whatever we needed. It is no coincidence. God placed just the right person on the bleachers next to me years ago, and providentially, he is here to rescue us.

Zack's nap is cut short when Taylor and Jessica bounce in the room. They pile on the bed and fill him in on the latest school gossip. Zack decides we should take another walk. He wants to play them in Chinese Checkers, so we head to the gym. Over the last week, Zack has grasped the concept of the game and plans his moves ahead. Now, he easily beats them both and keeps me at a distance, so I don't cramp his style with the ladies. I trail them around the campus, figuring this won't be our last walk of the day, but I can't let Zack run off without me.

I lumber along, 10 feet behind, as he leads them back to the room. He turns on the CD player, and pop music drifts down the hall. I now have to be the sound monitor, since each new song becomes a favorite, requiring the volume to be jacked up. When "Hollaback Girl" comes on, Zack can't contain himself and jumps out of his chair to dance. His moves become more exaggerated, and soon, we are laughing so hard that tears run down our faces. I look up to see Nurse Dana standing in the doorway, also entertained by his gregarious dance. When the song ends, he flops back into the recliner, pleased to be the center of attention. He tells the girls that he was supposed to start school Monday, and it sucks because they won't let him go. Taylor glances at me, and I shake my head to let her know that it's only wishful thinking on his part to be out of here by Monday.

Another group of friends arrive, and the dance party continues. I perch on my chair in the corner, trying to disappear, so Zack can enjoy his friends and not feel like he's being chaperoned by his mom. I consider how fortunate we are that so many visitors have kept him busy all day. Without much of a nap, he should be exhausted by bedtime. I feel strange thinking that my 16-year-old son requires a nap like he is two, but our visitors understand. This path God has chosen to set us on has been a blessing. Forced into a situation beyond our control has taught us how to trust God. When you see your need for God, you see Him more clearly. Our prayers have been answered in ways we never imagined.

Zack is alive, even though we were told he wouldn't survive. I remember how badly I wanted to see him move a thumb or a toe, and now, he walks and walks and walks. I look forward to the day when he walks in church and stands next to me, lifting his hands in worship as we sing, "God will make a way, where there seems to be no way. He works in ways we cannot see. He will make a way for me."

Mrs. Funderburg graciously volunteered to work with Zack this morning, so our family, including Rita— who has been stepping in on Sunday mornings—could attend church together. I hope she wore comfortable shoes, since he is sure to plan numerous treks around the campus. As soon as breakfast is over, he announces, "Let's go," and they stroll down the sidewalk outside before heading to the gym. He does some light weightlifting to show her how he is regaining strength in his right arm before heading back to the room for his lessons. They work for an hour on object identification, opposites, and number values, but Zack closely watches the clock.

Once his 60 minutes are up, he is ready to put in a CD and show off his dance moves. Deciding that an audience of one wasn't suitable, he trots to the nurses' station and returns with several staff members. He's certainly not shy and quite the entertainer. As his spectators break away to tend to other patients, he decides it's time for another walk, but insists on taking his Walkman, so they can listen to music. The morning sunlight bounces off the windows as they wander around the block, his music the perfect companion. Zack sings the lyrics, and they watch themselves dance in the reflecting mirrors outside the parking garage. They stop in the hospital gift shop just to nose around and a patron compliments him on his beautiful eyes.

Scott had promised Zack a surprise this morning, so he slides out of church and prances into his room with Waffle House. Zack covers his stack with syrup, and the three of them have a feast. Before she leaves, Mrs. Funderburg leaves me a note about their excursion to the gift shop and the compliment he received. She wrote, "His eyes are beautiful, but there is something more awesome and beautiful behind those eyes. Zack is my reminder of how fearfully and wonderfully we are made." I consume her words and store them in my heart as I gaze lovingly at my son.

I feel as though God is creating Zack all over again, and this time, we get to see it happen. As Scott is leaving, a minister from Southeast Christian Church comes to give Zack communion. His daughters accompany him, and my hormonal son is distracted by one in particular. As soon as they walk out the door, he tells me, "That one girl was tight." He wants to find out how old she is. Fearing what awkward conversation might develop, I stop him at the door and offer to find out myself. I catch up with them in the hallway, explain that Zack thought she was attractive, and ask how old she is. Returning to report that she may look older, but she was only in eighth grade, I expect him to be disappointed. He peeks out the door and watches as they turn the corner, replying that he likes eighth graders. It's painfully obvious that he appreciates pretty girls, so I hope God backs off with the testosterone a bit.

Sunday always brings plenty of visitors, and once Kathy exists, a large group of teenagers swoop in. Knowing we will be chastised for entertaining this many in our room, we move to the conference room, and an exciting game of hot potato ensues. Eight kids spread out in a circle and quickly pass around eight balls of various sizes. I'm allowed to referee and announce when to switch directions. It's amazing how engaged they are, playing a childish game and arguing over who causes a ball to drop.

Winded from laughing so hard, they take a break, and Zack announces, "My friends don't think Dad is a good supervisor, so we will have to find somebody else." Andrew immediately goes on the defensive, claiming that no one has mentioned Scott, so I tell him that I will supervise. Zack raises his eyebrow, exclaiming, "Just you?" I ask him if he thinks we need more chaperones, and he looks around the room. "Well, yeah, look how many people we have." I guess he is planning a party and doesn't think his dad will be patient with their rowdy game of hot potato. I'm content to play the role assigned to me, but Scott likes to have his son to himself.

Deciding that he's hungry, our army marches to McDonald's, with Zack leading the way. He orders a Big Mac and chooses a table in the back of the restaurant. Kids gather around and talk about school and the friends who are no longer there. I feel almost invisible. Sitting off to the side, I listen to gossip and watch the dynamics of teenagers interacting. Most parents would love to be a fly on the wall during these intimate conversations. We walk back to Frazier, taking the long way outside, past the Heart and Lung Building. All of the security guards know him and wave to Zack from across the street. They holler greetings to him, and he struts in the front door like a celebrity.

As we say goodbye to this group of friends, another batch arrives. Trey, Nick, and Chas want to play Texas Holdem, and I'm impressed that Zack remembers how to play. He wins several hands before the cards are put away, and the discussion turns to the female visitors who were here earlier. They compliment Zack on his tennis shoes that the girls signed and gave him for his birthday. Nick asks Zack if he can "have um". He replies, enunciating his words, "I know what you're saying. Can I have them?" We all howl with laughter at Zack correcting Nick's grammar. Mrs. Funderburg will love that.

The boys are curious over what girls are frequent visitors, since many come from different schools. They ask if he has a girlfriend, and when he says yes, they want to know her name. He smiles mischievously and says, "Personification."

Trey chimes in, "Wow, big word. Can you define that for us?"

He doesn't miss a beat with his response. "Yes, a person plus an onification." Another round of hysterics. He may have aphasia, but he certainly knows how to use it to get a laugh.

When the last of his guests leave, Zack is ready to climb in bed. Busy most of the day with visitors, he never took much of a nap. He falls asleep quickly, and I reflect on our day. Someone gave me the lyrics to the song he listened to on his walk outside, and I read them as if I can hear Zack sing:

I will never be the same again,

I can never return; I've closed the door. I will walk the path, I'll run the race And I will never be the same again. Fall like fire, soak like rain, Flow like mighty waters, again and again. Sweep away the darkness, burn away the chaff, And let the flame burn to glorify Your name.

I know I will never be the same again. I have witnessed the awesome power of God first-hand. I can testify that that our cries have pierced the ears of heaven, and our prayers are answered.

Zack wastes no time preparing for his morning walk around campus. After a quick breakfast, he showers, gets dressed, grabs my hand, and heads out the door. We barely make it to the elevator when we are interrupted by Dr. Mook, making his way to our room to discuss discharge plans. By the time our conversation is over, there is no time for a walk before speech, and Zack is perturbed. Kathy calms him down and gently asks what he did over the weekend. This is a loaded question to test his short-term memory. He grins and says he went surfing, quickly following up with, "Do you believe me?" She is too savvy to play guessing games and turns her attention to the wall plastered with pictures of his friends. They have reviewed these posters before, but she points to each one and asks who they are, grimacing as he makes up silly names.

When Donna slips in, he refers to her as his sitter and claims he doesn't know her name. He has more difficulty today with matching objects to the written word, and it upsets him when he chooses incorrectly. He is less impulsive when making his choice, but his aphasia is a major roadblock. It is even more apparent when he fails to correctly identify several objects. After several wrong selections, he gets agitated and complains, "I stayed up late last night." In search of the objects that she hid, he goes to the exact location, looks right at them, but still can't find them. When they are pointed out, his reply is disheartening, "That was sad. You got me on that one." I feel as if there is a vision issue that hasn't been identified, but Kathy blames it on aphasia. He can't find an object if he doesn't know that's what he is looking for. Overall, in both memory and cognitive function, speech was a disappointment.

Once in the gym, Zack proves his stamina is improving substantially by extended time on the treadmill and stationary bike. However, when Amy asks who Donna is, he replies, "My sister-in-law," still unable to recall her name. Impatient when Mary Beth is late, he stares at the clock and keeps asking questions. "How do you know what time it is? How do you know when Mary Beth is coming?" It bothers him that he can't tell time, and he desperately wants to learn. It is baffling how some skills seem to come back and then disappear again. Only a few days ago, he accurately answered questions about time with Mary Beth. Now, he glares at the clock like it is a foreign language. He is becoming more aware of his deficits, which is the first step to recognizing and conquering aphasia. However, it also increases his anxiety.

Once Mary Beth gets him settled, he fares better with writing his name, date, and what he did over the weekend. Without help, he wrote, "I played Texas Holdem with my train," and when questioned, recognizes that train is not correct. Given the "f" sound, he finally pulls "friends" out of the cabinet in his brain that still seems so disorganized. Mary Beth understands his frustration and wants him to leave therapy feeling successful at some task. She pulls out a hammer, large carpenter nails, and a block of wood. Instructing him how to hold it, she explains he has to nail it flat to the wood, without bending the nail. This is a risky exercise, since he could easily smash his finger, but he expertly finishes three nails with no incidents. Two weeks ago, he couldn't manage one nail before it was bent beyond use. These victories are crucial to boost his confidence and give him a sense of accomplishment. Physically, he has made substantial progress, but by comparison, his cognitive deficits are magnified.

When he returns to the room for lunch, he announces, "I'm going to flavor in my room tonight." When it is pointed out that one word is wrong, and flavor doesn't make sense, he corrects himself and says, "I'm going to stay in my room tonight. I did good." He wants so badly to correct his mixed-up words. Memories flash across my mind's eye of when he was a little boy, learning to read. He was exceptionally bright and identified the words for numbers, colors, and animals, well before starting kindergarten. I recall him snuggling in my lap as we read book after book, with him filling in the words he could pick out. I considered digging out some of those books, but feel it might be humiliating. My 16-year-old would not want his friends to know he is reading *Goodnight Moon* with his mom.

Our meeting with Dr. Han requires a trek to University Hospital, where I have to fill out mountains of paperwork. Once complete, it was hurry up and wait for over an hour in a stuffy waiting room. Zack was getting tired, so I ask if there was a place for him to lay down, and we were escorted to an exam room. This was more comfortable for him, but not so much for me, now perched on a stiff plastic chair. After 30 minutes, with Zack's patience wearing thin, he sits up and declares, "Suspension of this would be good." Fortunately, Dr. Han sweeps in with his charts at about the time Zack is ready to escape. He is not able to report whether Zack's bone flap has been contaminated, so we don't know where the surgery will occur. If he requires an acrylic flap, we will be sent to Norton Hospital; otherwise, we will be back at University, where it all began.

Regardless, surgery will not occur until Zack is released from Frazier, and Dr. Han is already scheduled two weeks out. After a four-day stay in the hospital, he will be able to start speech and OT, but no physical therapy for two weeks. The stitches will remain for 10 to 14 days, which leads to my request for a plastic surgeon. That appeal is denied, and Dr. Han says he will be doing the closing. He explains that a plastic surgeon would want to remove too much scalp, which would create a new wound as a potential infection site. He is more concerned about getting a good seal on the bone flap and if we were concerned about a visible scar, we could enlist a plastic surgeon when it was fused together and completely healed in 12 to 18 months.

While in the building, we drop into Neuro ICU to see the staff that took care of Zack in the beginning. Christy cries when she sees him, revealing that we gave her the incentive to keep working in ICU, a department with a high turnover. We greet Yolanda, who was astonished to see him walking in, and Karen, our first physical therapist who gave us so much hope during desperate times. Presented with copies of the pictures I took of Zack with each of them when he was comatose, we took new pictures to show his amazing progress for their bulletin board. As we leave the hospital, we meet Dr. Densler on the sidewalk, and he embraces me immediately. This is the surgeon I was told never hugs anyone. He is delighted to see his patient doing so well and poses for a picture. Zack shakes his hand, thanking him profusely when I explain that this is the surgeon who removed his bone flap. Dr. Densler is so enamored with his progress that he asks if Zack and I would speak at the Brain Injury Survivor Reunion next year. They better be prepared for a God-filled message. As we walk back to Frazier, Zack remarks how good it was to see Dr. Densler again, but when I ask if he remembers him, he just laughs, *"No way."* He will not remember the accident or his time in ICU, another blessing from God that all that pain is long forgotten. At least, for Zack. It will forever be embedded in my memory.

At the entrance to Frazier, we run into Amy, and we tell her about our visit back to ICU. When we walk away, he says, "Who is that lady?" I tell him he has worked with Amy in the gym every day since he arrived. He glances back and explains that he knew her, but he didn't know who she was. This is what short-term memory loss does to someone recovering from traumatic brain injury. He has her stored in the file for gym and can't place her on the sidewalk. While we make our way back to the room, Zack says something and mixes up his words. I suggest getting a tape recorder and record him talking so he can hear himself. He is not receptive and becomes upset, saying it would kill him if I taped him. He reveals he doesn't want to hear himself messing up and is near tears at the thought of it. He crawls in bed and finally gets a long-awaited nap before dinner.

Friends start sauntering in after dinner, and he turns on the music to dance. His guests enjoy his routine as much as Zack loves the attention. When visiting hours are over, we escort them to the lobby, and he strolls down the hall with a girl holding each hand. I trail behind, my grin testifying to my amazement at his ability to attract female interest while adorned in a rubber helmet. Any teenage boy would be envious at the parade of ladies that come to see him every day. He may mix up his words, but I still mix up their names. Exhausted when he finally settles in bed, he falls right to sleep. I check my notebook, marking down dates on the calendar, and smile at my slumbering son. I am resigned to the fact that I will be tending to his incision at home after surgery. I would much rather come back to Frazier with nurses fussing over him, and Dr. Mook checking things out, but insurance doesn't work that way. I conclude that I have had enough experience now, and God will take over where my knowledge ends.

There is nothing worse than rush hour traffic on 64W in the pouring down rain. Even though I am running late, Zack is still asleep when I walk into his room. His breakfast is getting cold, but he insists on showering first. He pulls on jeans, a t-shirt, and his new, white sneakers. I hand him his helmet, and he shakes his finger at me, picks up his baseball cap, and places it on his head. A lively discussion unfolds over why he has to wear his helmet, even if he was just sitting in his room. Picking at his eggs and sausage, he agrees to let his therapist decide.

Kristi arrives with a U of L student and introduces us to Billy. She takes her seat, and Zack wastes no time in trying to enlist her opinion of his clothing choice this morning. Pulling on the brim of his Yankee cap, he grins and says, *"Do you think I look good in this? My mom won't let me wear it."* She glances at me, leans forward, and tells him to put his helmet on. He thinks twice about asking Billy, but accepts the helmet, glares at me, and places his cap in my hand. Loosely fastening the strap, he politely asks Kristi if she had worked with him before. Unsure of where the conversation is going, she says she has worked with him several times. He smiles to win her over and reveals that he remembers her. It appears as if he is flirting, so she won't be mad about the hat. She starts to ask questions and some of his answers are impulsive. When asked what he sleeps on, he replies "pistol", but when given the beginning sound of the correct word, he answers "bed". Same with his choice for what do you shave with? "A computer", before he gets to "razor". He thinks about his answer when she slows him down, but the struggle to overcome aphasia is real.

Another U of L student is shadowing Amy in the gym. Zack now has an audience, as Stacey joins in observing his therapy. Word of his unusual recovery has made its way around campus, and all of the students want to study him. He is a unique case. Wanting to prove worthy of their attention, Zack increases his time on the treadmill and adjusts the difficulty on the stationary bike. After physical therapy, Zack insists that he hadn't had breakfast, and Billy walks with us to the cafeteria for a banana. He talks baseball with Billy, who seems fascinated with his progress and the support we have received. The two of them hit it off, and I can sense a challenge coming when we return to the gym.

Mary Beth starts with a memory game on the computer that requires him to remember pictures as they flash across the screen. She keeps increasing the number of pictures while increasing the speed at which they are shown. Whether it was having an audience or his natural recovered ability, he gets them correct each time. He taunts Billy to beat his record. When he misses one, Zack howls with laughter.

Exiting the confined room as the self-appointed champion, Zack wants to continue his interaction with Billy, so Mary Beth gets him a football. They toss it back-and-forth, until Billy spies a hula-hoop and teases him to see if he can throw it through the hole. Determined to prove himself, Zack spirals the ball towards the hoop and makes it on the second try. His competitive spirit is ignited having a guy to show off his skills to. When our session is over, Billy is reluctant to end his observation. Captivated by what he perceives is an amazing recovery, he continues asking questions on the way to our room. He appreciates the need for more male therapists, since boys are twice as likely to incur a traumatic brain injury than girls. I explain our progress through University Hospital, and he looks through the photo album as I point out the timeline. He keeps glancing from the pictures to Zack, almost as if he can't believe it's the same person, and becomes overwhelmed with emotion. Revealing that he's a Christian, he believes that God is answering our prayers and vows to come back again to see Zack.

Having missed his morning journey around the Frazier campus, Zack is anxious to take a walk after lunch. One of the security guards had told me about an outside balcony with a great view, so Donna and I take Zack across the street to the Heart and Lung Building. The rain has stopped, and the Ohio Valley humidity threatens to choke us in the noon-day sun. I thought Zack would enjoy gazing out over the city, but once the stuffy air hits his face, he declares he's not impressed. He decides he would rather walk to McDonald's, but we have another speech session scheduled.

Kristi is waiting for us when we shuffle into the room, and Zack complains that I made him late just to look at the roof. I'm sure at sunset, he would feel differently about our view, but unfortunately the balcony gets locked at 5:00 p.m. She pulls out letters, jumbles them up, and asks him to spell the object. He spells it properly, but can't identify the object. To help break through the aphasia, she has him write the word three times and say it out loud. When she hands him common objects, he is able to identify the purpose of some, but looks at others like he has never seen them before. This language disorder is frustrating his recovery, and it is a mystery how to help him.

Missing a nap, Zack's concentration in the afternoon is affected as Amy works with him on path finding, showing him the directory where his room is located. She drills him on his room number, name, and address, but he is tired and not paying attention. When Mary Beth brings out the seek-n-find puzzles, I fear he may fall asleep at the table, but he is able to circle all of the words she asks him to find. His grasp of math is steadily returning, and he masters all the simple problems easily. On the way back to the room, Grandma Rita asks what his best subject was in school, and he agrees that it was math. When she inquiries about his worst subject, he replies "jacuzzi." She prods him, asking what is hard about jacuzzi. He looks at her incredulously and answers with a straight face, "Saying it." Rita wants to continue their amusing conversation, but Zack can't wait to jump in bed.

He doesn't want to get up for dinner, but I remind him his food gets cold if he waits. Curious about his accident, I explain what happened, emphasizing that he snuck out of the house. He asks, "How did I get that stupid?" There is so much wisdom in that statement. I think we can all relate when we consider the foolish decisions that haunt us. When we play a word game, I discover that if I show Zack a written word, half of the time he can't identify it, but if I spell the word out loud, he gets it every time. I drill him on spelling words, and he does exceptionally well. All of the information is in there; it's just filed wrong. Pulling out my little notebook, I mark down a reminder for Kathy to test him verbally before moving to the visual exercises.

McDonald's seems to be on the agenda when Dan and Andrew make an appearance. It hasn't been that long since dinner, but Zack still wants fries and a milkshake. He selects our table in view of a group of Amish folks in bonnets and long beards. I caution him not to stare, but he admits, "It's hard." I try to distract him with questions and ask where he thinks they are from, but his response, "somewhere messed up," just draws more attention to our table when his friends start to giggle. I'm embarrassed until I notice one of the Amish boys seems just as curious about Zack in his helmet. When Brittney joins our entourage, he forgets all about our unusual neighbors and announces it's time to go. He wants to get back to the room, turn on some music, and dance.

Previous performances were more repetitive, but tonight, I can really see his rhythm coming back. He varies his movements to the beat of the music and extends his hand to Brittney. The boys sit back and watch. An occasional laugh escapes when Zack gets silly, but I imagine that they are envious of his uninhibited expression that seems to appeal to the ladies. I meld into the wall, trying not to cramp his style as I daydream about the day he can finally attend a school dance.

I have no doubt there will be plenty of girls vying for the opportunity to have him as their escort. I hope I will be able to release him to the care of his friends, but I will likely volunteer to chaperone every event. Monitoring his every movement over the last months, I feel like the umbilical cord has reached out like a vine, binding us together. His friends say goodbye, and Zack hightails it to his bed. He is worn out from today's activities and is asleep soon after his head hits the pillow. I imagine the first weekend that Zack comes home, I may be able to sleep in a little longer, but tonight, I am grateful to leave by 10:00 p.m. There have been many obstacles he has overcome—learning to breath, balance, right-side neglect, keeping food down (though, I don't miss the vomit), his dizzy spells, and now the monster of aphasia. I am at peace with our situation: no regrets, just hopeful prayers. I know that there is no mountain so high that God cannot level it. He is the way maker, miracle worker who keeps whispering in my ear, "Just wait until tomorrow."

Holly steers us to the nurses' station after our morning stroll, so she can update Zack's weight in the chart. I'm not surprised, with our frequent trips to McDonald's, that he is steadily putting on pounds, now up to 143 pounds at six feet tall. He is still a little scrawny, but he is building muscle and could stand to gain 15 more pounds. When Kathy arrives for speech, we discuss his aphasia and my finding that he identifies words much better if I spell them. She explains that his auditory comprehension is good, but he has "anomia", one of the components of aphasia. Anomia is the inability to recall the names of common objects, so the goal of speech therapy is to rewire the brain by using exercises that practice retrieving words. He also has a problem recognizing symbols, which makes reading difficult. She shows him a picture and instructs him to find various objects within it. Requiring lots of hints, he indicates it is hard, but he is patient and polite; deep sighs are his only indication of frustration. When he fails to locate the cup, and she points it out, it's like a light bulb goes off, "Oh, that's a cup." He needs a lot of rewiring.

While he works on balance with Amy in the gym, the recreational therapist stops by to remind us that she is scheduling an outing for next week after 5:00 p.m. Kari won't confirm that it's a trip to the bowling alley, but her secret grin leads me to believe that's where we will be going. Dr. Mook also searches us out to report that Zack is going home October 1st and is scheduled to start outpatient therapy at Frazier East on Monday, October 3rd.

Going home! How we have prayed to hear those words. It was nine weeks ago today that I was told at University Hospital to start looking at nursing homes, yet here we are, planning his outpatient schedule. His voice drifts back into my daydream. "Judy, our pediatric coordinator, will contact Christian Academy to coordinate a program to wean him back into school." My mind goes down all kinds of rabbit holes now. Zack can't pick out a cup in a picture, so how on earth will he identify proteins in science or grasp algebra II, when we haven't gone past addition and subtraction?

Panic starts zipping through my heart, and I feel as though my morning coffee may come up into my throat. Suddenly, these walls don't seem so confining, but more like a safe cocoon where my butterfly has not yet grown wings. "Mrs. Hornback?" I slowly sink into a chair as I try to wrap my mind around what he is saying. "Insurance will allow three days a week for outpatient rehab, so we are discussing a tutor through Jefferson County Schools. They could possibly come to your house on the days he's not with us, most likely on Tuesday and Thursday." He waits for my reply, but all I can manage is a half-hearted smile, nodding my head as I stare off in the distance. Dr. Calvary's words during the family meeting echo in my ears… "his injury is difficult to understand, and teenagers can be cruel in their ignorance." I defended his friends and our school system, but thinking of him sitting in class, trying to comprehend new material, has me terrified. I remind myself to breathe and feel my heart slowing down to a normal pace. Breathe. God has moved mountains. He can handle school.

Mary Beth has him shopping again at the Frazier grocery store. She instructs Zack to get four items: ice cream, tomatoes, chips, and cereal. He remembers two of them, so she writes downs the missing items and sends him back with the list, but he still can't find the tomatoes and ice cream. She gives him four new items, and he reads them from the list before searching the store. He comes back emptyhanded, and five minutes later, can't even read the list, confessing, "This is hard." Mary Beth comments that his aphasia confuses her, because it's never consistent.

After lunch, while Zack takes a short nap, I click on the link that Judy gave me regarding services offered through Jefferson County Schools. His brain injury falls under disabilities and an individual education plan will be created based on his needs after he is evaluated. I recognize that we aren't just being thrown to the wolves. There are programs in place that allow him to continue his education with accommodations. I tap the link for forms and realize it will take weeks to complete them all.

Rousing Zack from his slumber, he is sitting on the side of the bed when Kathy returns for our afternoon session. I inform her that we have a release date, and she asks Zack how many days before he is leaving. My mouth opens to answer, as I count out the days on my fingers, but Zack replies, "Nine!" his face lighting up in anticipation. Wow! He figures some things out immediately! I guess when my mind was in a panic over school, he was already counting down the days. Kathy continues with her questions and asks him why he is here. Grinning, he replies, "To see you." She's flattered, but that's not the answer she seeks. "No, what happened that you are here?"

His voice is more somber, "An accident. We hit another car." I guess it doesn't matter that there wasn't another car involved, and Kathy doesn't know the details of the accident anyway. However, I can clearly picture the mangled guardrail that shattered the windshield and collided with his precious head. I imagine the girls screaming in the backseat when they realize Zack is pinned in the car and see his face covered with blood and glass. The sirens from the fire engine racing to the scene and the chopping blades of the helicopter that whisked him to the hospital ricochet through my mind, even though I wasn't even there. They are the sounds that wake me up at night.

Pathfinding with Amy seems like a critical skill to master now that I envision him trying to find his classroom or his locker amongst a sea of grey metal cabinets lining the halls at Christian Academy. She gives Zack several locations to find on the directory, and then, trails him as he wanders through the halls looking for offices. He knows how to get to his room, the gym, McDonald's, and the lobby, but the maze of corridors is confusing, even if you don't struggle with a brain injury. She lets him drift into dead ends and the locked doors of secured staff areas, so he recognizes where his impulsive choices lead them. When they return to the gym, he apologizes for getting aggravated with her when they got lost. He is so sweet.

Since it's an in-service day, the girls are out of school, and Rita brings them by just as Zack fills up buckets with water to wash the Frazier car. Mary Beth agrees to let Logan and Kyle help him, and minutes later, he is cackling as he sees his little sisters covered with suds. He tells them it's funny that they would spend their day off from school washing a car that doesn't even work. Mary Beth asks him what kind of car his dad drives, and he answers, "A truck, black, Mercedes." Kyle knows that's not right, and says it's a black truck, but thinks it's a Ford. A Mercedes truck is wishful thinking on his part. With their help, he finishes the car with time to spare and empties the buckets into the tub.

Mary Beth suggest that his sisters can help him with a puzzle, and they quickly take over while she watches how he interacts with them. He jokes around and gladly lets them complete the puzzle. Riding up the elevator on the way back to our room, he asks about my mom, who is 87 years old. "What are we going to do with Nana?" I have no idea why he would think of her, other than an elderly woman was getting physical therapy on the other side of the gym. Kyle pipes in and inquires what he thinks we ought to do with her, and his response makes me smile. "I don't know, as long as it isn't fishy." He loves my mom and is concerned that she needs a cane to walk now.

When dinner is over, Zack selects a CD and dances with his little sisters. They are enchanted to be included in his dance party, but I know when his friends arrive, he will not want them hanging around. As he twirls Logan in circles, he catches a glimpse of himself in the mirror and decides he needs a shower before his buddies show up. He heads to the bathroom, and Rita agrees to take the girls home, so I can catch up with messages. Dr. Han left a voicemail, reporting that Zack's bone flap had been cleared and the surgery is scheduled for early October. He requests that I call his office for the exact date and get the pre-op instructions. Frazier East has requested his surgery take place prior to beginning therapy, so it looks like we will have to move his start date out another week. I respond to emails and check things off my list, doing my best to be prepared in advance for that glorious day when Zack comes home.

Beginning to master his morning schedule, Zack is up before breakfast to shower, so he can have time for a patrol around campus. He may not be able to verbally express the time, but he watches the clock and knows when Kathy comes for speech. I've noticed on the days when he feels in command of his time, he also performs better in therapy. After a roam around the halls, he is more focused. Kathy drills him with questions, object identification, and reading. He accomplishes more than he has all week. His determined energy continues in the gym, when Amy adjusts the incline and speed on the treadmill, doubling his time from a week ago. Since mastering his signature, Mary Beth has modified her technique as well. Taping paper to the walls, Zack has to print his name and write his signature correctly on the vertical surface, which requires more control than writing on the table.

He moves across the wall, filling each paper as if he's competing for a prize. Computer games have become a favorite, and although Zack does well snowboarding virtually down the snowcapped mountains of Colorado, he improves his score on each attempt at driving a car. Most of his friends have their driver's licenses, and had he not been in an accident, he would possess a permit as well. It's a secret goal each time he plays this game to prove he is capable of driving a car. Mary Beth won't be the one listening to him beg to drive once we go home. She also won't miss getting trounced in Blackjack, since Zack has definitely regained his card skills, consistently beating her.

After lunch, Zack informs me that he needs to take a shower before we return to the gym. The timing is not good, and I remind him he had a shower this morning, but he is fretting over his appearance. He pulls me in front of the mirror, "Look at these pistols on my face." I explain that he can't mean pistols, because that is something that you shoot to kill someone with, and he must mean pimples. "Yeah, the pimples are killing me." It's hard not to grin at his choice of words, which seem to fit the situation perfectly in his mind. It's also a gentle reminder that he is getting back to normal teenage behavior, frequent showers, and obsession over acne.

The clock convinces him another shower is out of the question, and we rush to Kathy's office. His reading comprehension and sentence completion is improving. He completes more than half the work independently, but aphasia still makes word retrieval his biggest challenge. Word of his dance moves made it around the Frazier staff, and Kathy wants a demonstration before we leave. A mischievous grin slides across his face as he shuffles his feet to imaginary music, gyrating at the end for effect. He invites her to our room later, promising a much better performance to actual music. Her compliments provide a boost to his confidence that carries him into the gym, where Amy tosses him a football. She produces a large balloon and asks Zack if he could rest his foot on it without popping it. She demonstrates, resting her shoe on the balloon and asks him to throw her the football. Not to be outdone, and to prove he has as much balance, they switch places. With each catch, I cringe, expecting him to bear down and pop the balloon, but he shows amazing restraint. She moves him to various surfaces, and he balances like a flamingo, never falling.

His swagger leaving the gym reminds me of how he walked in his first cowboy boots. We lived in California, and I had found these tiny, black boots that he had worn everywhere. My two-year-old had strutted around like John Travolta in those shoes, often wearing nothing else as I chased him around the house to get dressed. Now, he struts up to the nurses' station and looks for Emily, the cute brunette receptionist. He leans his elbow on the counter and with his most flirtatious tone asks, "Do you want to give me a shower?" The crimson creeps up her neck and spreads across her face. Several nurses within earshot giggle as I take him by the arm and direct him towards our room. "Come on, Romeo. I think you need a nap." He grins and salutes, like some sailor leaving the dock. Plopping in bed, still sporting a cocky smirk, I'm sure my toddler didn't fall asleep as fast as he does now. Kerri, from recreational therapy, interrupts his slumber when she delivers our outing schedule. She has arranged for lanes at Lucky Strike on Fourth Street Live, so he will be going bowling next Thursday. Zack loves to bowl, and the atmosphere at this downtown alley will be an exciting experience.

During dinner, Dan and his Mom stop by, and Zack decides that McDonald's sounds better than finishing the meatloaf on his tray. He needs no help finding his favorite restaurant and chows down a second meal, taking it seriously that he needs to gain 10 pounds before we leave. When we return to the room, it is full of visitors, and he is surprised that so many of his friends came to see him tonight. He turns on the music and pushes a chair out of the way to create a larger dance floor. I stand at the door, talking with moms who came along to witness his hip hop parties that are gaining notoriety. Normally, my only conversation is with polite teens who feel obligated to include me once in a while, so to have fellowship with other moms is a treat for me. They whisper to each other how Zack's situation has impacted their families.

Teenagers are talking about prayer and the astounding realization that God is in control. Parents are in awe, witnessing a recovery against all odds. We walk with the last visitors to the lobby, and worn out, Zack announces that as soon as he gets home, he is going to sleep. It's ironic he refers to his room as home, but it won't be much longer. Dr. Han left a message at the nurses' station that his bone flap surgery is scheduled for October 5th at University Hospital. I will return to that same, second floor surgery waiting room, where God's plan had been set in motion. This time, I won't hold the tattered, bloodied clothes from the accident, but rather, the image of my son recreated.

God's perfect plan continues to unravel and amaze me. I consider His promise in Isaiah 48:18—

"Do not remember the former things, nor consider the things of old. Behold, I will do a new thing, now it shall spring forth; shall you not know it? I will even make a road in the wilderness and rivers in the desert." Our wilderness was the ICU, and Frazier is the desert he flooded. I have an unshakable faith that God is at work on a new creation in Zack and I can't wait to see what springs forth.

$Z$ack is up early and has already showered, dressed, and eaten breakfast by the time I arrive. As we head out the door for our morning jaunt around the halls, Dr. Mook and our case worker stop in to discuss his release and upcoming surgery. Sarah says that someone from the Centre for Neuro Skills is coming to speak to me about their program. This is a one-of-a-kind facility in Dallas, Texas that incorporates independent living with intense therapy. Apparently, Dr. Kraft has closely followed Zack's progress and has reported his findings to the Centre.

When their representative arrives, she reports that Zack is the perfect candidate for their program: a good student, no behavior issues, cooperative, actively participates in therapy, and has a high level of rehabilitative outcome. I thumb through the slick brochures, full of smiling patients and engaged therapists, that offer outcome-driven therapeutic rehabilitation. Frazier has referred him, and he has been accepted, but now, we have to get insurance approval. I have been through this battle before, but something else is gnawing at me. Walking to the gym to catch up with Zack, my mind is pouring over details left unanswered. Would Zack go to Dallas alone? Could we afford a leave of absence from work for me to go with him? How long would he stay there? The thought of sending him hundreds of miles away and only talking with him by phone leaves me feeling physically ill. I sink into a chair in the hallway, take a deep breath to calm myself, and examine the business card she handed me. They offer extensive life skills for those with traumatic brain injury but … where is the family?

I peer down the corridor, trying to get a glimpse of their perfect candidate, and I see my son concentrating as he balances on the incline ramp. The lump in my throat pushes the tears out of my eyes, and a steady stream falls of the vinyl floor between my legs. Uncurling my fist, I look at the card now crumpled in my hand, and smooth it out on my knee. Am I denying Zack an opportunity for the best outcome because I can't bear to be away from him? I feel selfish as I consider not even pursuing the insurance approval. I close my eyes, squeeze out the last tear, and listen for God's voice. If this is part of your plan, Lord, please let me accept that my role in his recovery will be at a distance. Then, I start compiling a mental list of friends who might offer me their frequent flier miles.

Plastering a smile on my face, I enter the gym, determined not to let my negativity rub off on Zack. He finishes a game of solitaire on the computer, turns, and proclaims, "I whipped that lady." I fight back tears, thinking I won't hear about these tiny victories in Dallas. When we get in the elevator, he asks where I was when he was working with Amy.

Knowing how badly he wants to go home, I decide it's best not to mention the Centre and ignore his question with one of my own. "Did you have to balance on a balloon again?"

His reply made me laugh, since I'm certain that Amy didn't sit on it till it popped. Once in the room, I clear off the table for his lunch tray, hiding the brochures beneath the papers on my desk. While he is eating lunch, he keeps one eye on the clock, swallows the last bite, and announces he is taking another shower. I am thankful we are not paying the water bill, since he is back to three showers a day. He also changes his clothes each time, generating heaps of laundry, making me indebted to my neighbor, who still volunteers for this task.

Sporting another outfit, he struts to Kathy's office for speech, throwing peace signs to the residents as we pass their room. Leading the way, he has traveled this path so often he could likely find her blindfolded. He does surprisingly well unscrambling letters to spell words of objects he must search for in a picture. She changes course and has him describe what is in the picture, expecting aphasia to hamper his expression. Word retrieval may come slowly, but she is impressed as he describes flowers as colorful, you get them for a surprise, and they smell good.

When we get to the gym, Mary Beth challenges him to a spider walk race. She is no match for my competitive, determined athlete, and he easily beats her across the gym. I watch him collapse in laughter and notice the weight gain is starting to show. Muscles have regained their shape, and I think if he stood next to Andrew, his lanky best friend, he would actually appear more physically fit. Unfortunately, his muscles don't help when they move to the Frazier grocery store. He has difficulty finding any of the items on the list, but after several hints, he is successful. Zack never went to the grocery store before the accident, so I wonder if the outcome would be different if he was searching the shelves for things that interested him. Maybe we should try sports equipment or have him locate different brands of sneakers. I know grown men who are lost in a grocery store.

Frazier Rehab is located in Jewish Hospital, which is part of a larger campus of hospitals and medical office buildings. We have exhausted most of the corridors within our building and search for new trails to blaze. After dinner, we walk to Norton's cafeteria to get a slushy and watch the commuters in the traffic outside our window. Our small talk turns to Zack's aspirations, and he states that he's not sure what he wants to be yet. We narrow it down to a doctor or a preacher. Intrigued, I ask him what he would preach about, and he replies, "I will preach the Word, and the Word is God." I comment that it would be a short sermon, and he says that's all the people need to know. If only it were that easy to convince people the truth of the gospel.

As we continue our stroll to the parking garage, I imagine what an amusing preacher he would be with aphasia. Our walk takes us to the roof, and we look out over rush hour traffic. I point out various landmarks, University Hospital, the river, and finally, the direction of our home. We stand silently, staring east, lost in our own thoughts as the sun paints a glorious sky behind us. Up here, looking down upon the world, it doesn't seem as threatening. I think that way beyond that horizon is Dallas. I set my chin and vow not to get weepy. If God chooses that path, I will figure out how to fly there often.

Zack's legs are getting restless, and he heads towards the elevator. We maintain an almost marathon pace as he leads us around the building to the main lobby. He is concerned that his friends might be waiting in the room and is disappointed to find no one there. I coax him into a game of golf. This is a card game that requires strategy, planning, and math skills. He actually taught me how to play the year before his accident, and now, I have to refresh the rules as I deal out six cards. After the required nine hands, with no mercy from me, he beats me fair and square. He may not be able to go to the grocery store, but he certainly knows his way around a card table.

While Zack is gloating over the score of our game, pointing out his win by circling the score several times, my friend, Teri, drops in with her daughter, Kirsten. With school back in session, they haven't seen him in nearly two weeks, and Teri is yakking in my ear, amazed at his progress. Sometimes, I forget that only a month ago, he was barely speaking, so his evolution is remarkable to those who haven't been here. Zack decides that he's ready for McDonald's, so they join us for his second dinner. Following him down the corridor, I brace myself for the bruises as Teri hits my leg to emphasize her amazement. He leads us into the restaurant, politely holding open the door before picking out his favorite table in the back. Kristin chatters on about cheerleading, and Zack slurps up every last drop of his vanilla milkshake. We walk them to their car before taking the long way back around the building.

The streetlights start to flick on, warning of the time, and the guard in the lobby taps his watch as we enter. I realize we should have cut through the building, since they don't want him outside after visiting hours. As soon as we cross the threshold of his room, he heads to the bathroom for another shower. Worn out and relaxed from the warm water, he is asleep by 9:30, leaving me to ponder the events of the day.

The quiet is interrupted when Scott calls, and we discuss Dallas in hushed tones. He hears the uncertainty in my voice and reminds me to accept whatever happens, because we know that God has carefully orchestrated it from the beginning. We have learned that our plans can change in an instant, and we have to look ahead with hope, regardless. I hang up, convicted that the past should not be a place where we live, but something we learn from. My boy sleeps peacefully unaware of the tug of war going on with my heart and Dallas. I touch his cheek, afraid that if I kiss him goodnight, my emotions will spill out over his pillow. I whisper to myself that God is in control… just breathe.

Weekends have become a validation of how well I pay attention during the week to his therapy exercises. With only minimum therapy on Saturday and Sunday and no real schedule, it is up to me to reinforce what skills Zack needs to master. Kathy often provides a folder of worksheets that we can review, and she encourages card games. This morning, we have OT scheduled in the gym with Angela, so Zack sleeps in until after 9:00 a.m. He is still snoozing when I arrive, and his breakfast is getting cold. Waking him up is a morning treat for me, since he always greets me with a sleepy smile. He doesn't get serious about the day until he has his shower, and I persuade him into eating first, so we can talk about his schedule. Recreational therapy is scheduled in the conference room. I'm not sure what that will entail, but I hope it's better than our experience with art therapy.

PT with Angela starts out slow, just checking out his finger dexterity by having him thread a metal hose through wooden holes. This exercise is easy for him, but when she checks her notes and heads towards the grocery store, I know he will be challenged. It is not his concentration or short-term memory that makes shopping difficult, it's the aphasia that prevents him from recognizing the items on the list. Even when he personally writes them down, he still can't find them on the shelves. He stares at the salt as if it's not there. I'm still not convinced that there isn't an issue with his vision, which further complicates this exercise. Imagine being sent into a room to retrieve objects that someone requests in a foreign language. Bring me getreide, seife, and kartoffel. Would you be able to find corn, soap, and potatoes? Sooner or later, you hope to learn the language, but with aphasia, the next time you seek out those items, it's in Japanese, instead of German. Zack knows the purpose of each object; he just doesn't know what they are called.

There are four other patients in the conference room when we arrive and find two seats together. This room contains more than just a large table, and we find ourselves near the upright piano, which never seems to be in use. The purpose of this meeting becomes apparent when one of the therapy dogs pads in and makes his way around the room. Many survivors of traumatic brain injury have decreased social skills, so bringing them together in this type of environment helps them adjust to leisure participation. Zack has no trouble in the social area, since we have been conditioning him with visitors since day one. He does have somewhat of a fetish with clean hands. He willingly pets the gentle Golden Retriever, but once the dog licks his hand, he is done with recreational therapy. Keri reminds us of our bowling outing next week, and we head back to the room.

Tiffany arrives just as Zack decides he needs to get up and move. The hallway seems like the perfect spot to work on Amy's foot drills, so he starts out walking backwards around 4South. At first, he doesn't trust us to not let him run into things and keeps glancing over his shoulder to avoid a collision. But when Tiffany turns to walk backwards beside him, it's a contest to see who can go faster. They circle the nurses' station, with Zack enlisting a cheering section. After the first lap, they switch to sideways walking, and then, the grueling physical challenge of lunges. He groans, turning the final corner, and Tiffany gives up completely, but our exercise is not over. The last lap is skipping, and I tease him that I hold the record for my fourth-grade class. You can imagine the sight we make, prancing around the hallway, being cheered on by the nurses. Refusing to concede that I had beat him, he collapses in his bed, complaining how badly his legs hurt from the lunges.

Spying the cards, I shuffle the deck and proclaim he can seek his revenge at the table. He jumps into his chair and reviews the rules of "Golf" for Tiffany. This time, I mark the paper with columns and instruct him how to keep score. After each hand, he has to add up our individual points and counts the cards like a pro. With nearly flawless strategy, he beats us both twice, but I am more amazed at how quickly he adds up our cards to register the scores.

With his legs recovered, and the sun beckoning us outside, we walk to University Hospital to visit the nurses in Neuro ICU. Several staff members were missed on our jaunt earlier in the week, and I was hoping to see Dr. Mutchnick. Members of the Critical Care Team and Nurse Tom are delighted to see him walking and astounded with how well he has recovered, but Dr. Mutchnick is nowhere to be found. I have imagined his bewildered reaction when I present the patient who was doomed to linger in a nursing home and has now risen like Lazarus from the grave. That won't happen today, since he fails to respond to the page.

On our trek back to the room, we play a memory game, where we each add an item that we are taking with us on a trip. As the list grows, Zack gets tickled trying to remember his bizarre choices. He doubles over, holding his sides and laughing until it hurts. His glee is contagious, and I nearly pee my pants searching for a restroom. Depression seems like a fleeting memory, but these moments of sheer joy are embedded in my soul. Even the security guard chuckles as we enter the lobby, and he has no idea why.

Claiming exhaustion, Zack jumps in bed and asks me to find the football game on TV. I click through the channels, unable to find the game that interests him. I'm about to give up and hand him the remote when Dale and Lauren slide in. Another avid fan, Dale conveniently brings up the college game, and I get a moment to rest myself. By the first commercial, Zack announces we need to play "Golf" again, and we gather around the table. They catch him up on the latest gossip at school and reveal that tonight is the homecoming dance. That magic word brings out the CDs, and music draws Zack out of his chair to show them what moves would be gracing the floor, if only he could go. Behind the smiles, I sense that Lauren regrets bringing up this favorite event, knowing that they will walk out the door and leave him behind. He walks them to the elevator and reminds them that he will be home soon.

Staring at the door as it slides shut, he tells me how badly he wants to leave with them. No doubt, the thought of dancing in the high school gym, festooned with balloons and plenty of partners, seems like a dream come true. He sulks into bed, barely interested in the football scuffle still in progress on TV. Perched in my chair, I wonder if any more friends will visit tonight, since most will be attending homecoming.

It isn't until Scott struts in with pizza that I finally see him smile again. Dad knows just how to elevate his mood as he tunes in the U of L game and divvies out the slices. Zack relaxes in the recliner, pizza sauce dripping down his chin and cheering on the Cardinals. Sitting quietly in the corner, I feel grateful that the game has overshadowed missing out on the dance. I look forward to the day when Zack can enjoy normal activities with his friends; then, I realize that things will likely never be normal again. I have a strange sense of peace about that. God has taught me not to dwell on the past, but to embrace the idea that his future will be even better. Normal is overrated anyway.

The rain this morning slows us down as I make my way to Frazier after Sunday service with Dylan, Kyle, and Logan in tow. Mrs. Funderburg and her husband graciously step in again to allow our family to attend church together, and Zack drags her through the corridors, looking for *"that place"*. She is so patient with him, and after roaming the halls, she finally asks where they are going. Smiling, he responds, "Kroger," but immediately starts laughing, since he knows that isn't right. Finding the Wall Street Deli and the gift shop closed, Zack decides they better return to the room before "that man" (Mr. Funderburg) gets tired of waiting for them. As a typical teenager before the accident, he wasn't really concerned about whether he was being inconsiderate of adults, but now, he seems so polite and thoughtful.

Cardiopulmonary is required to monitor Zack's heart for 24 hours to ensure he doesn't have any more issues with orthostatic hypotension, the low blood pressure that was causing his dizzy spells upon standing. Katie attaches the silver dollar-sized electrodes to his bare chest, where wires lead to the monitor the size of a small camera that is strapped around his waist. Zack is curious and cooperative while Katie explains how to record his activities in the journal, so they can compare the differences in his ECG readings. She is enamored with his charm and flirtatious grin, which seems to be a frequent response from the staff. Once he is all hooked up, he elects to show off his card playing skills and beats Mrs. Funderburg in Blackjack. Not to be left out, Mr. Funderburg shows him how to play table football with paper folded into a triangle and fingers as the goal post. Zack is delighted to have another game to master, and promptly beats his new adversary.

Listening to the Master's Men belt out beautiful melodies as our church service begins, I lean over to Scott and whisper that if Zack doesn't go to Dallas, he might be sitting here with us next Sunday. The thought that we could be worshiping together as a family again, that our son would finally be out of the hospital, is overwhelming, and tears track silently down our faces. We sit lost in our own thoughts, both praying that God will give us peace with his plan.

When our brood arrives at Frazier, a volunteer from Southeast Christian Church is there to give Zack communion. Mr. LaFan gathers us around the table, and we bow our heads as he offers a prayer. Midway through his plea, he is overcome with sentiment and has to pause to regain his composure. It reminds me of how tragic our situation can seem, but we feel blessed with remarkable recovery. It is apparent to believers that God's hand has been guiding us, and He is in control. His pause gives me a second too long to bring Dallas into the picture in my mind, and I am once again wiping away tears. I sense two pairs of eyes carefully watching me. The girls aren't aware that their brother could end up hundreds of miles away, or they would be crying, too.

Off to McDonald's for lunch, and our crew heads to the pedway, to avoid the rain. Zack jokes with his little sisters, occasionally pointing out that, "This one here doesn't know where she is going," as Kyle tries to lead the way. Aphasia makes name recall especially difficult, but it is obvious from our conversation he knows who his siblings are, and he reminds them that he will be coming home soon. Our meal seems so familiar with the boys stealing fries from one another, and me trying to hush their voices, so as to not disturb the other patrons. Soon, my giggles join their celebration, and I'm less concerned about the scene we make, grateful not to be eating in a hospital cafeteria. A month ago, I would have never imagined such an ordinary activity was possible, and now, I dare myself to dream up dinners at home again. I suspect next week we will either be planning a cookout at home or stuffing my heart in a suitcase as we pack him for Dallas.

Our trek back to 4South is peppered with skipping races, and Zack gets silly with his answers when questioned about what he does in therapy. The cards come out in the room and a game of "Golf" ensues as his friends start to sweep in. When Trey and Nick arrive, the challenge turns to Texas Holdem, and another familiar tune sweeps across my mind as Zack informs me the little kids can't play. Clearly disappointed that they no longer have their brother's attention, I'm charged with entertaining the girls while Dylan is allowed to watch the card game.

Zack talks about going home and how much he looks forward to returning to school. More than once, I have to caution guests not to ask about Dallas, since we haven't discussed that possibility with him. The cards are traded in for a plethora of balls, with Dylan and the girls being allowed into the hot potato circle. I lean in the doorway, taking in their escapades, and their laughter echoes through my veins. My mind wanders, and I find myself staring at the raindrops gently pounding our window. If he doesn't go to Dallas, I still have work to do to prepare for him to come home. How can we put him back in his bedroom in the basement with that window beckoning like a bad dream for him to escape? Would Scott be comfortable sleeping on the floor outside his door, or should we consider putting Zack on a pallet in our room?

Andrew's voice breaks through my daydream. He reminds Zack that he only has a week left and asks if he is ready to come home. "I've been ready!" elicits cheers from everyone but me. I'm frozen in the realization he may not remember home. Is home just anywhere outside of these walls that have kept him captive the last two months? He knows his friends, but not their names. If he walked into our house, would he even remember where his bedroom is? Does it matter?

Kyle fiddles with the CD player and a slow ballad has Zack twirling Kara on the dance floor that makes up the center of his room. As I watch the scene unfold in front of me, I picture him all gussied up in a suit and tie, prancing around the floor at Winter Ball. Would he be at Christian Academy for that special occasion, or is Texas going to swallow up my son for months on end? My racing thoughts are interrupted when Scott slips in to take over for the evening. I review the journal entries, cautioning him not to forget to record all activities, so the ECG readings are accurate. Rounding up the rest of my kids, we head to the parking garage, and the bickering begins over who will get the front seat. Logan moves close to take my hand, apparently the only child who notices my indifference to their seating arrangement, which is uncharacteristic. The drive home has me miles away, conjuring up pathetic scenes with Zack alone in Dallas, while his friends commemorate without him.

It hardly registers when my phone rings, and I answer it absentmindedly. Donna picks up on the forlorn nuance in my voice and responds to my sadness over what Zack is missing out on. She reminds me that he will experience things that his friends will never share, and one day, will speak before his classmates on how God rescued him. He will recount his recovery at the Brain Injury Survivors Reunion next summer and embody a symbol of hope. He has encountered dedicated, compassionate staff at Frazier and conquered battles that his friends can only imagine. Now, my tears are a reminder of how brave, strong, determined, cooperative, polite, and kind my son has become. I don't know if I could have described him that way before the accident. I'm beginning to comprehend the depth of character that Dr. Kraft identifies in his patients with brain injury. I think of the comparisons he offered and contemplate how Zack's injury has refined his moral fiber. I loved my son from the moment he took his first breath, but now, I admire the new creation God has given us. Revelations 21:5— "Behold, I make all things new."

Several accidents on I64 interfere with my progress, and I arrive much later than usual. The breakfast tray is empty, and Zack is already in the shower with Jennifer standing watch outside the bathroom door. She reports that he removed his heart monitor upon waking, announcing to the staff that he wore it long enough to prove he was alive. Dr. Mook must agree, because he discontinued the medication he was taking for low blood pressure. The door swings open, and Zack smiles at me while declaring I am late. Accepting my apology, he nods to Jennifer, "Thanks for watching me."

Sunshine floods though the window, and he is anxious to get outside to feel it on his face. He has taken care to match up his clothes and checks out his reflection in the lobby window. He comments how his head would look much better in a ballcap and threatens to throw his helmet in the garbage can. Bumping fists with the guard, he heads out the front door, and we lap around the building. The changing season adds an invigorating breeze to our morning walk, and he stands at the crosswalk, breathing in the sweet fall air.

When we return to the room, his case worker is waiting. When Sarah mentions the Centre, I pull her into the hallway for a private discussion, explaining that Zack is unaware of the potential of more rehab out of state. She reveals that we did not have insurance approval on Dallas yet, but the Centre was coming for an in-depth evaluation on Thursday. Last night, Scott and I agreed that when it came time to tell Zack, he would be the one to break the news. Perhaps that bomb should drop tonight.

We are being shadowed by a U of L student. John introduces himself to Zack. Pursuing a connection, he asks Zack about the sports he played and picks up his baseball. The paraphernalia adorning our room indicates that he was an athlete, but Zack doesn't remember playing any sport. John understands the complexity of his injury when Kathy begins speech with object identification. Although he can spell the word with ease, he cannot identify the item in a picture. Aphasia strangles his attempts to complete four-word puzzles, and he is stuck on the word "eclipse", using it repeatedly.

When we walk to the gym, John studies Zack intently while I answer questions about his accident. Like most students who shadow us, he is staggered by the progress achieved in such a short time. His education continues when he is drawn into physical therapy and tosses a medicine ball with Zack. There is a genuine smile engulfing Zack's face, but John's looks more like a grimace as he struggles to keep up with him. Amy is attuned to the affect a male competitor has on Zack's determination, so she has John challenge him in badminton with a balloon. He does not disappoint, playing as if defending a Wimbledon title, and again, John is the one huffing at the end of their game. He has a chance to recover when Mary Beth moves Zack to the computer to type sentences. Now, the encounter is no longer physical, but a cognitive trial that prompts frequent requests for help.

Lunch is followed by a quick nap, and when Zack wakes up, he complains his arms are sore. Forgetting about tossing the medicine ball, he rubs his shoulders remarking, "Did you beat me up this morning?" When John walks in with Kathy, Zack doesn't remember him, explaining, "I was sleeping during that." Unfortunately, it was not a dream. Short-term memory loss is amplified when he is tired. Kathy demonstrates the frustration of his language disorder with another exercise. She selects two items—a belt and a sock—and asks Zack to point to the belt. No problem. She places a spoon next to the sock and ask which one is a spoon. He points to the sock. Then the aphasia kicks into high gear, and he cannot identify any of the objects by name, but can show what each one is used for. At least he won't try to eat with a sock.

When the session is over, we walk with John to the elevator. He shakes Zack's hand, wishes him good luck, and steps into the cab. The look on his face as the door slides shut is one of resignation; the patient he spent half a day with won't remember him tomorrow.

Grandma Rita joins us after physical therapy and questions Zack on how he would respond if Dylan tried to sneak out of the house. "I'd smack him. A big, large hand of smack'em." Well, that's a message I won't interfere with, and one he definitely learned the hard way. Rita wraps her arms around him and whispers how much she loves him. I have given up trying to prevent her from slipping him forbidden candy. He associates the sweet treats with the woman from his childhood. Perhaps that's why he never forgets who she is, since after each visit I find the wrappings that are left behind. She has always indulged her grandchildren, but now more than ever, she wants Zack to enjoy life's simple pleasures. In her mind, that must include candy.

Scott arrives after dinner, and Zack acts silly when the nurse comes to take his blood pressure. His dad instructs him to settle down, and the authoritative tone gets his attention. When I ask him who is the boss, he looks at me, but immediately points to his dad. That's just as well, since after I leave, Scott will break the news about Dallas. Andrew and the guys drop by and fill Zack in on the latest happenings at school. The comedian in Scott, always interested in an audience, seems to have disappeared, and he is more preoccupied with how to approach his mission tonight. Zack ushers his friends to the elevator, which gives me a moment alone to offer advice. Scott waves me off, revealing he has thoroughly rehearsed his presentation and really just wants to get it over with. The tremor in his voice indicates he is not as sure of himself as he wants me to believe. An encouraging hug, and I'm out the door, not envious of the conversation he's tasked with.

Once they are alone, he praises Zack's efforts in therapy and says that he's a rock star among the staff. He asks him if he still gets frustrated and whether he wants to learn how to use his words right again. Describing a place that sounds more like going off to college, he explains that there is a Centre in Dallas that has offered him a scholarship. Brilliant! At first, Zack reveals that he is scared to go, but his dad promises he will graduate after only a semester. They talk about the weather in Texas and agree that a cowboy hat will look much better than his helmet. When he tucks his son in bed, he reminds him that no matter where he is, he is not alone. The God that carried him through therapy at Frazier will rustle cattle with him in Texas.

I have a sense of peace as I drive into Frazier this morning and reflect on how Scott presented the possibility of more rehab in Dallas to Zack. To consider this move as if he is continuing his education, makes it an exciting opportunity and not so fearful. Believing that God has carefully choreographed my son's recovery means that I must trust His plan, even though it might separate us for a time. As Zack maneuvers through his morning speech, PT, and OT sessions, I keep one eye on the clock, preparing my heart for his evaluation just before lunch. He is more concerned about his outing this evening to Lucky Strike and trash talks with Amy, vowing to beat her in bowling.

A clinical nurse evaluator from the Centre for Neuro Skills introduces herself and addresses her queries directly to Zack. She asks him a variety of questions about his abilities, and he answers them all correctly. The aphasia kicks in at times, but she is aware of his deficits and needs to see the extent that it impacts his responses. Instructed to draw a floor plan of his room, he works on it carefully, and I can identify the bed, even if the rest of his furniture is obscure. To evaluate his cognitive skills, she has him answer some more thoughtful questions. "What would be the reason a letter would be returned to you?"

His reply, "The Lord," was not what she was looking for, but made me smile. As she finishes checking off her list, Wendi confirms that he is the ideal candidate for their program and will be finalizing the request to our insurance company. She has to provide a written evaluation of what the Centre would do to address his needs that couldn't be done here and expects a reply tomorrow. As soon as she leaves, Fox 41 News Team arrives to interview us. Word of Zack's accident, severe injury, and miraculous recovery is just the sort of inspirational story they like to feature. This gives me an opportunity to explain that we feel led by God to inform other teenagers how simple decisions can change their lives forever, and that through therapy and prayer, amazing things can happen. Stephan Johnson is touched by Zack's determination and positive outlook, promising to stay in touch for a follow-up story. The evaluation and interview cut into his nap time, so the reporter is barely out of our room when Zack jumps in bed.

The anticipation of a bowling outing prevents him from sleeping, and Zack decides he wants to shower, instead. He carefully selects his clothes and struts to the nurses' station to see if they approve. Taking advantage of a captive audience, he shows off his dance moves, finishing off with his version of a Michael Jackson moonwalk. They are delighted and reveal that no other patient has entertained them with such joy. In the gym, Mary Beth sets up plastic bowling pins, instructs him how to stand and when to release the ball. Once he gets the timing down, he starts to throw strikes and pick up spares. She points out that his right wrist is still weak, and he should use a lighter ball at Lucky Strike. High-fiving Amy, she reminds him of their challenge, and Zack reveals that he likes dancing better than bowling. Perhaps he's pushing for a disco outing to seek his revenge in the event that she beats him on the lanes.

As we wait for recreational therapy to announce our departure time, Zack prepares as if he's going on a date. Brushing his teeth and examining his face, he comes out of the bathroom without his helmet. He casually walks to the dresser and puts on his ball cap, gazing at himself in the mirror. I shake my head and explain that he cannot leave his room without his helmet. "I cannot bowl in that thing. My balls will not be strikes if you make me wear it." He plops down in the recliner, and I decide to let his therapist answer this complaint. Amy arrives with Karri, and without argument, Zack trades out his hat for the helmet.

Rita is surprised when she learns we are walking the five blocks to Fourth Street Live, but it is a beautiful day, so Grandma agrees to make the trip with us. The guard in the lobby sends us out the door, promising to inform any visitors of our destination, and Zack steps into the sunshine, grinning ear to ear. Initially, he sets a fast pace as we make our way down the sidewalk, but I notice he keeps slowing down and glancing over his shoulder. When Amy asks him why he is walking so slow, he looks back and replies, "Because of that lady back there." Rita has been walking with us, but couldn't keep up and has fallen way behind. My sweet boy was slowing down, so his grandma could catch up.

Striding into Lucky Strike, Zack inhales the atmosphere, his eyes lit up with excitement. Amy helps him select the right ball, and we exchange our sneakers for bowling shoes. Zack bowls first and starts off with a spare. By the time we get to the second frame, his friends start to arrive, and Amy shoots me a knowing look. Seeking to avoid unnecessary distractions, they had requested that we keep our group to just the family, but she knows that's hardly possible. Before the first game is over, at least 10 teenagers are cheering him on from the sidelines. Each strike is met with roars from the gallery and his occasional gutter ball elicits chants to stay focused. Each time, he is careful to check the scores, and he battles for the lead with Amy, losing by five pins in the final frame. He poses for pictures with his friends and is reluctant to leave when the event is over. Rita hitches a ride with Andrew, who promises Zack that the festivities will continue in our room. As we walk back to Frazier, his friends pass us on the street, honking their horns and attracting attention from other commuters. He relishes in his newfound celebrity, and my heart dances as he waves to the strangers who have joined in.

Dinner is waiting when we get back to the room, and his friends start to arrive before Zack has finished eating. Several classmates missed him at the bowling alley and want to join in the party that typically occurs every evening in our room. The cards come out, and Zack deals while I go over the rules of "Golf" to a few who haven't played. I watch, still amazed at his strategic skill, as Zack wins hand after hand. When this group of players prove not to be a challenge, he hops in bed, and half his friends end up piling in as well.

I reach for my camera to record him perched among five teenage girls all vying for his attention. Brooke wears a button that she made with a picture of him at last year's homecoming, and several girls have "I love ZH" written in magic marker on their hands. There is giggling and whispering before someone asks him how he got to be so hot, and he replies, "My mom and dad made me this way." Now they include me in the conversation, chanting "Hot Mamma Hornback," which drifts down the hall to the nurses' station. When nurse Holly peeks in the door, I am already rounding them up, announcing that visiting hours are over.

Tonight, I get no protest from Zack, and he doesn't even walk them to the elevator. It has been an exhilarating day, and he is already preparing for bed. Our release date has been set for Oct 5th, when we will transfer to University Hospital for his bone flap surgery. With no complications, he will recover in a couple of days and either come home or go to Texas. Our lives are about to drastically change again. Whatever path we take, I know that God is in control, and His plan is perfect. God is our redeemer and restorer. He can redeem the past and restore what was lost. We must trust Him to do those things. We can never move out of the present, into the future God has in store for us, if we cling to our lives of the past.

Friday, September 30th

This morning, Zack is dressed and waiting for me to arrive, announcing that he wants to go swimming. Fairly certain that there is not a therapy pool within our complex, I agree to help him search the hospital on our morning walk. We trek down several corridors for staff only, opening doors to labs and utility rooms, but our quest to find a pool is futile. We make it to Kathy's office just in time for speech, and Zack complains that they don't have the right accommodations. She is as perplexed with this sudden desire to swim as I am. When he's questioned, he states matter-of-factly that "Some of these places have pools." As she sets him up on the computer, I run through images in my mind of the Centre in Dallas, wondering if perhaps they have a pool and he had seen the brochures. In the gym, he quickly forgets about swimming and embraces his new title. Apparently, most of the staff saw our interview on Fox 41, and now address him as "Hollywood".

After lunch, we head to University Hospital for his pre-op appointment. We stop by the Information Desk to visit with our prayer warrior, and Linda greets Zack with a warm embrace. She looks him over and keeps repeating "Ain't God good." We check into the second floor and see other staff, who remember us from our time in Neuro ICU. They are flabbergasted that Zack is the same boy who left here unable to hold up his head. As we wait to be called back for bloodwork, the surgery doors slide open, and Dr. Mutchnick strides out with other residents. Since we are seated at the end of the row, facing the surgery doors, he can't help but see us.

I introduce him to Zack, and he is visibly amazed. Crossing his arms, he rubs his chin and studies the teenager standing before him. He asks about his deficits, and I explain that physically, he is nearly back to normal, that aphasia is our biggest battle. Revealing that he will be taking care of Zack when we return, he shakes his hand and heads off down the hallway. Before disappearing, he glances back with a smile on his face, and I toss him a thumbs up. While we fill out mounds of paperwork, several strangers approach us about the story on the news. Each time, Zack grins and offers a handshake. No doubt if they asked for his autograph, he would have probably signed it Hollywood. After he is weighed and has his blood pressure taken, we meet with the anesthesiologist, who informs me that he is to check-in October 5th at 6:00a.m.

Back in the gym for OT, Mary Beth has him complete a memory game on the computer. We are both impressed with how well he performs, but then, she changes the program to object identification. His aphasia runs rampant, and he misses nearly half of the questions. It doesn't seem to bother him, and he even laughs at his own wrong answers. There is no frustration, and this amazes his therapists, but alarms the psychologist. Dr. Calvary expects him to respond like other patients who become depressed when they recognize their deficits. She is an educated, intelligent woman who can't seem to grasp that Zack is unlike any patient she has ever had with traumatic brain injury. When his session is over, he instinctively signs out, requiring no instruction. He is a child of the technology age, and computers are like a second language, unaffected by aphasia.

Unable to take a nap this morning, Zack is anxious to slip in bed before dinner. His head barely hits the pillow when Teri arrives with her daughters, and they coax him out of bed. They get the balls out and start a fast game of hot potato, switching directions on my command. Childish laughter zings around the room until Zack is doubled over, holding his sides. Can you picture how a baby laughs with his entire being? That is the gregarious way my son expresses happiness. His eyes dance, and his face beams with joy. I feel as if I could watch this game all evening, but it is interrupted when his dinner arrives.

Our guests leave, and when dinner is over, Zack wants to go outside. My choice of footwear today is not conducive for long walks, and I chastise myself for wearing boots. A blister has already formed from our jaunt to University, but I comply, and we make our way to the lobby. As we stroll around the building, I limp, trying to keep up with his usual fast pace. We discuss his surgery, which doesn't seem to alarm him. He is far more concerned about the shape of his head and is self-conscious about taking his helmet off in front of people. He understands that when his bone flap is replaced, his head will be symmetrical again. Complaining that his hair looks bad, I tell him he won't have to worry about that much longer because they will shave it off for surgery. Since he has sported a buzz cut for baseball, being without much hair doesn't bother him, as long as his head isn't misshapen.

When we get back to the lobby, we are greeted by friends of mine. Kelly, Dana, and Shane haven't seen Zack since he left University Hospital. Tears immediately spring to Kelly's eyes when Zack shakes their hands as I make introductions. She has watched him grow up, visiting us in California soon after he was born. She remembers how he loved his little cowboy boots and the ridiculous amount of baseball caps. With my feet protesting, we walk the long way outside to McDonald's, as they profess their amazement at his miraculous recovery. Following his progress online just doesn't give you the same sense of how far he has come. Zack is polite and charming, holding the door open and cleaning our debris from the table.

When we return to the room, it's time for another game of hot potato. This time, he has four adults laughing hysterically as we attempt to make the others drop the balls. Zack is even able to teach adults how to have fun with simple games. It's hard not to get caught up in the revelry when he is obviously having so much fun. I will miss him so much if he goes to Dallas. We still do not know if we will get approval from our insurance company. Sarah left a message this afternoon that the Centre hadn't submitted their report, so a request has not been filed. We will have to wait until Monday and then scramble to make arrangements. As I say goodbye to my friends, and Zack collapses in bed, I feel blessed for every moment I get to spend with my precious boy. Right now, I would walk the 800 miles in these aching boots all the way to Texas to hear him laugh.

With minimal therapy on the weekend, there is no reason for Zack to be up early, so I have to drag him out of bed when I arrive at 8:30. Halfway through his breakfast, he announces, "When I'm through with this, I'm getting back in that bed." Before he has a chance, our nurse arrives to take his blood pressure. He is experiencing the opposite effect of his dizzy spells. Now, when he stands, his blood pressure rises and then levels off before going back down to normal. Dana applies the cuff to his upper arm and records the reading in his chart, noting the rapid changes. When she leaves, he comments, "I suck at doing that for her." I explain that he can't control his heart rate, but he wants to do well at everything, apparently viewing this as a skill to master. He plops in bed, and I remove his helmet, so I can rub his head. His eyes are closed, and the side of his mouth is quirking upwards. When I stop, his eyes pop open, and he pleads, "You can stay and keep rubbing my head." I imagine it feels pretty bizarre on the right side, where his bone flap is missing and only the thin scalp covers his brain. It kind of creeps me out.

Scheduled for occupational therapy just before lunch, we meet with Trina in the gym. Her little brother had a traumatic brain injury four years ago, and he transferred to the Centre in Dallas after his initial therapy at Frazier. She explained how much he progressed in their program, and he wasn't as far along with recovery as Zack. It is no coincidence that the first weekend therapy session we have with Trina, she is able to set my mind as ease with the possibility of additional rehab in Texas. God places just the right person in our path at the most opportune time. She continues to describe the advantage the Centre provided for her brother while setting Zack up on the computer memory game. Amazed at how well he does, she sets it up to play against him. When he exceeds her with more correct answers, she decides this program is too easy and moves to object identification. Aphasia takes over, and she is stumped. This language disorder is difficult to understand, and the Centre has a program of intense therapy specifically designed to reduce impairment.

After an hour in the gym, Zack is too hungry to wait for his lunch tray to be delivered and insists we go to McDonald's. After multiple hikes yesterday, I was smart enough to select comfortable sneakers to wear today. As we head out the door, Kelsey and her dad arrive and walk with us to his favorite fast-food joint. He talks with Kelsey about school and tells her, "I'm going back to school after this next three." I am initially puzzled by the comment, until Kelsey inquires how long he will likely stay in Dallas. Just yesterday, our case worker remarked that the Centre will likely request a three-month rehab program. Zack remembered her comment, and I didn't even know he was paying attention. As they continue their conversation, he inquires, "How long have you been in this period?" This took us longer to decipher, but after further discussion, we determine he wants to know what semester this is in the school year. I doubt there has been another teenager so anxious to return to school.

Back in the room, our guests bid farewell, and Zack is able to take a much-needed nap. This gives me the opportunity to pour over the brochures on the Centre and check out their website full of smiling faces of recovering patients. I calculate that a three-month stay would put him in Texas for Christmas and look up the cost of airline tickets. If I start saving now, I reason that our family could be together for the holidays if we forego gifts. My children have all they need in material things already, and I know Grandma will fulfill any last-minute wishes. I settle in my chair, daydreaming of surprising Scott and the boys with Cowboys tickets. When I google the cost of pro football tickets, I find myself wishing that Santa were real.

As soon as his siesta is over, Zack announces he is starving and wants another meal at McDonald's. Expecting his dinner to arrive at any time, I talk him into waiting 30 minutes. He glares at the clock and tells me he knows when 30 minutes is up, so I better be ready. I am relieved when two friends arrive to take the pressure off his constant time announcements. When he deals out the cards, he decides that I can't play, because I make him eat hospital food.

His tray arrives late, and when we see what's for dinner, he makes his point. He has become a much pickier eater, but I'm sure after weeks of mystery meatloaf, mashed potatoes, and peas, I would prefer other options myself. A month ago, he would have eaten anything, so I attribute his newfound palate as a sign of recovery. Disgusted that I made him wait, and now, he considers his tray unworthy, so I promise his dad will bring him pizza.

He forgets that he's mad at me when Rick Thompson pops his head in our door. He has been away at WKU and hasn't seen Zack in over six weeks. Giving me a huge embrace, he whispers in my ear a common reaction, "What a miracle." With Dan and Trey in tow, there are too many to continue the card game, so they ruffle through CDs. Zack has learned many of his smooth moves from Rick, so now a dance competition ensues. Rick may be the only guy less inhibited than Zack, and before long, several staff have gathered in our doorway to enjoy the entertainment. The words to the song seem to flow from Zack automatically, and now, I understand why music is frequently used as a teaching tool. I feel so grateful for these teenagers who spend prime time on a Saturday evening visiting their friend. They are in part responsible for how quickly he is recovering, because they bring normalcy and stimulation to the inevitable boring times in his room. These are the moments that Zack will miss most if he ends up going to Texas.

Scott arrives with pizza, and I walk with his friends to the lobby. I field a million questions about the Centre and head home to spend time with Dylan and the girls. There is a cookout with the football team tonight, and it will be the first time since his accident that I get to socialize with other Christian Academy families. Everyone is interested in the latest update on Zack's progress and excited for the opportunity the Centre offers. These are the folks who have supported us with dinners, encouragement, service, and prayers.

As the night winds down, I lay on a blanket with Logan and look at the stars. She has heard about Texas and wants to know how far away her brother might be. As I explain that it is too far away to drive by car, the tears well up in her eyes, which brings a big lump in my throat. I point out the brightest star, and remind her that no matter how far away he is, they would be gazing at the same stars at night. Her tiny voice exposes another fear that I may be going with him. After assuring her that I am staying home, she snuggles next to me and reveals that her prayer is God will keep him here. We turn silent. The crickets sing in the distance, and my thoughts take me back to Frazier.

Without therapy scheduled, Rita allows Zack to sleep in while we are at church. When he finally rises, it is nearly noon, and he wants to go jogging. Pulling on shorts and sneakers, he goes out into the hallway to stretch. Rita announces that she has to go with him, and he finds that particularly amusing, since she couldn't keep up with us walking to the bowling alley. Once outside, she convinces him that a fast walk would be better, but she still struggles to keep him in sight. Grandma is relieved when I come strolling down the sidewalk to take over, and we head back to the room for lunch. We pass a new patient in a helmet slowly inching his way down the hall, held up by the gait belt around his waist.

Zack comments that the guy is really messed up, and when I reveal that he was worse than that when he first arrived, he doesn't believe me. He doesn't remember his condition two weeks ago, so I am not surprised he questions his condition two months ago. I remind him that he was in an accident, spent three weeks in ICU at University Hospital, and when he arrived at Frazier, he couldn't hold his head up, walk, or talk. With furrowed brow, he glares at me incredulously and shakes his head. Reasoning that the staff may offer some insight, we approach the nurses' station on 4South. Jennifer is reviewing charts and glances up when her favorite patient leans on the counter. Explaining that Zack doubts my recollection of his tenuous condition upon transfer to Frazier, I request that she fill him in. She points to the empty wheelchair parked haphazardly in the hallway and asks if he recalls using one to get to the gym. He frowns, "I didn't have that."

Pulling up his t-shirt, she shows him the pink scar where his feeding tube was located and explains that was how he ate. He throws his head back and laughs. "No, that's from football." She grows quiet and places her hand on top of his. Misty-eyed, she reveals that he won't remember her after he leaves. Zack promises he will, but she reiterates that he will likely not remember Frazier at all. Perhaps he could recall bits and pieces of therapy, but specific people on the staff will fade from his memory. Understanding how difficult it must be to care for someone for months only to have them forget you within days of departing, I place my arm around her shoulder. I vow to never forget her and promise to come back to visit often. The staff grows close to patients, since many reside here for months. They have become our family, and it will be an emotional parting.

Compiling a photo album that has chronicled his recovery, I realize I can prove to Zack with pictures just how far he has come. Before we have a chance to get back to the room, I spy my sister Colleen, ushering my mom down the corridor. In her 80s, my mom should be using her cane, but complains that it makes her look old and often refuses to use it. Today, she clings to Colleen's arm and waves when she recognizes us standing in the doorway. Embracing Zack for a long time, she wipes away tears when he finally pulls away. She frequently expresses how it grieves her to think about him trapped in a hospital room. Now that she's here, it's time to play "Golf", and Zack deals out the cards. His love of cards is definitely inherited from my side of the family, and my mom hates to lose. He chuckles each time Nana squeals when he outplays her. Her competitive spirit won't allow her to cut him any slack, but he doesn't need any pity points. Multiple hands later, he is declared the rightful champion.

Scott has promised to bring Zack a steak, but when his dinner tray is delivered, he is too hungry to wait. His plate is nearly empty when Scott bounds in with Dylan and the girls. It is amusing to watch Zack close his eyes, lean back in his chair, and chew each tender bite of ribeye with exaggerated expression as he finishes every morsel. With our trips to McDonald's, frequent slushies from the cafeteria, and three complete meals every day, Zack is nearly back to the weight he was before the accident. When he stands up, he is taller than his dad, but still seems fragile to me. I think it must be the helmet, signaling that he's been broken, a constant reminder of how delicate life can be. Without his friends to occupy his time, he is content to play ball with Dylan, and even allows Kyle into their game. After they leave, I convince Zack to take a walk, in order to keep him out of bed.

As we head out the door, several friends arrive, and I take advantage of the extra hands to carry items out to my car. I am beginning to clean out his room in preparation for our transfer back to the hospital. He has accumulated a lot of stuff in 66 days, and our early surgery appointment will leave little time for packing. With additional muscle, it only takes one trip to load up my trunk. The guys find the Nintendo cart and prepare teams for video games. At times, the laughter becomes too loud, and I have to quiet them down. These are my favorite times: watching my son enjoy the company of his friends and know that they don't feel I'm intruding. I'm in a unique position, being allowed into the hallowed surroundings of teen companionship. Most evenings, I sit in the corner and just watch. Their whispers aren't even hushed anymore, and I am privy to gossip that most parents would relish. I will definitely miss these nights hanging out with Zack and his friends. When we walk them to the lobby, several guys tell me that they are planning on using their parent's frequent flier miles to go to Dallas if Zack ends up there. They don't intend to let the miles stop them from visiting, although it won't be as often.

With his guest gone, Zack is quick to jump in bed, announcing how tired he is, since I prevented his nap. I continue to pack up his belongings and slip out to get more plastic bags. Passing the room of the new patient we saw earlier, I notice he is alone. I quietly move towards the bed, hoping for an opportunity to speak with him. His eyes are closed, and the steady rise of his chest indicates he is asleep. He appears older than Zack, but has the same familiar accessories he sported when we first arrived. Without his helmet, I observe his swollen head where the skull is missing and his trach that is still held in place with stitches. Vivid images parade across my mind, and my throat tightens as the tears begin to fall. I reach out to take his hand, intending to comfort this stranger, when his nurse returns. Surprised, she cautions me that policy doesn't allow me in his room, and I make a quick exit.

Zack is asleep when I slide next to his bed. His hand is mine to hold, and I bring it to my lips for a gentle kiss. I melt into the chair and stare at his profile. This angle obscures the disfigured portion of his head, and he resembles the clever teenager that beat curfew the night of his accident. I consider that in a few days, we will be sitting in that second floor surgery waiting room at University Hospital; only this time, we will have assurance of a positive outcome. We won't be waiting for a thumbs up, but rather, his beautiful smile and a "What's up?" as he comes out of anesthesia. Overcome with emotion, I plant my forehead on his shoulder and weep. I cry for the stranger alone in his room, for the fearful mother

I was in ICU, for the broken father Scott was in the emergency room, and for my precious son pinned under a guardrail. My halting breaths bring me back to reality, and I lift my head, wondering how Zack could sleep through my sobbing. His shirt sleeve is soaked with my tears, and I attempt to wipe them away, my hand tracing up to his face. I whisper a prayer, thanking God for His ever-present hand, and His promise in scripture: "If anyone is in Christ, he is a new creation, old things have passed away; behold, all things have become new." 2 Cor. 5:17

Our normal morning schedule is interrupted when an aide informs us that Larry is being transferred to another facility. An accident victim from another state, he also has a traumatic brain injury and has been in the room next to us since his arrival weeks ago. With little family support, his recovery has been slow, and now he is being relocated to a nursing home. My heart aches for this man who will likely linger in a facility for years with minimal therapy. I know very little about Larry, except that he was married and has a little boy in Tennessee who will never know his dad. I met his mother when they first arrived, and teary eyed, she showed me a picture of her grandson, who Larry doesn't remember. I never saw another visitor.

As we head to the gym, we pass by the other patient who grieved me last night, and I peek into his room. Again, he is alone, and thoughts start swirling through my mind that bring tears to my eyes. If only the loved ones of these TBI survivors understood the message I received from Dr. Kraft: the difference that family support makes in the recovery process. I'm preoccupied all morning as I consider the fate of these two men.

During lunch, we talk about Dallas, and Zack informs me that he is not going. He wants to come home and start back at Christian Academy with his friends. It's a difficult discussion as I explain that even if he comes home, he won't be going back to school this year. I remind him that he struggled this morning identifying objects and how aphasia steals his words. His math skills are rapidly improving, but he is only at a third grade level. I reveal that we don't have approval yet for Dallas, but if he has the opportunity to go, it would be the best thing for him. The grimace on his face softens when I bring up Larry and how thankful I am that he never had to go to a nursing home. He stares past me towards the door, and a gurney takes our neighbor to the waiting ambulance. Curious, he walks to the hallway and watches as they load Larry into the elevator. An aide carries several plastic bags that contain all his possessions, and under her arm is the framed photo of his young son. It has taken me days of packing all the stuff Zack has accumulated, and our walls are still covered with posters and cards. Larry's life seems summed up with that one photo.

At afternoon speech, Zack works as if he has something to prove. When aphasia strangles his choice of words, he recognizes when he's wrong and corrects himself. Each time he gets a right answer, he does a little dance in his chair and makes up a rap song about the object. Kathy gives him four letters, A T H W, and asks him to spell a word. He moves them around to create HATW. When she explains that it's not a word, he grabs the W and hides it under the table. She laughs and agrees that HAT is a word, but what about the W? His faked innocent expression as he raises empty hands and the W falls on the floor is priceless.

As we leave, he does a little farewell dance, and Kathy addresses me, "You really got your hands full."

Zack replies, "I know," and walks out the door. His stride down the corridor is one of confidence as he leads me to the gym.

My packing continues as Zack eats dinner, and when he's through, he offers to help. Meticulously folding even his boxers, he empties his dresser drawers. After selecting clothes for the next two days, he decides it's time for a walk, and we head outside. My mom had mentioned yesterday that they had stopped by the nursery, so now he wants to go to Norton Hospital and see the babies. A block away, we check out the hospital directory and proceed to the maternity ward. He is disappointed when there is only one baby, but a nurse holds the crying child up to the window for Zack to see. I watch as his eyes light up, and he taps on the glass, grinning ear to ear. Another trait inherited from my mom—he loves babies. He explains that it is good that the baby is crying, because that means he is alive. Crying certainly is an emotion attributed to the living.

We stop by McDonald's on our way back for a milkshake, and I get a call from the nurses' station that we have visitors waiting. When we get to the lobby and pass the information desk, they also inform us that several guests have been directed to our room. Zack is curious and asks if they are his friends, but she replies they are adults. Confused, he asks me what she means, and I explain that they are grownups, like me. Disappointed, he puts me in my place, "You mean they are all old."

Our room is full of people. Aunt Penny and Uncle Jay are talking with several guests I don't recognize, and they introduce themselves as fans from University Hospital. Kristy Noland has brought her mom, who was having surgery when Zack was in ICU. Vicky Wolfe saw us in the second floor surgery waiting room also came to meet the amazing boy they had been following online. They wanted to see for themselves just how far he had come in such an unbelievably short time. I'm flabbergasted that so many strangers have become attached to our story. We are privileged to meet some of the finest people through this tragedy. While they snap pictures with Zack, Jill Ramsey arrives to shave his head. Knowing that the surgeon would only have his right side shaved for surgery, I didn't want him leaving the hospital lopsided.

Not since he was a toddler has getting a haircut been so exciting. We gather around the chair as her shears buzz off all his hair, and we take turns rubbing his bare head. When he looks in the mirror, he is more concerned with the remnants scattered across his shoulders. Announcing that he needs to take a shower, he says goodbye, and I walk our visitors to the elevator. Relieved of the hair and in clean clothes, he lies in bed and asks me questions. "What's this called?" and points to his mustache. "I want to take it off." I get him a razor and watch as he carefully removes the whiskers from his face. "What are these called again?" He is examining his fingernails. "I want to cut them off." Using the clippers, I show him how to trim his nails. He goes through a whole grooming exercise before climbing into bed to watch the Packers game.

Knowing it may be their last chance, several nurses stop in to say goodbye. It is bittersweet. Dana tells Zack how far he has come since the first night she took care of him. She reminds him that before he could speak, she fell in love with his eyes. Melissa makes Zack promise to come back to visit and kisses his cheek. Kendra brings him a popsicle and hugs me without saying a word, emotion written all over her face. Once alone, Zack continues to watch the game, and I return to the note that Rita handed me earlier. Zack had said he wanted to write a letter. He wrote something to Scott, his brother, his sisters, and me. Then, he wrote a letter to Jesus with a sentiment that we find profound— "Dear Jesus, even though your things went fast, you still saved a bunch of people. You do really good. I love you. Goodnight."

Our last day at Frazier Rehab starts out very hectic, and Zack is obliged to go to therapy without me, since my car won't start. After 45 minutes of frantically trying everything, I am rescued by a neighbor. Carey Donovan from Swope Auto brings me a loaner, and my car is towed for repairs. Needless to say, I am stressed out over the whole ordeal, knowing that I miss my last meeting with Dr. Mook during rounds. Reminding myself that God is in control, I wonder what lesson he is trying to teach me.

Zack's final assessments reveal his balance and endurance in physical therapy show little measurable deficits. He keeps asking Amy where I am and gives her instructions, "While I'm in here, I want you to go up to my room and get my mom and bring her down here." It was a clear, well thought out request. Mary Beth records that his fine motor skills, dexterity, and resistance between the right and left sides show minimal difference and projects that his right side will continue to improve. When requested to type a sentence on the computer, he makes a statement, "Tomorrow is a special day, because I am leaving." They look at pictures of him when he first arrived and how he wrote his name, which allows Mary Beth the opportunity to commend his progress.

She reveals that hundreds of patients come through Frazier, and there are a handful that you remember…Zack is one of them. When it's time to say goodbye, both therapists get emotional as Zack sings "Amazing Grace". How I wish I could have witnessed him belting out, "Amazing Grace, how sweet the sound, that saved a wretch like me!" A grand old hymn that we have sung many times in church, but not one I would have thought Zack would remember. He clearly understands that God saved him. I am blessed that Mary Beth sought me out to reveal that it was the perfect way to end his time with her at Frazier.

Arriving in time to attend his final speech session, I'm disappointed that Kathy is off, but Zack is not. Kristi works through his assessment, and he thinks she is cute. Whenever she isn't looking, he makes goo-goo eyes at her. He answers all her questions correctly and does his best ever in speech, even correcting himself when he calls her by the wrong name. When we return to his room, a nurse comes to draw blood in preparation for surgery and records his vital signs. It becomes very real that our time at Frazier is ending when even the transport and nutrition staff stop in to say goodbye. Some people I don't recognize, but they have seen us roam the halls or had brief contact with Zack during the last 66 days. The impact that his recovery has had on strangers and staff is obvious when a woman from housekeeping slips in for a hug. She whispers, "Praise Jesus," and I'm certain it's the first time I've ever seen her.

Scott arrives with Dylan and the girls, so we head to the conference room for a feast provided by a business associate of mine. Kathy Brown brings in lasagna, salad, and apple pie for the first dinner our entire family has enjoyed together since the accident. As he says grace, Scott gets choked up, and the room falls silent. Zack's eyes dart from me to his Dad before proclaiming, "Praise Jesus" and digging into his food. Today has been stressful for me, worrying about surgery, wondering when we will hear about Dallas, and anxious over leaving our safe little room at Frazier. Twice, I have been rescued: Carey with a car, and Kathy with a meal.

Perhaps God's message is that my problems are no longer a matter of life and death, but what ordinary folks face every day. Or maybe, He is reminding me to trust him with even life's simple aggravations. After dinner, several of his friends arrive to spend their last evening here with us. They help me remove all the pictures from the walls and pack away mementos, commenting that they will miss their trips downtown. Mark Key arrives with Pat Day, who presents him with a shiny silver helmet. He autographs it with the sentiment, "God loves you, Zack. John 3:16." This famous jockey is a devout Christian who believes that God has a message to reveal through Zack. He prays with us and teases Zack that he really came to see him dance. The CDs come out, and little Fred Astaire shows off his moves.

We continue listening to worship music while we pack away memories. Occasionally, I hear in the depths of my mind the click, click, click of a roller-coaster. I look back at pictures of Zack at University Hospital and catch a glimpse of my son laughing with his friends. My breath is strangled as I come face-to-face with the reality of what God has done. His words, "Just wait until tomorrow," echo in my ears, and I sneak into the bathroom to be alone. My back against the door, I slide down to the floor, and the tears begin to flow. Tears of gratitude, reflection, and awe at how faithfully God answered prayers. How he carried me when I couldn't breathe and orchestrated the perfect plan for Zack's recovery.

When I am finally able to peel myself off the floor, I walk into a room that looks very different. His walls are bare, and the chairs moved out to make room for my bed. I will sleep here tonight to ensure we are at University Hospital by 6:00 a.m. Sleep won't come easy as I think about the four-hour surgery that lies ahead. After we walk his friends to the elevator, Zack saunters up to the nurses' station. I was expecting him to dance for them or maybe rap the 23rd Psalm, but he only offers hugs. When we are finally settled in bed, he reveals that he's not scared, but he can't sleep. Facing each other, we stretch out our arms and hold hands.

We drift off to sleep, claiming God's promise in Mathew 17:20, "I tell you the truth, if you have faith as small as a mustard seed, you can say to this mountain, 'Move from here to there,' and it will move. Nothing will be impossible for you."

As expected, I had a fitful night's sleep. I was anxious about surgery, and now, my back aches from a terribly uncomfortable hospital bed. Nurse Holly woke us at 5:00 a.m., so Zack could take the required shower, and once he's out, he wants breakfast. I explain that he can't eat before surgery or even swallow water while brushing his teeth. Of course, he strolls to the nurses' station to check the validity of my instructions and returns, complaining that he will starve. Applying a little reverse psychology, I pick up the phone to order breakfast and tell him we can cancel surgery if he agrees to stay at Frazier until they can reschedule it. He gets the point.

Scott picks us up, and we check into University Hospital at 6:00 a.m. We are bumped from our scheduled 7:30 surgery, due to another head trauma. The helicopter pad is visible from our window, and I watch as emergency staff unload the gurney. It is eerie to think that the same helicopter delivered Zack to this very hospital. As a lump forms in my throat, I explain to Zack the reason his surgery is delayed reclines on that gurney, and we take an opportunity to pray for this faceless stranger. Dr. Lenhardt, the attending anesthesiologist, and Dr. Janjun, the resident neurosurgeon, come to prep us on what to expect. Zack reveals that he's not nervous or afraid, but he is very hungry. Dr. Janjun informs us of the risk involved: the scalp has to be separated from the brain, which carries a chance of brain damage or stroke. There is also a risk of infection, and the chance that the bone would not be absorbed by the body. I'm presented with consent forms that list other risks, including death.

Once alone, my fingers curl around my son's, and I pray for God's hand to be present during surgery—that He will give the surgeons wisdom if confronted with the unexpected. Together, we pray the 23rd Psalm, and I am comforted that Zack's voice is strong and confident. At 9:45, they take him away, and I return to the second floor waiting room.

Scott doesn't do waiting well. Unable to sit still, he makes frequent visits to the smoking area outside. Nervously watching the clock, I pass the time playing cards with Rita and Donna. I search the room, trying to determine if the head injury that bumped our surgery might have someone waiting here. At 11:30, Dr. Janjun slips out to update us on their progress. His brain looks great, separation went as planned, and reattaching the bone went well. Everything is going smoothly, and he doesn't expect any complications. When the surgery doors slide shut, and he disappears, I inhale sharply and whisper a prayer of thanks with my exhale. I check the clock and tell Scott we have less than two hours now.

Glancing around the waiting room, my eyes land on a woman sitting alone, nervously wringing her hands. She looks to be in her mid-30s, wearing a Harley t-shirt and a tear-stained face. I approach cautiously and take the seat next to her. Speaking softly, I ask if she was here with whoever was stat-flighted. She eyes me suspiciously and leans away, so I clarify. I explain that my son was stat-flighted with a traumatic brain injury on July 8th and was only wanting to offer hope and encouragement.

A tear slips slowly down her cheek as she explains that her boyfriend was in a motorcycle accident, and she didn't know what other injuries he might have sustained, but he lost his leg. I pat her knee and ask if I can pray with her. She bows her head and folds her hands together, almost like a child. Praying for a successful surgery and God's comfort as she waits for results felt awkward. When I finish, she thanks me, jumps up from her seat, and walks towards the elevator, fingering a pack of cigarettes. I didn't have enough sense to ask her boyfriend's name or tell her Zack is recovering.

Reluctant to leave the waiting room and having no breakfast, my stomach was growling for lunch. Donna had just left for the cafeteria to get me a sandwich when the surgery doors slide open, and Dr. Janjun reports that everything went as planned. He also revealed that he was able to close the area in the front, where scar tissue prevented hair growth, something I had asked of Dr. Hann. The bone flap fit perfectly in the front, but his head had continued growing these last three months, so there would be a slight divot where the flap came together in the back. Nothing would be visible, but Zack would be able to feel it with his finger. I find it bizarre that his head would grow enough in three months that the bone wouldn't fit perfectly back together.

After an hour in recovery, we would be able to see him. I breathe a sigh of relief, knowing that the worst is over and pray that there is no regression in his recovery. Secretly, I hope that his aphasia will disappear as the anesthesia wears off. As we anxiously wait, I receive a call from our case worker at Frazier, saying that insurance had denied our request for rehab in Dallas. She explains that Frazier has already requested a peer-to-peer review and gave me a number to call to start the process. Even though I was heartsick at the thought of sending him to Texas, I had promised myself I would do whatever gave him the best chance of complete recovery. Convinced that three months wasn't that long and having several friends offer frequent flier miles, I dial the number and speak to a special inquiry representative. She refers me to the Board-Certified Doctor of Internal Medicine who will review our case and promises an answer tomorrow.

As we talk, I have three pair of eyes staring a hole through me and hanging on my every word. Of course, Grandma Rita wants Zack to stay here, and Scott would prefer that, as well. He didn't even want me to pursue it if initially denied. Donna is my voice of reason, reminding me that if God wants him in Dallas, he will open doors to make it happen.

Finally, at 3:45, we are ushered into recovery. I am apprehensive when we first walk into his room, until he opens his eyes, "Hi, Mamma." My eyes drink in every inch of him, and my heart leaps upon hearing his voice. I tell him how good he looks, and his response makes us all chuckle. "Do I really look that good?" Pointing to Rita, I ask if he knows who she is, and he puckers his lips in a kiss. "My Grandma." She can't contain her joy and nearly pulls him out of bed with her hug. I am relieved he knows her, because yesterday, he kept calling her Donna. When I ask if anything hurts, he complains about his stomach, and the nurse reveals he is likely nauseous from the anesthesia. Touching his swollen lip, he says it hurts as well, and she explains that the tube down his throat had irritated his mouth. I flash back to when they had tried to suction him the first time, and Zack bit his lip to prevent anything from going into his mouth.

Throughout the evening, friends form a line to wait for their 10-minute visit. At one point, I call Scott to tell him I wasn't feeling well, and Zack strained to look around his visitors to where I was sitting. "Are you okay, Mom?" He is so darn sweet. He just had his head cut open, and he is worried about me. Scott had left to pick the kids up and bring them in to see their brother. Our family reunion at University Hospital is much happier this time.

I can still picture the terrified look on Logan's face the first time she saw Zack here after his accident. This time, she bounces around the room until I threaten to put her in the corner. Fortunately, Kaitlyn and her mom offer to take the kids to dinner, so Scott can stay here, and I can ride home in quiet thankfulness.

God has carried us through the valley, and now I seek to praise Him from the mountain top. I will sleep well tonight, knowing that Zack is resting peacefully. God answers prayers.

This morning, Zack was moved to Neuro ICU, the same unit that took care of him after the accident. He is very hungry, but only allowed a clear liquid diet, so nurse Kathryn orders his breakfast. His tray is delivered with Jell-O, milk, and Cream of Wheat. Wolfing down the Jell-O, he tentatively takes a bite of Cream of Wheat and decides it's disgusting, even if you're starving. Every time Kathryn comes into the room, he professes how hungry he is until she finally gives in. She comes back with graham crackers and a 7Up, which he devours in a matter of minutes. If he keeps it down, we can order a regular lunch off the menu, with no restrictions. Zack is so sweet and doesn't want me to bother her again, especially since she gave him something to eat, but his head hurts. He says it's not like a headache, but feels as if someone hit him with a brick. I notice that he is still very swollen at the temple, so we have Kathryn request a doctor come check it out.

Dr. Mutchnick is not concerned. He explains that it is fluid from surgery, not uncommon, and will eventually be absorbed into the body, but it could take weeks. After thoroughly examining his head, he decides to clean up the stitches and has Kathryn bring some supplies. My heart starts to race as I remember the last time I witnessed him scrub my son's head like an old boot. He tells Zack it will sting and motions for me to hold his hand. It is painful for me to watch and excruciating for my boy.

Before long, Zack is howling in pain and sweat is pouring off his body. I clasp both hands and try to comfort him, as Donna has her hand on my shoulder comforting me. My tears soak his arm as I mumble that it will be okay. Through his tears, he keeps apologizing for crying out. I glance up and see Kathryn standing in the doorway, wringing her hands, her eyes spilling over.

After what seems like eternity, Dr. Mutchnick claims the stitches look great and wraps his head in a turban. Zack calms down quickly, says he has to go to the bathroom, and tries to get up. Discovering that he still has a catheter, Dr. Mutchnick decides to remove it as well. With little warning, he tells Zack that it will sting a little and yanks it out. Kathryn produces a portable urinal, but he decides that it hurts too bad, so he just won't go to the bathroom. I get him settled in bed and wipe his face with a wet cloth. It's hard to imagine another 16-year-old who has been through so much and handled it with such grace.

When Zack drifts off to sleep, I take the opportunity to call the insurance case worker to see about the approval for Dallas. She informs me that after a conference call between Dr. Mook at Frazier and the medical director at Anthem, we were denied. No explanation, just conjecture that he could receive the therapy he needs at Frazier East as an outpatient. I hang up, relieved to finally have an answer, and then, panic eases in as I realize that now he is coming home, and we are not ready.

As if on autopilot, I rush out to the car and drive around, trying to figure out what we need to do. I feel silly merging into traffic downtown, but the chaos of rush hour matches my synapses all firing at once. Of course, I accomplish nothing, and while I am gone, Stephan Johnson from Fox 41 stops by the hospital. He delivers a copy of the story they did on us at Frazier and brought his wife to meet Zack. I was disappointed to miss them, but Zack greeted me with a glowing grin. Grandma told him he was not going to Dallas, and he couldn't be happier. "Mom, remember what I told you? I'm not going to that place." Sliding next to the bed, I kiss his cheek and reveal that God answered his prayer.

We are playing cards when Dr. Mook arrives. I tell him Dallas is out, but of course, that's why he is here. He says he has a plan and is petitioning the insurance company for more outpatient benefits, since the 20 visits in my plan will not suffice. All of his therapists will write detailed reports on exactly what Zack requires, and they will be faxed to the medical director tomorrow. He explains that Anthem is willing to consider more outpatient benefits if they can make a compelling case.

Once he leaves, I call Scott with the news, and he is over-the-moon that Zack is coming home. As I begin to run through my list of things that need to be done to prepare, he assures me that everything will be fine, and God is still in control. Zack confesses he is tired and ready for a nap, so I tell him I need to run an errand and head back to Frazier. I have cards and pictures for his therapist and had also left some things behind. The brisk walk gives me time to mull over the mental list I start.

When I reach the lobby, the guard is surprised to see me without Zack. I assure him this is a social call, and his favorite patient is recovering nicely after a successful surgery. Everyone knew that Dallas had been denied, and they were already working on their reports. They promise that Zack will get the therapy that he desperately needs here in Louisville. I return to University and talk with Zack about coming home. It's hard not to get caught up in his excitement, but I reveal that we aren't prepared. He's not deterred. "It's okay, because I'm ready for home." Visitors begin to arrive, and the news of his homecoming spreads. I knew his friends would be elated, and suddenly, my desire to have everything perfectly prepared fades away.

The ICU visiting schedule is strict, and at 7:00 p.m., our nurse says all visitors must leave until the staff does reports and change shifts. Several friends had been patiently waiting their turn, so I accompany them to the second floor waiting room. We kill time playing cards and talk about Zack coming home. I am reluctant to return Zack to his bedroom in the basement with an entire floor between us. There's a schedule of medicine that I will be responsible to administer and stitches in his head to care for. As I voice my concerns, I'm struck by the puzzled faces around me. "What?"

It takes me a few seconds to embrace what Andrew points out. "You've got this." I have trusted God through the most difficult part of Zack's accident and recovery. Now, He is fulfilling the prayer that I cried out from the beginning. That my son will come home. It doesn't matter that I'm not prepared or that I feel ill-equipped to care for any medical issues that might arise. God's perfect plan will not fall apart.

Late last night, Zack was moved to a private room on the ninth floor, since he doesn't need enough medical attention to stay in Neuro ICU. I brought some of his own clothes, so our nurse asks if he would like to get cleaned up. He heads to the bathroom, and before we know it, he was in the shower. She is concerned about contamination and instructs him not to get his head wet. Immediately, the water stops, and he comes out of the bathroom in his boxers, apologizing as he pats his head dry. She examines the drain that was still in place from surgery and determines that everything is intact. It is mid-morning when Kim Meyers, nurse practitioner for the neurosurgeons, arrives to remove the drain. I echo the concern on her face when she can't budge it, so she calls for Dr. Janjua. Unfortunately, he's in surgery, so we have to wait at least an hour.

Playing cards with Zack keeps me occupied, but I do take note of the time. It's the longest hour ever when Dr. Janjua finally sweeps into the room at 3:30. He tugs at the drain, which should slide out relatively easy, but it won't dislodge. Approaching it more aggressively, he yanks at the tube, and Zack yells out, his eyes filling with tears.

Stepping back, Dr. Janjua states that they will have to go back into surgery to remove it and walks out the door. I was not expecting his response and am left standing there with no explanation, only concern that we are going back into surgery. Before I have a chance to process this latest update, Dr. Janjua returns with the attending neurosurgeon, and they attempt to remove it again. More pain, and this time, the tears belong to me. I feel as if the entire neurosurgery staff is ready to line up and take their turn torturing my son. Just when I feel my mamma-bear claws beginning to descend, Dr. Meyers agrees that surgery is the only option.

They check for an operating room and inform me that they will take him in two hours. Without alarming Zack, I start making phone calls to Scott, Rita, and Donna, to inform them that we are headed back into the operating room. Although I witnessed how firmly embedded the drain is, I'm still uncomfortable with the whole surgery option. I head to the nurses' station, intent on getting questions answered. To my good fortune, I see Dr. Meyers, who explains the procedure. The tube is stuck just beneath the scalp, not under the skull. He says that four things need to be in place for this surgery: a patient, a doctor, an operating room, and an anesthesiologist. Right now, we have a patient and a doctor, so we are waiting on the room.

After reviewing his chart, he concludes that Zack can't be put to sleep, because it hasn't been eight hours since he has eaten. If an operating room becomes available before the required eight hours, they will attempt to remove it with only a general anesthetic to numb the area. Then, it will be up to Zack on how much pain he can tolerate. If he becomes distressed, they will stop, wait the eight hours, and try to have all four pieces in place. "How much pain he can tolerate" reverberates in my mind as I wring my hands and return to the room.

Having nothing since breakfast, Zack complains he is hungry, and I have to explain why he can't eat. He patiently complies, and while we wait, I hear the chopper landing on the rooftop pad. Now I know a 6:00 p.m. surgery is unlikely to happen, and he will have to wait even longer before getting fed. Just as I am about to call Scott and fill him in, my phone rings. Jude Thompson, President of Anthem, confesses that he personally reviewed Zack's case and was the one who ultimately denied our request for Dallas. He explains that he wants to do what is best for our family and believes that means keeping us together. Understanding that family support has made the biggest impact on Zack's recovery, he vows to approve the additional outpatient hours. He knows that Zack did not want to go to Dallas and not to worry, because he would get whatever he needs at Frazier East.

I am speechless and thankful that we have Jude in just the right place to make the best decision for our family. Zack has been listening and at the mention of Dallas, his face is full of concern. I declare there is no cause for alarm, he is still coming home, but Jude Thompson wanted to confirm his decision. Reminding him that he played basketball at Christian Academy with Jude's son, I reveal that he was the one who denied Dallas. A grin spreads across his face, "I always liked him." Yep, me too.

Zack is taken down to surgery at 9:30 p.m. Dr. Janjua says he will be put under anesthesia, and the procedure will take only an hour. I sit alone in the second floor waiting room, which is eerily quiet. There are no other people waiting, which seems almost planned. I have no distractions and think about all the people God put in just the right place to see us through. This accident has happened for many reasons, but today, a new explanation comes to surface in my mind. God needs to show us how he intends His church to work. As Christians, we are all members of His family, and He wants us to love one another as He loves us. We have experienced that firsthand, and feel honored that God is using our tragedy to lift up his church. He sits on his throne and proclaims, *"Watch my people."*

Teenagers have fallen to their knees, encountered God, and experienced the power of prayer. Strangers have heard of a miraculous recovery and recognize that the Great Physician can do much more than we ever hope or imagine. I personally have learned to embrace not only a faith that God will work, but one that trusts in how he will work. Countless times, my prayers were not big enough. God's perfect plan continues to unfold and amaze me in untold ways.

Just shy of two hours, Dr. Janjua slips out to tell me they just finished. He had to open the incision to remove several pieces, and since it was so late in the day, he doesn't want to release him tomorrow. Zack will still be groggy from the anesthetic, so it would be safer to keep him another night. I explain that we need to leave early, because I intend to take him to church on Sunday. He promises to have his papers ready by 7:00 a.m., so we can attend our regular 11:15 service at Southeast Christian Church.

As I watch him walk away and melt back into my seat, I inhale and close my eyes. I picture a homecoming that has us walking into God's house to give him praise. It won't matter what the sermon is, it will be emotional to have my boy finally sitting next to me in church. I'm startled when an aide touches my arm and nearly jump out of my chair. She apologizes, but just wants to let me know I can go back to see him now.

In recovery, Zack's face lights up, and he tells me he is going home tomorrow. I reply that it is very early on Saturday, so yes, he is going home tomorrow. He's perplexed, and I can see him thinking about it. "Is it Saturday already? Then, I'm going home today!" Choosing my words carefully, knowing he's not going to like my answer, I explain that because his surgery was so late, he can't go home until Sunday. He grimaces. "Mom, if I don't get to go home today, I'm going to be pissed off." There is not a lot I can say, but I'm sorry, and I promise that his friends will be here today to keep him company. Then, I describe my plan of taking him to church on Sunday and what a glorious vision it will be. That pacifies him for the moment, but I know he will badger me again when he wakes up.

It is 1:30 a.m. before he is back in his room, and this long day has worn me out. Only one more day, and this rollercoaster will slide into the station. That thought keeps coming to mind as I walk to the parking garage. My imagination paints a rickety wooden track. It runs from University Hospital, loops around Frazier, screams through a scarily blind tunnel as it passes Aiken Road, where a mangled guardrail marks the accident scene and smoothly lands beneath the portico at Southeast Christian Church. "All aboard," the conductor shouts from heaven. "This is the ride of your life."

Zack slept soundly last night, still groggy from anesthesia. I stumbled home at 2:00 a.m., and Scott was waiting up to head to the hospital himself. Now in the homestretch, we want to continue being vigilant advocates, so he will spend the night, in case Zack gets sick. Dr. Janjua has started an antibiotic as a precaution against infection, but everything seems to be going as planned. Zack complains that his head hurts on the outside, which is to be expected after the trauma of surgery. He's given a mild pain reliever and drifts back to sleep. Several of his friends have asked how many stitches he received, and ironically, the surgeons reply is "one" … one long continuous stitch.

When Zack wakes up after lunch, he grins, remarking that he is going home today. I had prepared for the barrage of protests, so I move to his bedside and examine his face. His right eye is very swollen, and I gingerly caress around his temple. I feign apprehension and remind him that they won't release him until Sunday, because they have to be sure his whole face doesn't blow up like a balloon.

Now I have his attention as I appeal to his vanity. His fingers creep up to his face, and he traces along the curve of his forehead and down his cheeks to his chin. Studying my composure, his eyes narrow, expressing doubt in my explanation, but I continue the ruse. Gently tapping the area around his eye, I study his face and actually become genuinely concerned. Deciding a doctor needs to take a look, I head to the nurses' station, intending to have Dr. Janjua paged to our room.

As I scurry down the corridor, I see a familiar form chatting with one of the nurses. Dr. Densler, our initial neurosurgeon the night of the accident, is on rotation at another hospital, but had stopped in to pick up files. He recognizes me immediately and welcomes the opportunity to check on his famous patient. As we stroll back to the room, I fill him in on Zack's progress and realize it's been exactly three months since we started on this journey. Dr. Densler takes on a professional, serious demeanor as he explains why Zack's eye is so swollen, qualifying that it will get worse. He describes that when the bone flap is replaced, the scalp is peeled back from the top of his head down to his ear, exposing the whole surface. This causes trauma to the entire area, with fluid building up around the right eye. We should expect bruising and the inevitable black eye. No wonder my son complains that his head hurts on the outside. He recommends a cold compress and says Zack looks great, so I shouldn't worry. His face softens, and that beautiful smile welcomes my hug.

Keeping Zack occupied with a challenging card game helps keep his mind off of the desire to go home. As we battle it out through a game of "Golf," I get a phone call from Rita, who has found a deal on a sectional couch. We want to create a pleasant place for Zack and his friends to hang out, so we are upgrading the family room in the basement. Teenagers have visited every day at Frazier, and we want them to continue to feel welcome once he has come home. I make some phone calls to arrange a truck to pick up furniture. Once they are on the way, I head to the house to organize the décor. Planning helps me maintain some control over this next phase of recovery, and I still hold firm to the belief that his friends are instrumental for the best outcome.

Once the furniture is positioned to allow for a dozen teenagers to gather comfortably, I make my way through rush hour traffic back to University Hospital. I feel energized now that I have crossed things off my list in preparation for tomorrow's homecoming. When I bounce into his room, I notice that Zack's eye is completely swollen shut, and a purple bruise is forming on his cheek. He looks like he's been in a fight, and I ask if it hurts. He says it just feels weird, and his fingers move carefully over his face. I scurry to the nurses' station to ask for a cold compress, but there is no one around. Deciding it will be faster to make our own ice pack, I soak a washcloth in a plastic pitcher full of ice water and apply it to his engorged face. He shivers each time I rewet the cloth, and after 10 minutes, decides he's had enough.

Visitors stream in after dinner, and since we no longer have strict ICU rules, our tiny room starts to fill up. There are only two chairs, so kids lean against the wall, and the chatter carries out into the hallway. At times, it feels like Zack is on display, sitting up in bed with all eyes fixated on him. As the crowd thins out, he is no longer groggy and gets up to sing and dance to music from Kaitlyn's phone. It's a bizarre scene. His shaved head exposes the fresh stitches that run from the top of his head to the back and around his ear. The right side of his face is puffy and discolored, his swollen eye now clearly sports a shiner.

But there is a magnificent grin plastered across his face, as he makes up silly songs to entertain us. People slow down as they pass our door, peering in to see who commands such a commotion. An elderly woman leans in our doorway and asks Dan what is wrong with Zack. I'm certain it's difficult to grasp why someone who looks so horrendous would have any reason to act so joyful. I slip out into the hallway and explain that he is thrilled to be going home tomorrow. Describing his accident, surgeries, extensive rehab at Frazier, and the challenges he still faces, I reveal how God carried us to this exuberant moment. Her wrinkled hands grasp both of mine while tears spill down her cheeks. She professes that the good Lord worked a miracle in my boy, and he will be a blessing to me until I take my last breath. Shaking my head in agreement, I watch as she shuffles down the corridor. I look at the celebration going on in our room, and my heart dances with joy.

As we say goodbye, Kaitlyn's mom hands me a package, explaining that she made this for Zack after reading one of my posts. It is a thick, black t-shirt with "Thunder" emblazoned in white letters across the chest. It's perfect and I hold it up for Zack to see. I clarify that when our prayers our answered, sometimes God whispers, and sometimes he sends thunder. Pointing at him, I declare, "You are thunder!" He smiles and replies, "I like being thunder." I must confess I half expected to hear it roar outside. When our guests are gone, Zack wants to finish our earlier card game, so he can beat me before he goes to sleep. We only make it halfway through one hand when he tells me he's tired and ready for bed. Our party tonight must have worn him out because he is asleep in no time. I slide out to the nurses' station to discuss what needs to be done in order to leave in the morning, and then, decide to go home to put the finishing touches on his room.

Walking to the parking garage, I know I haven't been this happy in a long time. Earlier today, I found myself skipping down the hall, clicking my heels and singing, "We're going home tomorrow." I ride home in silence, thinking of the sonic shock wave that set us on this path. I voice my pleas to God, thanking Him for bringing us to this point. I believe He heard my prayers every morning and sent thunder as his answer. I have faith in Psalm 3:3, "But you are a shield around me, O Lord, you bestow glory on me and lift my head. To the Lord, I cry out aloud, and He answers me from his holy hill." Great is His faithfulness, deep in His mercy, and mighty in His power.

Zack will never be the same, and neither will we. We are better with our hearts laid bare to receive God's blessings in whatever form He chooses. We have learned to listen for his whisper, appreciate His thunder, and believe His plan is perfect. We will begin a new day, a new life, and how fitting that it will start on Sunday.

Like a child anticipating a morning trip to Disneyland, I had a difficult time going to sleep. I expected Zack to be dressed, anxious to finally be released into the world again, but found him sleeping when I arrive at 7:00 a.m. Sliding into the chair next to his bed, I greedily drink in the sight of my son with wonder. His eyelids flicker as I reach up to caress his face, and the corners of his mouth turn up in response. The first words he utters are to remind me that we are going home today. I order his breakfast and stare at the clock, wondering why we haven't seen Dr. Janjua or Kim Meyers with our paperwork. When an aide comes to take away his tray, I ask if I missed rounds this morning, and she looks at me as if I'm speaking a foreign language. I head to the nurses' station seeking anyone who can provide accurate information on what time the doctors make rounds, only to learn that on "the floor", there is no schedule.

Finally, Dr. Janjua arrives with our prescriptions and care instructions. After two family meetings at Frazier, I expected more fanfare, but he is sending us home with very few directives. Follow the directions on the bottles, if the stitches start leaking or if he runs a fever, bring him to the emergency room and come to the clinic on Thursday to have the stitches removed. That's it. He has had brain surgery, and I get more instructions when I take the kids to the doctor's office for flu shots. Frankly, I was dumbfounded. I had my little notebook out, poised to jot down a plethora of commands, but all I get is "read the bottles". He signs the release papers, hands me a copy, and says someone from transport will be here shortly with a wheelchair.

Zack pulls on jeans, his Thunder t-shirt, and the white tennis shoes his friends gave him for his birthday. He had asked that I bring him a ball cap to cover his stitched-up shaved head, but Dr. Janjua cautioned against anything too tight. We decide on a straw cowboy hat, because it would partially shield his swollen black eye, but first, I needed to protect the incision from any contamination. With a clean, black silk scarf, I wrap his head like a pirate, loosely tying it at the nape of his neck. When the cowboy hat is placed on his head, you can barely see the scarf beneath.

Zack studies himself in the mirror, lowering the brim of the hat until he's satisfied. He looks perfect, dashingly handsome, in spite of the puffy bruising. I doubt most people will see past that glowing smile. Now that he is dressed, I lean in the doorway, glancing both ways down the corridor in search of our transport. I remind every nurse and aide that passes that we are ready to go. After 30 minutes, just as I threaten to walk him out of here myself, our chariot arrives. We stop by Neuro ICU to say goodbye to the staff that lovingly cared for him for 21 days after the accident. To most of them, he has risen from the ashes, a walking Lazarus that they won't forget. In the lobby, we are blessed to find Linda at the information desk, the same spot where Scott first encountered her. He clung to her promise that God would answer our prayers, and now she embraces Zack with tears in her eyes. I leave him in her care and race to the garage, honking the horn as I pull up to the curb.

When he slides into the passenger seat, Zack looks at me, grinning, "See how easy it was to get out of here. You said I couldn't leave until I got my words fixed." Laughing, I comment that they will fix his words when he continues therapy at Frazier East. The smile dwindles, and he looks at me, surprised that he's not going back to school. I explain that he's not quite ready for the demanding agenda at Christian Academy, but Frazier East will get him there. Before he can argue, I reveal that all his friends will be meeting us at church, and he proclaims, "I knew my people would be there."

Sunday morning traffic on the I-64 is light, and the sun shining through the window captures our mood. Zack feast his eyes on the sights around him, his face cracked in a perpetual smile. Christian rock flows from the radio, and he taps his foot, keeping beat to the music. In the rearview mirror, I can see University Hospital and Frazier Rehab slowly fading in the distance. I never allowed myself to get to this moment when we were at University. I survived one hour at a time, dependent on God to get me through to the next hour, not thinking about a future beyond the next day.

Seeped in gratitude, I inhale the words to the song, "Praise You in This Storm", that fills our car. Zack fumbles through some of the verses as he tries to remember the words, but he clearly embraces the message: "And I'll praise you in this storm, And I will lift my hands. That you are who you are, No matter where I am. And every tear I've cried, You hold in your hand. And though my heart is torn, I will praise you in the storm."

The lyrics flow through my veins, validating that God heard my cry and whispered, "I am with you." Our momentary bliss is interrupted when my phone rings, startling both of us. Ruth Schenk, a reporter with the *Southeast Outlook*, wants to get pictures as we walk through the door. I promise to call when we arrive and feel my heart racing with excitement as we get closer to our destination. Then, I spot the cross, rising 40 feet above the gleaming copper roof that marks Southeast Christian Church.

I swallow the lump in my throat, gleefully announcing, "There it is!", like we are approaching the eighth wonder of the world. Trailing the line of traffic, we pull into the parking lot, and I call Scott, who is waiting with Ruth in the atrium, announcing our arrival. As Zack steps out of the car, he checks his reflection in the window, adjusts his hat, and turns around, grinning ear to ear. We proceed to the main entrance, and I notice his swagger as he pulls at his pants. Dang. In my rush to get out of the house this morning, I forgot his belt, and now his pants, which are still too big, keep falling down. He laughs, confessing that if he keeps his hands in his pockets, he can hold them up.

A greeter holds the door open as we walk into the atrium. Beneath his notable hat, a smile explodes across his face as he makes a grand entrance to the cheers of his friends. They are all here, clapping and calling him Thunder. Their faithful support never wavered, and they joyfully celebrate his homecoming. Ruth is snapping pictures as Dave Stone reaches out to shake his hand, clarifying that he and Sam get the first golf game. Scott takes note of Zack clinging to his pants and offers his belt to solve the problem.

Logan and Kyle fight their way to their brothers' side, and Grandma Rita envelopes him in a bear hug dripping in tears. I fall back, content to take in the scene, but my quivering chin and rapid blinking betray me. My heart races, and my body feels buoyant, as if I'm walking on clouds. Euphoric contentment warms me down to my fingertips. I glance at Scott, his arm around Dylan's shoulder, wiping his cheek with the back of his hand. There was a time, only three months ago, when we thought this day may never come. Our entourage heads towards the sanctuary, drawing attention from strangers who notice the commotion. Several people stop us to congratulate Zack, confessing their daily obsession as they followed his recovery on the blog.

As we cross the threshold of the worship center, Zack pauses to take in the massive sanctuary of over 9,000 seats. Many of the individuals filling these seats have walked along beside us and now bear witness to the power of prayer. His eyes drift upward, slowly trailing the edge of balcony until he lifts his gaze to the ceiling. He stands there staring heavenward, thanking God for bringing him home. Family members wave to get his attention, drawing him towards the section where they have our place reserved on the first floor. We slide into our seats, Zack between Scott and I, our family filling in beside us while his friends take up several rows around us.

The worship team begins the service, and I watch for signs of overstimulation as the lights on the stage pulsate to the beat of the music. Belting out the lyrics of the songs he knew, Zack is content to listen and read the words on the screen for the ones he didn't recognize. He isn't anxious during the sermon and doesn't even shake his leg tensely, as he would during speech therapy. He seems completely at peace. Peering around him, I whisper to Scott that our prayers have been answered, which fills his eyes with tears.

Congregants continue to stop us on our way back to the atrium after the service. Some I recognize from Christian Academy, but many identify themselves as people who heard about the accident and prayed for his recovery. Zack shakes hands and hugs strangers, beaming as he relishes his new celebrity status. Andrew whispers that we need to take our time getting home to give his friends time to prepare. Scott takes Dylan with him, and the girls insist on riding with their brother. Their non-stop chatter in the backseat seems to normalize our extraordinary homecoming. We stop at Walgreens to get his prescriptions filled and finally pull into our subdivision.

The trees lining the main road hold colorful hand-made signs with sweet sentiments. Welcome … Home … We love you. As we pull onto our street, his friends are lining the sidewalk, cheering as he exists the car. Everyone piles onto the front porch, and I snap a picture to memorialize this special occasion. Zack checks out his bedroom for the first time in three months, and I point to the ominous window that he climbed out of on the night this all began. "Stay away from that window!" I wrap my arm around his waist and lay my head on his shoulder, my tone softening. "Welcome home."

Guiding him into the lower level family room, we proudly show off his newly furnished hang out and before long, he is playing pool with his friends. I'm content to serve snacks and listen to the sounds of raucous teenagers, tuning in multiple artists as they battle over the music. I find it amusing that they can't seem to listen to a complete CD. They move outside to throw a football in the backyard, and my antenna is on high alert, threatening anyone that throws a ball to close to Zack's head. I perch on the deck, wringing my hands with each toss, until I realize I am overreacting and relax.

Scott places burgers on the grill, and soon, the deck is crowded with famished teens devouring our simple picnic. By the time I'm able to grab a plate, there is nothing left but potato chips and a withered hotdog with no bun. Ironically, it suits me just fine. I'm satisfied to feast with my eyes, watching my son cavort in the backyard. Once his friends leave, Zack is content to play basketball with Dylan and Kyle. I cuddle Logan in my lap and watch the sun sink slowly behind our neighbor's house, painting the sky in brilliant hues of pink and orange. Wrapping my arms around my youngest, I feel a piece of heaven has fallen right here in our backyard.

With the sun gone, the air begins to chill, and we head inside. Logan goes to bed with no complaint, the excitement of the day having worn her out. I remind Dylan and Kyle that they have school tomorrow and grab clean towels for Zack. I gather sheets and a blanket for the temporary mattress on the floor in our bedroom. This is where he will sleep until I'm comfortable enough to put him back in his bedroom in the basement.

While he showers, Scott and I have our first minute alone all day. We sit in the family room, looking at each other, unable to speak, knowing that our voice will be flooded with emotion. I scoot next to him, resting my head on his chest, each lost for a moment in our own thoughts. Scott begins to pray, but chokes on a sob, and returns to silent contemplation. Zack finds us huddled together on the couch, tears of joy streaked across our faces. He's a sight to behold. From his shaved head, down to his SpongeBob pajama bottoms, he looks like an overgrown four-year-old. With a smile that lights up his face, he announces he's ready for bed. As he heads to the basement, Scott explains that he's sleeping upstairs for a little while and shows him the pallet on our floor. He doesn't protest, and as we tuck him in, he starts to laugh uncontrollably.

When he is finally able to speak, he reveals that he is deliriously happy to be home. I second that! I climb into bed, and before long, I can hear his steady breathing. A rumble of distant thunder cloaks me in God's promise to never leave me or forsake me. Knowing that His perfect plan is still unfolding, I drift off peacefully.

A loud crash, like an explosion of glass, a shrill scream followed by a multitude of phones ringing, jolts me awake. I bolt upright, my heart pounding out an erratic rhythm as my eyes adjust to the darkness. I'm panting, lightheaded, clutching the covers with both hands. The familiar sound of Scott snoring finally drowns out the terror echoing in my ears. I squint and make out the silhouette of Zack sleeping nearby. Wiping my sweaty palms on the sheet, I ease myself onto the pillow, and slowly, my heartbeat returns to normal. I stare into the shadows, scared to close my eyes, until a gentle voice from heaven whispers… "Breathe."

Zack started outpatient therapy at Frazier East on October 10, 2005. At that time, he was barely reading at a kindergarten level and struggled every minute with aphasia. He had overcome his physical deficits as an inpatient; conquering right side neglect, abnormal tone, and regaining his strength to the point that physical therapy was no longer a focus. Outpatient treatment consisted of speech and occupational therapy with active participation in group therapy. It was an adjustment for both of us, since I was no longer with him to monitor his progress. Frazier East expects their clients to be independent, carry their own schedule, know where they are supposed to be, at what time, and how to get there. This required Zack to take notes, which he carried in a binder with his weekly schedule.

Leslie, his speech therapist, incorporated his textbooks from Christian Academy to improve reading speed and comprehension, math skills, and memory, in preparation for his return to school. Suzanne, his occupational therapist, continued instruction with everyday life skills, which included frequent walks to the Kroger grocery store. She was also tasked with reviewing all the information, symbols, and laws in the state driver's manual, in preparation for Zack to get his license. Other than returning to school, learning to drive was a daily preoccupation for Zack. Both of his therapists agreed that Zack was very intelligent and were baffled by his aphasia, which made every task more complicated. Within the first few weeks, Leslie noticed that Zack was having "cognitive return", where the chemicals in the brain are stabilizing. As they stabilized, his memory improved, as well as the aphasia and other cognitive skills.

Group therapy was interesting for Zack, since he was, by far, the youngest patient. Most of the other clients were recovering from strokes, and he had little in common with them. They would play games that emphasized deductive reasoning, problem solving, concrete verses abstract thinking, recognizing similarities and differences, organizing thoughts, and recognizing relevant information. Circles involved each patient explaining their injury, resulting deficits, and ongoing struggles. These social settings created an awareness that, despite their age difference, he was recovering just as they were. His involvement made a great impact on the other patients. One elderly gentleman told Zack "meeting you opened my mind to what I can achieve."

Frazier East was where we met Dr. Perri, neuropsychologist, who approached Zack in a different way. They frequently spent time throwing a baseball outside while they explored the emotional side of his brain injury. Zack's use of humor to compensate for his language disorder endeared him to most of his therapists, but he formed a unique bond with Dr. Perri. He seemed honestly fascinated with Zack. Where most of the staff was nervous when they saw me taking notes, knowing that information might be recorded on the blog, Dr. Perri embraced the idea, and even used it as part of his therapy. They would read the blog entries and discuss the accident and his struggles in rehab. His therapist agreed that Zack had a good attitude, worked hard, and was cooperative, but he also didn't recognize his deficits, or blew them off as insignificant. It is a blessing that he wasn't depressed, but in order to compensate and correct deficient areas, you have to recognize that they exist. Hours of conversation with Dr. Perri helped Zack acknowledge that he would struggle with some deficits for a long time. Zack showed Dr. Perri a resiliency and fierce determination that would overcome many obstacles while using humor to stave off depression. Examining the depth of his injury and unpredictable recovery, Dr. Perri recognized that Zack was one in a million. Through the years their relationship evolved from doctor/patient to an enduring friendship that lasts to this day.

It was Dr. Perri who discovered that Zack had retrograde amnesia. He did not remember the person he was or events that occurred before the accident. I had my own experience with this a few days before Christmas when, in casual conversation, Zack mentioned he didn't remember any holidays. I was broken-hearted thinking of all the precious memories he had lost. Then, on Christmas morning, as the kids sat on the floor of the family room, opening presents like we had done every year, something changed. Sitting in the midst of torn wrapping paper, a strange expression came across Zack's face. Suddenly, he looked up at me with a smile and exclaimed, "I got an airsoft gun for Christmas last year!" Apparently, many of those precious memories came flooding back when he experienced our family tradition again. We had this situation occur again a few weeks later, when Zack pointed out the ocean on a movie and said he had never been to the beach. For years, our family had vacationed in Hilton Head, South Carolina, and Zack spent many summers there with his grandparents. After our Christmas morning revelation, I was excited to plan our spring break. The following April, I waded in the surf, waves lapping our ankles, waiting for any sign of recognition. After ten minutes of walking on the beach, Zack suddenly took off running towards an outcropping of rocks. When I finally caught up to him, his eyes were bright, and he danced around, confessing, "We use to sneak over here and smoke cigarettes." We have had several similar experiences, but, in most cases, Zack can't remember past people, places, or events, only how they made him feel.

After only two weeks as an outpatient, Suzanne and Leslie confirmed that Zack had a vision deficit they identified as a "field cut." This is where a portion of his visual field is missing, but it doesn't manifest as a blank spot, but, rather, his brain fills in what should logically be there. This is not an issue if he is looking at the sky, because his brain just fills in more sky. However, it becomes a problem when trying to read, since his brain doesn't always fill in the correct letters. He was referred to Dr. Weinberg, a behavioral optometrist, for vision therapy to improve fundamental visual skills necessary for processing information. They believe that vision is a learned process that can be improved through progressive visual exercises. After his screening, the therapist noted that Zack's biggest issue was eye movement. A normal fixation should be 96 per 100 words. Zack was at 356, which meant all of his energy was focused on just trying to stay on the line he was reading. He could read, but it was extremely hard; like trying to read while someone jiggled the paper around. This also presented a problem when learning to drive. His field cut was where a parked car would be in his line of vision. He has 20/20 eyesight, but his brain does not perceive what his eyes see in that area. Zack had eight months of vision therapy, where he learned tracking, focusing, and scanning techniques that enabled him to compensate for his vision deficit. There is no surgery or glasses to correct a field cut, since the problem is in his brain.

In order to return to school, Zack had to take a neuropsych evaluation, which would clearly identify his cognitive deficits, so an individual education plan could be developed. It was an important step in his recovery enabling Frazier to formalize the remaining portion of his therapy to focus on specific weaknesses. A lot of what was discovered in his first evaluation was not surprising. Reading and verbal comprehension was impacted by aphasia. The test showed deficiencies in processing speed and attention to visual detail. His visual perception problems impacted his performance across tests requiring visual acuity. His immediate memory was impaired, with retention of auditory information a bigger problem than visual memory. The amazing finding was that his working memory was very strong. Working memory is the ability to hold several facts or thoughts temporarily while solving a problem or performing a task. Often referred to as the ability to think on your feet, it is an important memory system, and one that most of us use every day. He demonstrated above average attention and concentration, and was strong in perceptual organization and reasoning. He scored above average in a category that involved novel problem-solving that is not dependent on academic training. He easily and quickly developed strategies to use in situations required to solve problems. Zack's injury is very unique. Most survivors of brain injury struggle with attention, concentration, and working memory. Zack has no problems in these areas; however, his aphasia presented a challenge for his therapy team.

After four months of outpatient therapy, Zack returned to school part-time, taking classes that he passed as a sophomore. School became an extension of his therapy, getting him accustomed to organizing notes, studying for tests, and maneuvering through crowded hallways to find his locker. He was also back with his friends who had supported him throughout his recovery. In addition to World Civilization, Computer, Algebra, and Bible, he spent four periods working with Carol Britton, an education therapist. Carol was another person who God carefully orchestrated to be part of Zack's recovery. The only licensed therapist in our county for Rhythmic Writing and Instrumental Enrichment, she just happened to work at Christian Academy. Rhythmic Writing is a visual-motor task that improves mental calculation, working memory, sequencing ability, and tracking. Instrumental Enrichment is a process-oriented program that focuses on different cognitive skills that engage students in problem-solving by developing their ability to understand and elaborate information. If Zack had attended any other school, at any other time, he would not have been exposed to these programs. Carol became an advocate for Zack within the school system, and these therapies helped build new neuro pathways to access the information his brain had stored. Zack returned to Christian Academy full time in the fall of 2006, having only missed one year of school. Against all odds and defying what many professions said would be impossible, he graduated from an academically challenging school, never earning less than a C.

The first year of his recovery, Zack achieved many milestones. In addition to getting his driver's license and returning to school, we became First Contact Volunteers with the Brain Injury Alliance of KY. Meeting with families of teenagers struggling with traumatic brain injury, we provided needed information and encouragement. Helping survivors who are going through the same experience is the mission field that God has placed us in. Zack relished returning to University Hospital and Frazier Rehab as a beacon of hope. He is the first to ask people if they believe in God and the power of prayer. We were also invited to speak at multiple schools and youth groups. Hearing about Zack's accident firsthand drives home the message to teenagers that one decision can change your life forever. Discussing his amazing recovery allows us to introduce them to a merciful God and inspire them to embrace the power of prayer.

We have seen many examples of what Dr. Kraft told me would be a "deeper appreciation of life". Zack takes notice of the world around him, and has taught me to reflect on simple pleasures. The first snowfall brought him to the window, where he pointed out how the rays of sunlight touched an icicle dangling from a tree branch. He said it looked like the finger of God reaching down to warm the earth. Many mornings, he would drag me outside in the cold to see the sunrise, and he still texts us pictures of sunsets. Zack has a unique perspective, and I marvel at his enlightenments. He told me that he thinks God made different time zones, so that not everyone would be sleeping at once, and there would always be someone praying. He sits on his deck in the morning and talks to God. In church, he worships with his hand raised to heaven. His understanding that he is closer to God is worth more than any honors degree he might have earned before his accident. His short-term memory is impaired, but his feelings are sharper than ever, and he expresses them often. What the accident took away, God replaced with something better: sincerity, gratitude, contentment, compassion, faithfulness, and hope.

Zack still struggles with aphasia, but has no problem getting people to understand him. Those who don't know him think he has a unique sense of humor and don't realize that his choice of words is out of necessity. He works with Scott in the family tile business, and they frequently end their day on the golf course. He bought a condo not far from where we live, and I often find myself on his deck playing cards. His accident left him with an imperfect brain, but a renewed heart for God. We know one day, God will restore Zack fully. It may not be this side of heaven, but it will surely happen to His glory. Gods hand has been masterfully orchestrating our lives. He turned the most tragic experience into a wonderful testimony of His power. How he can take the darkest moment, make you dwell in it just long enough so that when he brings you into the dawn, his light shines so brilliant you can't ignore it. It is only through these moments that we can come to fully understand his mercy, his grace, and his unfailing love.

Psalm 31:14 "I trust in you, O Lord...My times are in your hands."

# WHERE HOPE DWELLS

*When you enter the room,*
*You are surrounded by pain*
*You see a struggle to conquer death*

*Click...click...click...*
*The machines beat like the consistent tick of the clock,*
*But they're not keeping time,*
*They are maintaining life*

*Tubes...wires...cords...*
*Like snakes entangled among each other*
*With the sole purpose of winning the battle*

*Your skin is chilled*
*White sheets stretch out like snow*
*There is no warmth or hope here*

*Motionless sorrow and despair*
*Wounded body...eyes swollen shut*
*Mangled and defeated, like a warrior who lost his battle*

*Shaved head...grossly misshapen*
*A train track of staples charting the path of the surgeon's hand*
*Wounds aching to tell their story*

*Blank stare...like no one is there*
*A twitch of the fingers...uncontrolled*
*Thoughts, but no statements*

*Discarded dreams thrown in a heap with bloodied gauze*
*Tears of agony dare not hope for too much*
*Prayers pierce even to the ears of God*

*Who can save the broken when misery is overwhelming?*
*Fear is the enemy of faith*
*God conquers fear and gives hope for a new beginning.*

**Zack Hornback**
*May 20, 2007*

Having survived a parent's worst nightmare, Eileen Hornback chronicled her son's miraculous return from the brink of death as he struggled with traumatic brain injury. Overwhelmed with the need to provide medical updates to friends and family, she was inspired to blog throughout his recovery. It became a cathartic platform that enabled others to grasp the power of prayer that sustained her when faced with life and death decisions. The blog became the outline for this book that provides hope and encouragement to other families dealing with their own personal tragedies.

Becoming a First Contact volunteer with the Brain Injury Alliance of KY was a natural transition for Eileen as she sought to reach out to other families. As a speaker for Fellowship for Christian Athletes, her message allows hundreds of teenagers to understand the impact of their decisions and meet God in powerful and personal ways as she unfolds the story of her son's amazing journey.

Married to Scott for over 35 years, she is a mother of four who spends her spare time as an interview coach for young women competing in pageants. As a board member for the Dream Factory of Louisville, she embraces the mission to grant wishes for children who have life threatening and chronic illnesses. You can connect with her at www.eileenhornback.weebly.com

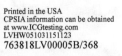
Printed in the USA
CPSIA information can be obtained
at www.ICGtesting.com
LVHW051031151123
763818LV00005B/368